Immunology: The Making of a Modern Science

Immunology: The Making of a Modern Science

Edited by

Richard B. Gallagher
Senior Editor Europe, Science, *Thomas House, Cambridge, UK*

Jean Gilder
Stazione Zoologica 'Anton Dohrn', Naples, Italy

G. J. V. Nossal
Director, Walter & Eliza Hall Institute for Medical Research,
The Royal Melbourne Hospital, Victoria, Australia

and

Gaetano Salvatore
President, Stazione Zoologica 'Anton Dohrn', Naples, Italy

ACADEMIC PRESS
Harcourt Brace & Company, Publishers
London   San Diego   New York
Boston   Sydney   Tokyo   Toronto

ACADEMIC PRESS LIMITED
24/28 Oval Road
LONDON NW1 7DX

United States Edition published by
ACADEMIC PRESS INC.
San Diego, CA 92101

A catalogue record for this book is available from the British Library

ISBN 0-12-274020-3

Typeset by Servis Filmsetting Ltd, Manchester, UK
Printed in Great Britain at The University Press, Cambridge

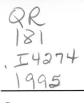

Contents

List of Contributors

Baruch S. Blumberg   770 Bierholme Avenue, Philadelphia, PA 19111, USA.

Jean Dausset   Human Polymorphism Study Centre, C.E.P.H., 27 rue Juliette Dodu, 75010 Paris, France.

Mark M. Davis   Howard Hughes Medical Institute and the Department of Microbiology and Immunology, Stanford University School of Medicine, Beckman Center, Room B221, Stanford, CA 94305–5428, USA.

Shuichi Furusawa   Department of Pathology, New York University Medical School, 550 First Avenue, New York, NY 10016, USA.

J. L. Gowans   75 Cumnor Hill, Oxford OX2 9HX, UK.

Eva Klein   Laboratory of Tumour Biology, Microbiology and Tumour Biology Center, Karolinska Institute, S–171 77 Stockholm, Sweden.

George Klein   Laboratory of Tumour Biology, Microbiology and Tumour Biology Center, Karolinska Institute, S–171 77 Stockholm, Sweden.

Ian R. Mackay   Centre for Molecular Biology and Medicine, Monash University, Clayton 3168, Victoria, Australia.

Jacques F. A. P. Miller   The Walter and Eliza Hall Institute of Medical Research, Post Office, Royal Melbourne Hospital, Victoria 3050, Australia.

Joseph E. Murray   Harvard Medical School, Brigham and Women's Hospital, 108 Abbot Road, Wellesley Road, MA 021812, USA.

Alfred Nisonoff   Department of Biology, Rosenstiel Research Center, Brandeis University, Waltham, MA 02254, USA.

G. J. V. Nossal   The Walter and Eliza Hall Institute of Medical Research, Post Office, Royal Melbourne Hospital, Victoria 3050, Australia.

Joost J. Oppenheim   Laboratory of Immunoregulation, Biological Response Modifiers Program, Division of Cancer Treatment, National Cancer Institute – Frederick Cancer Research and Development Center, Frederick, MD 21702–1201, USA.

Zoltan Ovary   Department of Pathology, New York University Medical School, 550 First Avenue, New York, NY 10016, USA.

Felix T. Rapaport   State University of New York at Stony Brook, Transplantation Service, Department of Surgery, Health Sciences Center, T-19, 040, Stony Brook, NY 11794–8192, USA.

Noel R. Rose   Department of Pathology and of Molecular Microbiology and Immunology, The Johns Hopkins Medical Institutions, 615 North Wolfe Street, Baltimore, MD 21205, USA.

Ronald H. Schwartz   Laboratory of Cellular and Molecular Immunology, National Institute of Allergy and Infectious Diseases, National Institutes of Health, Bethesda, MD, USA.

Arthur M. Silverstein Institute of the History of Medicine, Johns Hopkins University School of Medicine, Baltimore, MD 21205, USA.

David W. Talmage Department of Immunology and the Webb–Waring Lung Institute, Health Sciences Center, University of Colorado, Denver, CO 80262, USA.

Susumu Tonegawa Center for Cancer Research, Massachusetts Institute of Technology, 77 Massachusetts Avenue, Cambridge, MA 02139–4307, USA.

Byron H. Waksman New York University Medical Center, and Center for Neurological Diseases, Harvard Medical Center, New York, USA.

Rolf M. Zinkernagel Institute of Experimental Immunology, Department of Pathology, University of Zurich, Zurich, Switzerland.

Introduction

Foreword

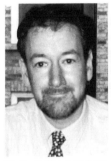 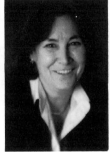 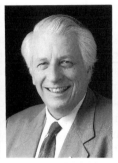 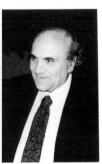

R. B. GALLAGHER   J. GILDER   G. J. V. NOSSAL   G. SALVATORE

Immunology has progressed in spectacular fashion in the last four decades. The progress predated, but was swept along by, the molecular biology revolution: studies of immunity both contributed to and benefited from the development of molecular tools for dissecting biological systems. There have been two strands to the development of immunology, which have often intertwined. One has been the study of the response to infectious agents, transplanted organs and tumours, with the ultimate aim of manipulating that response. The other has been the study of the immune system as a model system in molecular cell biology. This combination, plus the fact that the era began with such a rudimentary knowledge of the mechanisms of immunity, has attracted a continuous stream of the brightest theoretical and experimental scientists over 40 years.

This book is an attempt to convey the philosophies and approaches of some of the most successful of these scientists. It does so in the form of a series of narratives which describe the circumstances that led to a major discovery in immunology. Contributors were set the task not only of recalling an exciting period of research that helped shape modern immunology, but also of setting this in the personal context of place and time. It must be emphasized that this collection is not intended to provide a history of modern immunology – the title deliberately excludes the shackles imposed by the word 'history'. Nor do we make the claim that these are necessarily disinterested, dispassionate accounts of the development of the subject. On the contrary, they are passionately biographical, a series of essentially personal essays that provide an unusually intimate insight into the scientific process.

The book is in five sections: Introduction, Theories of Immunity, The Cellular Basis of Immunity, The Molecular Basis of Immunity, and Immunology

IMMUNOLOGY: THE MAKING OF A MODERN SCIENCE
ISBN 0-12-274020-3

and Medicine. It hardly needs to be said that these are arbitrary divisions, designed as much as anything to give some structure to the contents.

The origins of the book can be found in the eighth course of the International School of Biological Sciences at the Stazione Zoologica 'Anton Dohrn' di Napoli, held in the early summer of 1992. The event brought together immunologists and historians to learn each other's language and to respond to each other's central questions. The Stazione has been organizing similar International Schools of the History of Biological Sciences over the past 18 years. The enthusiasm generated at that meeting was the springboard for this publication, and many of the participants in the symposium have contributed to the book. Of course, it is possible to cover only a small minority of the important advances in immunology in a book of this size. Numerous critical contributions have been omitted, and for that we apologize.

All of us greatly enjoyed participating in this fascinating report of the Making of Modern Science, and if this volume conveys even a small part of the excitement that was generated during the meeting, we shall consider our task accomplished.

The Historical Origins of Modern Immunology

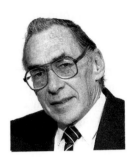

ARTHUR M. SILVERSTEIN
*Institute of the History of Medicine, Johns Hopkins University
School of Medicine, Baltimore, MD 21205, USA*

The purpose of the present volume is to bring together those investigators who helped to form and give substance to modern immunology. This chapter examines the historical factors that set the stage for the development of immunology following World War II. It will consider the two major eras in immunology that preceded the present biomedical one: the early age of bacteriology, with its emphasis on disease diagnosis, prevention, and cure; and its successor age of immunochemistry, with its concentration on the chemistry of antigens and antibodies. Special attention will be paid to the causes of these major directional changes in the discipline, and to the different theoretical frameworks and the new set of research questions and technical approaches that accompanied each change (1).

Scientific progress, in the classical formulations of philosophers and sociologists of science (2), was viewed as a smooth, progressive evolution toward the ultimate goal – a complete understanding of the physical world. But the logical and linear nature of progress implicit in this admiring view of the workings of science has been brought into question during the last few decades. Indeed Peter Medawar, from his own long experience, has argued that progress in science is neither logical nor illogical, but rather *non*-logical (3). It has come to be recognized that, whereas progress in a science may be evolutionary and linear during 'normative' periods, major revolutionary discontinuities may be accompanied by abrupt conceptual change and a burst of productive activity in the field (4).

Amost 60 years ago Ludwik Fleck pointed the way to an explanation of these shifts in a science in his book 'Genesis and Development of a Scientific Fact' (5). Fleck's description of those who govern a scientific field and determine its values and priorities (the *Denkkollektiv*) implied that replacement of these leaders by others with different backgrounds and interests might change the character of the discipline itself. In considering the two major conceptual

IMMUNOLOGY: THE MAKING OF A MODERN SCIENCE
ISBN 0-12-274020-3

transitions in immunology, it will be seen that each was accompanied by a *Denkkollektiv* replacement.

Early Immunology: the Bacteriological Era

The initial research programme

During its early years, the research programme of immunology was divided among six principal areas, each of which arose logically from the germ theory of disease, from developments in public health, or from chance laboratory observations. While closely interrelated, each component was concerned with its own questions and had its own technical approaches.

Immunization

Immunology was born as a science in the laboratory of Louis Pasteur, as the direct result of Pasteur's commitment to the germ theory of disease. Pasteur's earlier work on the agents responsible for diseases of silkworms and wine convinced him that each disease is the result of an infection by a specific microorganism. With Emile Roux, Pasteur discovered variations in the pathogenicity of different strains of a given organism, and devised techniques for the attenuation of cultures of virulent bacteria, working most notably with the organism responsible for the disease chicken cholera (6). Chickens that had recovered from a mild attack of chicken cholera induced by an attenuated strain were found thenceforth to be protected from challenge with more lethal strains. After more than 80 years, Pasteur had finally provided an explanation for Edward Jenner's success in the use of cowpox vaccine to protect against smallpox, and opened up an entirely new research programme of prophylactic immunization. Pasteur quickly applied this approach to anthrax, rabies and other diseases, and over the next quarter century scientists throughout the world endeavoured to develop preventive vaccines to all pathogens using Pasteurian methods.

Cellular immunity

Soon after Pasteur's first report, Ilya Metchnikoff sought to explain the mechanism of immunity with his cellular theory (7). Based upon purely Darwinian evolutionary principles, he suggested that the primitive intracellular digestive functions of lower animals had persisted in the capacity of the mobile phagocytes of metazoa and higher forms to ingest and digest foreign substances. Metchnikoff suggested that the phagocytic cell is the primary element in natural immunity, and is important also for acquired immunity. His theory had several far-reaching implications for biology and medicine. First, it introduced the notion that *interspecific* conflict might contribute as importantly to evolution as the classical Darwinian notion of *intraspecific* competition (8) – the struggle for survival is between the micro-organism and the infected host, with the phagocyte acting for the latter. The phagocytic theory also contributed importantly to the field of general pathology. Toward the end of the nineteenth century, most believed that inflammation was a damaging component of the disease process itself. Metchnikoff suggested that the inflammatory response was in fact an evolutionary mechanism designed to protect the organism.

Serotherapy

The next step in the expansion of the early immunological research programme came in 1890 with von Behring and Kitasato's demonstration that immunization with the exotoxins of diphtheria and tetanus organisms results in the appearance in the blood of soluble substances capable of neutralizing these toxins *in vitro* and rendering them harmless (9). Furthermore, these antitoxins can be transferred passively to protect a naive recipient from disease. Here was a remarkable new addition to the medical armamentarium, which offered great promise in the therapy of infectious diseases. In the 1890s, the new serotherapy stimulated an explosion of laboratory and clinical experimentation, in recognition of which von Behring received the first Nobel Prize in Physiology or Medicine in 1901.

It was while working on the standardization of diphtheria toxin and antitoxin preparations that Paul Ehrlich devised his side-chain theory of antibody formation (10). Ehrlich suggested that antibodies had evolved as cell receptors for nutrients and drugs. When these receptors (side-chains) are bound by injected antigen, an overproliferation is stimulated and the excess is cast off into the blood to appear as circulating antibody. Perhaps most significant for later developments in the field, Ehrlich attributed the specificity of antibodies to their stereochemical structure, and attributed their interactions with antigen to the establishment of strictly chemical bonding.

Cytotoxic antibodies

The fourth subject that helped to define early immunology stemmed from the demonstration by Jules Bordet in 1899 that antierythrocyte antibodies could cause the destruction (haemolysis) of red cells, in conjunction with the non-specifically acting serum factor complement (11). For the first time, the cells and tissues of the immunized host itself were seen possibly to be at risk by an 'aberrant' immune response against self-components. Scientists everywhere soon began to immunize experimental animals with suspensions or extracts of almost every tissue or organ in the body in an attempt to find cytotoxic antibodies that might be responsible for one or another local disease. The journals were quickly filled with reports of such experiments, and indeed much of the 1900 issue of *Annales de l'Institut Pasteur* was devoted to this question (12). It rapidly became apparent that *xenoantibodies* and *isoantibodies* were readily formed, and might show cytotoxicity against the appropriate target tissue or organ (13). However, *autoantibodies* were, with few exceptions (14), rarely produced. But for some years thereafter, the possibility was entertained that such cytotoxic antibodies might play an important role in the pathogenesis of a number of diseases, both as pure autoimmune phenomena and as secondary contributors to the lesions seen in such diseases as syphilis and ophthalmitis (15).

Serodiagnosis

A second consequence of Bordet's observation (16) on the mechanism of immune haemolysis came with the finding that *all* antigen–antibody interactions would result in the non-specific fixation of complement, and its disappearance from the test mixture (17). With the rapid development of techniques for measuring complement, it was apparent that if a given bacterial antigen were available, then the presence or absence of its specific antibody in a patient's serum could be assayed by measuring the effect of such a mixture on a standard amount of complement added to the system. A powerful new tool was thus added to the arsenal of the student of infectious diseases, who could now tell whether a patient had previously encountered the pathogen or, in certain cases, whether the patient currently had active disease. The first disease to which this new approach was applied, by August von Wassermann and his colleagues in 1906 (18), was syphilis. These serodiagnostic approaches were quickly applied to many other diseases, and the technique and its improvement provided a fertile field of activity for decades to come.

Anaphylaxis and related diseases

In 1902, the physiologists Paul Portier and Charles Richet reported a curious finding (19). Until then, the immune response had been viewed as a benign set of mechanisms, the only function of which was to protect the organism against exogenous pathogens; the discovery of cytotoxic antibodies had done little to alter this view. Now came Portier and Richet to demonstrate that a second exposure, even to innocuous antigens, could cause severe systemic shock-like symptoms. They termed this phenomenon 'anaphylaxis' in an attempt to distinguish it from the usual prophylactic results expected of the immune system. Then, in 1903, Maurice Arthus demonstrated that bland antigens could cause local necrotizing lesions in the skin when they react with specific antibody (20). In 1906, Clemens von Pirquet and Bela Schick demonstrated that serum sickness depends upon an antibody response by the host to the injection of large quantities of foreign protein antigens (21).

Here were observations that threatened the conceptual foundation of immunology, which had held the system to be completely benign and protective. It could not be argued that these were only experimental laboratory phenomena, since it was soon demonstrated that two of the significant curses of mankind, hay fever (22) and asthma (23), also belong to this same group of specific antibody-mediated diseases. These disturbing findings prompted many experiments to clarify the phenomenology of these diseases, and in particular to explain the paradox of how a system that presumably had evolved to protect, might give rise to the very opposite effect (24).

The fate of the original research programme

By the time of World War I, the young and highly productive field of immunology had begun to organize itself as a proper scientific discipline (25), with the beginning of a movement towards institutionalization. An institute devoted to the aims of immunology had been established for Paul Ehrlich in Frankfurt, and departments and services dedicated to the discipline had been formed within many of the leading research institutions around the world. Formal sessions devoted to one or another component of the immunology programme were to be found at International Congresses of Medicine or Hygiene, and an 'invisible college' (26) existed, involving informal exchange among its practitioners. The *Annales de l'Institut Pasteur* had long been devoted to immunological reports, and in 1908 the *Zeitschrift für Immunitätsforschung*, and in 1916 the American *Journal of Immunology* were founded. Finally, the commonality of interest of this subgroup of scientists and practitioners was recognized, at least in the USA, by the founding of the American Association of Immunologists in 1913 (27).

But immunology found itself at a crossroads during that second decade of the twentieth century. Each of the six components of the original research programme appeared to have been compromised. Preventive immunization had seen its great victories in the case of chicken cholera, anthrax, rabies, plague and several other important diseases. But increasingly, pathogenic organisms were being described for which it was proving impossible to prepare efficacious vaccines. These included such major agents of disease as the tubercle and leprous bacilli, the cholera *Vibrio*, the spirochete of syphilis, and the Gram-positive organisms, to say nothing of a number of newly described diseases of man and animals due to viruses and parasites. Thus, by 1910, the great early promise of Pasteurian immunization was no longer being fulfilled; new successes now came only rarely, and were achieved only with great difficulty. Work in this area very rapidly left the 'classical' immunology laboratory, and was taken over by bacteriologists, virologists, and parasitologists who were often interested more in organisms than in immunological mechanisms.

The study of cellular immunity and of Metchnikoff's phagocytic theory started its decline as early as the 1890s, at the hands of proponents of humoralist theories. Cells were much more difficult to work with than humoral antibodies; no such techniques as agglutination, the precipitin reaction, immune haemolysis, and the passive transfer of serum antibody existed in the field of cell studies. Indeed, the cell was still considered something of a mystery, whereas Ehrlich's pictures of antibodies and their specific combining sites could almost convince one that the antibody was a 'real' entity the structure and properties of which were readily understood. Thus, Metchnikoff's cellular theory of immunity fell into disfavour early in this century (to be revived in a somewhat altered form only some 50 years later), but not before its heuristic value had inspired many ingenious experiments and a wealth of important data, and not before Metchnikoff shared the Nobel Prize in 1908 with Paul Ehrlich.

Von Behring's serotherapy for the prevention or cure of disease suffered a fate similar to that of preventive immunization. After the remarkable demonstration of the efficacy of horse antidiphtheria and antitetanus sera in the treatment of these diseases, no significant further victories were recorded employing this approach. Although laboratories throughout the world continued to produce these two antisera (the Pasteur Institute helped support itself with its stable of immunized horses), interest in this approach waned, since there were so few other significant diseases caused by exotoxins, and thus amenable to this approach. When, much later, passive transfer of antibody would be employed, it would be by haematologists using human γ-globulin to prevent erythroblastoses fetalis, or by paediatricians employing sera taken from convalescents to deal with poliomyelitis.

The interest in cytotoxic antibodies proved to be ephemeral. Despite all attempts to implicate anti-tissue and anti-organ antibodies in the pathogenesis of disease, convincing proof was not forthcoming except in the case of Donath and Landsteiner's demonstration of the role of antierythrocyte antibodies in paroxysmal cold haemoglobinuria, and even this was soon forgotten. By 1912, the study of immune cytotoxic phenomena had left the immunology laboratory, to be pursued only within essentially unrelated clinical speciality areas such as ophthalmology, with its interest in sympathic ophthalmia and autoimmune disease of the lens (28). While an experimental pathologist such as Arnold Rich might later study immunocytotoxic events in the pathogenesis of tuberculosis (29), or a virologist such as Thomas Rivers might produce experimental allergic encephalomyelitis (30), these were far out of the current mainstream of immunology, and the results were generally published in journals other than those specifically covering immunology.

The sociologist of science would probably view the field of serodiagnosis as a more typical example of disciplinary differentiation. These techniques originated within the heart of a science interested in immunity in the infectious diseases. This required not only an understanding of disease pathogenesis, but also the ability to diagnose these diseases. Syphilis was the mainstay of the serodiagnostic laboratory, and investigators worked to perfect the technique and to extend it to other diseases. Very quickly, however, the technique became quite routine and immunologists interested in basic mechanisms soon lost interest in the procedure. Activity in the area was taken over by classical bacteriologists, and indeed those who devoted their time to this and other aspects of serodiagnosis soon began to call themselves 'serologists'. They worked principally in hospital diagnostic laboratories rather than in basic immunology research.

Soon after they were discovered, anaphylaxis and the other diseases related to it attracted the attention of immunology investigators. They were interested in the nature of the antibodies responsible for these phenomena, and in the mechanisms that resulted in disease. But after a short and not very successful struggle with the paradox of immunological disease, most immunologists soon gave up the field to others. Most of those who took up these interests were clinicians concerned with hay fever and asthma, which had just been identified as 'anaphylactic' diseases. It was this identification that was responsible for the establishment of clinical allergy as a medical subspeciality (31), and it was primarily in the laboratories of allergists that further progress was realized in sorting out the mechanisms involved and in developing skin tests and therapeutic approaches to the treatment of human allergies. In addition to these, however, the study of anaphylactic and related phenomena was of great interest to physiologists such as Sir Henry Dale (32), and to a group of experimental pathologists interested in the species variations of the lesions that accompany these diseases.

The Transition to Immunochemistry

Not only were basic scientists losing interest in the problems that had earlier defined immunology, but the original giants of the field were dying off. Pasteur and Koch were gone, and neither Ehrlich nor Metchnikoff survived World War I (although significantly, Ehrlich had long since given up immunology for chemotherapy, while Metchnikoff became preoccupied with digestion and philosophical speculations).

The seeds of the future interest in the chemistry of antigens and antibodies had already been planted in the 1890s by Paul Ehrlich. His side-chain theory of antibody formation claimed that antigen, antibody and complement were real molecules; their combining sites were pictured as being stereochemically complementary structures that would account for the specificity of their interactions. Most textbooks ascribe the paternity of the field of immunochemistry to the famous physical chemist Svante Arrhenius, since he coined the term in a famous series of lectures in 1904 (33). Like many other physical scientists, Arrhenius was attracted by the mysteries and by the confusion that existed in biology, and felt that he could bring some order to the chaos with the introduction of the rigorous laws of chemistry and physics. But Arrhenius' contributions were purely theoretical. They could not be adequately tested at the time, and had little apparent influence on subsequent events.

It was Obermeyer and Pick who showed the way by their demonstration that protein antigens could be modified chemically to alter their immunological specificity (34). Thus, when animals were immunized with nitrated proteins, the specificity of the resulting antibodies was directed at the added nitro groups rather than at the original protein. Then, in 1912, Pick published an extensive review showing that a number of different synthetic groupings (called haptens) might be joined to a carrier protein to serve as antigenic determinants (35). A powerful new tool was thus introduced into immunology, whereby the nature of immunologic specificity and the character of the combining site on the antibody could be studied, using the small molecules produced in the organic chemistry laboratory. No one exploited this approach more effectively than Karl Landsteiner. In 1917, he published two papers (36) which clearly showed the power of this new approach, and which helped to define both his own work until his death in 1944 (37), and much of the domain of immunochemistry as well. The physiological basis of antibody formation and the biological consequences of antigen–antibody interactions now became secondary to interest in the chemical nature of antigens and antibodies.

Yet a second approach to the study of antigens and antibodies was initiated in the 1920s by Michael Heidelberger. An organic chemist who had found work in a bacteriological laboratory, Heidelberger was able to show that, in addition to protein antigens, the capsular polysaccharides of different strains of pneumococci could also stimulate specific antibody responses (38). The well-understood structures of polysaccharides used as antigens helped to clarify the structure of the antibody combining site, in the pursuit of which Heidelberger developed a number of quantitative techniques that helped establish immunology as a more exact science (39).

The chemists' theory of antibody formation

During the early era of immunology, the first theories by zoologist Ilya Metchnikoff and physician Paul Ehrlich were strictly Darwinian. But after World War I, the chemically oriented investigators who entered the field found the old theories of little value in explaining the structure and origin of antibodies. New theories soon appeared to fill the void, dealing specifically with the question of how each member of an ever-growing universe of potential antigens could possibly lead to the formation of its own specific antibody. It will be remembered that this was the rock upon which Ehrlich's side-chain theory had foundered – the implausible suggestion that evolution could have devised a mechanism for the spontaneous production of so many different antibodies, most of which were directed against bland and even artificial antigens of no obvious evolutionary selective force.

It will not be surprising that the new chemical theories of antibody formation were quite Lamarckian in nature; if the molecules of the biologist have a long evolutionary history, those of the chemist generally do not. In 1930, the biochemist Felix Haurowitz proposed that only the antigen itself contains all of the information necessary for antibody formation, and imposes a complementary structure on a nascent protein by acting as a template for the synthesis of a unique sequence of amino acids (40). This was the first so-called 'instruction theory' of antibody formation. It explained in a plausible way not only the tremendous diversity of different antibodies, but also how so fine a specificity could be conferred on the antibody molecule. This instructive theory of antibody formation was modified in 1940 by the chemical physicist

Linus Pauling (41), who proposed that the antigen serves as a template upon which the nascent amino acid chain coils to form a protein molecule. So ingrained in the collective immunological psyche of the times were these neo-Lamarckian chemical ideas that even biologist Macfarlane Burnet, in his first two theories of antibody formation (42), felt obliged to adopt instructive approaches.

The immunochemical research programme

The use of synthetic chemical haptens and natural carbohydrates as antigens helped to define the structure of antigen and antibody combining sites, and to measure the thermodynamic parameters of their interaction (43). These studies were simplified when antibody was identified as a γ-globulin protein (44) (thus permitting its purification) and by the development of quantitative techniques for the measurement of antigen–antibody and antigen–hapten reactions. The nature of the research problems that interested many immunologists between the 1920s and the early 1960s is best epitomized by the leading monographs and texts of the period (45): Well's *The Chemical Aspects of Immunity* in 1924; Marrack's *The Chemistry of Antigens and Antibodies* in 1934; Landsteiner's *The Specificity of Serological Reactions* in 1937; Boyd's *Fundamentals of Immunology* in 1943; and Kabat and Mayer's *Quantitative Immunochemistry* in 1949. These were the reference books from which a generation of young immunologists learned their trade, and little attention was paid in any of them to the biological or medical aspects of the field.

This is not to suggest that all work along the six classical lines described above ceased during the immunochemical era. It has been pointed out that, '. . . research areas which have become well established take a long time to die out altogether. There is always *some* work that can be done' (46). Thus, as described above, the clinical allergists gave new life to the study of anaphylactic phenomena by redefining the field along new lines; continued progress was made in the preparation of better toxoids and better modes of immunization; serologists continued to improve and expand the application of serodiagnostic procedures; and, from time to time, an effective vaccine would be developed against one disease or another of man or animals.

True, there were other workers doing interesting experiments along newer lines during this period. Hans Zinsser (47) and Arnold Rich (48) studied allergic reactions to bacteria; Louis Dienes (49) and Simon and Rackemann (50) developed models of delayed hypersensitivity lesions to simple proteins; and Thomas Rivers developed an experimental model of allergic encephalomyelitis (51). But these studies seemed to interest only microbiologists and experimental pathologists, and otherwise excited little general interest. Only a later generation of immunologists more attuned to biological questions would retrospectively identify these contributions as landmarks in immunological progress.

The Immunobiological Revolution

Biological discontent with the chemical paradigm

The normative scientific activities of the immunochemical era between the 1920s and 1950s resulted in many interesting data. The chemical nature of both antigens and antibodies was now much clearer, and the structural basis and thermodynamic characteristics of their specific interactions had been well defined. Increasingly, however, biologists working on the fringes of mainstream immunology made observations, the explanations for which were not to be found in the received wisdom of instructionist theories of antibody formation. How, they asked, could antibody formation persist in the apparent absence of antigen? Why should a second exposure to antigen result in an enhanced booster response that is much more productive than is the primary response to antigenic stimulus? How can repeated exposure to antigen change the very quality of the antibody, in many instances sharpening its specificity by increasing its affinity for the antigenic determinant employed? Finally, how is it possible that immunity to some viral diseases appears to be unrelated to the presence of circulating antiviral antibodies? These and other biologically based questions began seriously to challenge the immunochemical paradigm, most notably through the writings of Macfarlane Burnet in his two books (52) *The Production of Antibodies*, in 1941 and 1949. Burnet complained repeatedly that the chemical theories, while quite elegant, failed to explain the more functional biological aspects of the immune response.

Then, as the result of wartime work with burn patients, Peter Medawar demonstrated that the rejection of skin grafts was a purely immunological phenomenon, but one apparently unrelated to humoral antibody (53). In 1945, Ray Owen described the curious finding that dizygotic twin calves were incapable of responding to one another's antigens (54). Burnet and Fenner suggested that, during ontogeny, a cell-based immunological tolerance develops to self-antigens (55). This was a daring hypothesis that Peter Medawar and colleagues (56) confirmed experimentally in 1953, and for which Burnet and Medawar shared the Nobel Prize in 1960. Yet another observation for which no ready explanation was available in classical theory involved the description in the early 1950s of a group of immunological deficiency diseases in man (57), the explanation of which would go to the very heart of the biological basis of the immune response. Finally, after a hiatus of some 40 years or more, interest in autoimmune diseases was reawakened by new interest in autoimmune haemolytic anaemias, experimental and human autoimmune thyroiditis, and allergic encephalomyelitis (58).

By the 1950s, the stage seemed to be set for a large-scale confrontation between the newer biomedical findings and the classical immunochemical tradition, such as has been described by Thomas Kuhn in his book *The Structure of Scientific Revolutions* (59). The older immunochemical ideas could no longer satisfactorily explain the newer findings, nor were its techniques applicable to the new questions being asked by a growing group of biomedical scientists. Only by the development of new methods could many of these problems be approached, and these were rapidly forthcoming. Immunofluorescent staining (60) and radioactive labelling of antibodies (61) permitted the tissue localization of antigen and of antibody-forming cells, while haemolytic plaque assays (62) allowed their quantitative enumeration. The techniques of passive cell transfer (63) and of cell culture (64), aided by the increasing availability of inbred strains of laboratory animals, permitted for the first time the detailed study of cell–cell interactions and immunocyte dynamics.

Theoretical underpinning

Thus was a true scientific revolution ready in the wings, requiring only the coming of a prophet to provide the text to be used against the old regime and its outmoded paradigm. That requirement was met by Macfarlane Burnet. In 1955, Niels Jerne revived the old Ehrlich theory of pre-existing immunological specificities based upon Darwinian evolution with his natural selection theory of antibody formation (65). In somewhat more modern terms, Jerne proposed that antigen does not instruct for antibody formation, but rather selects for the production of a few among all the possible specificities already present. Jerne's theory was imprecise in many respects, but its central feature, selection, was adapted by Burnet into his clonal selection theory of antibody formation (66). Not only was antibody formation defined in terms of cell receptors but, most importantly, it was now to be based upon the dynamics of cellular proliferation and differentiation. With its further refinement by Burnet (67) and by David Talmage and Joshua Lederberg (68), the clonal selection theory began to provide reasonable explanations for all of the hitherto inexplicable biological phenomena. Perhaps of even greater significance, the heuristic value of the theory quickly became apparent; it stimulated an explosion of new experiments and caused new questions to be asked that influenced a broad spectrum of biological and medical fields. It is interesting how, in immunology as in other scientific fields, there are continuous border negotiations between theory and technology. Theory sometimes drives the development of techniques and of progress in the field, while it is the application of technique that sometimes drives theoretical progress, in an ever-expanding interplay (69).

Within 10 years of its introduction, Burnet's clonal selection theory had proved its worth. The immunochemical paradigm had been completely replaced, except in the minds of a few diehard traditionalists (70). Many new young investigators were attracted to this rapidly moving and increasingly important field, but came now with prior training in biology, genetics, physiology, experimental pathology, and a variety of clinical disciplines of medicine. Immunology became once again what it had been 60 years earlier, an outward-looking discipline with much to offer to, and much to gain from, a wide variety of interdisciplinary ventures, as the large number of new subspecialty journals testifies.

Summary

There are a number of different reasons that might impel a scientific discipline more-or-less abruptly to change its research direction. One of these is the increasing failure of the old approaches to bring forth the impressive progress that attracts young students to its fold; another is splitting off of research areas into other subdisciplines. Both of these factors played a role in the shift of early immunology about the time of World War I from a medically oriented pre-occupation with bacteriology and infectious diseases to the study of more chemical aspects of antibodies and antigens. Thus, several of the components of the original research programme in immunology failed to maintain their initial high promise and went into decline: the development of new vaccines; serotherapeutic approaches; the study of cellular immunity; and the study of diseases mediated by cytotoxic antibodies. Two other research areas followed a different, though still productive, course. Anaphylaxis and related diseases passed primarily into the hands of the new field of clinical allergy, while the development and improvement of serodiagnostic techniques passed into the hands of the new discipline of serology. As interest in the old biomedical programme was declining, there developed a new and productive interest, led by a new group of individuals with a predominantly chemical approach to the study of antigens and antibodies.

The reasons for the second major transition in immunology, roughly during the late 1950s to early 1960s, is quite different. In this case, investigators (pre-dominantly biomedically oriented) from the periphery of the field (and some even from outside the field) made numerous observations that could not be explained by the reigning theories, nor investigated by the reigning techniques of the day. New theories and new techniques were quick to appear and, supported by a large influx of biologically and medically trained investigators, they substantially overthrew the prevailing immunochemical paradigm. Modern immunobiology had been born.

It is interesting to note how the changing nature of the discipline affected its relationship with other disciplines. The original immunology research programme had been extrovert; it had broad application to, and exchange with, many fields of biology and medicine. The new immunochemical programme of the 1920s to 1950s was more distinctly introvert, asking questions and obtaining results that were of little interest to those outside the field (71). With the advent of the immunobiological revolution, the field of immunology once again, and with even greater vigour, became one of the central players in the biomedical research enterprise, contributing both concepts and reagents to such fields as molecular biology, oncology, physiology, pathology, neurology and internal medicine.

Modern immunology demonstrates well yet another of the attributes of twentieth century science – the growing trend towards the unification of certain disciplines. In immunology, there occurred in the 1970s and 1980s a synthesis of the biological and chemical approaches (72). The immunochemists (who approached the system by studying the final molecular product, antibody) and the biologists (who approached it from the initial cellular interactions) found a common ground in the molecular biology of T- and B-cell receptors, of lymphokines, and in the structure and function of the immunoglobulin gene superfamily. Together they have clarified the major questions about antibody formation and cell–cell interactions. The broad implications of this unification into what has been termed the 'immune system' are discussed in detail by Moulin (73).

Notes and References

1. A more detailed analysis of these changes is given in A. M. Silverstein, *A History of Immunology* (Academic Press, New York, 1989) and 'The dynamics of conceptual change in twentieth century immunology', *Cell. Immunol.* **132**, 515 (1991).

2. See, for example, philosopher Karl Popper, *The Logic of Scientific Discovery* (Basic Books, New York, 1959) and sociologist Robert K. Merton, 'The normative structure of science', in *The Sociology of Science* (University of Chicago Press, Chicago, IL, 1973, p. 267 ff.).

3. P. B. Medawar, *Induction and Intuition in Scientific Thought*, Jayne Lecture, American Philosophical Society, Philadelphia (1969).

4. We owe this concept to T. Kuhn, *The Structure of Scientific Revolutions*, 2nd edn, University of Chicago Press, Chicago, IL (1970). There have been many critics of Kuhn's position. See, for example: I. Lakatos and A. Musgrave (eds), *Criticism and the Growth of Knowledge*, Cambridge University Press, London (1970); and F. Suppe (ed.), *The Structure of Scientific Theories*, University of Illinois Press, Urbana, IL (1971). The opposing positions are well summarized in: L. Laudan, 'Two puzzles about science: reflections about some crises in the philosophy and sociology of science', *Minerva* **20**, 253 (1984).

5. L. Fleck, *Genesis and Development of a Scientific Fact*, University of Chicago Press, Chicago, IL (1979). The original German version was *Entstehung und Entwicklung einer wissenschaftlichen Tatsache. Einführung in die Lehre vom Denkstil und Denkkollektiv*, Benno Schwabe, Basel (1935).

6. L. Pasteur, *C.R. Acad. Sci.* **90**, 239, 952 (1880).

7. I. I. Metchnikoff, *Virchows Arch.* **96**, 177 (1884). The theory is most completely expounded in his: *Lectures on the Comparative Pathology of Inflammation*, Kegan Paul/Trench Trübner, London (1893); *Immunity in the Infectious Diseases*, Macmillan, New York (1905).

8. Metchnikoff's Darwinian thesis is more fully described in: D. P. Todes, *Darwin without Malthus: The Struggle for Existence in Russian Evolutionary Thought*, Oxford University Press, New York (1989), pp. 83–103.

9. E. von Behring and S. Kitasato, *Dtsch. Med. Wochenschr.*, **16**, 1113 (1890); E. von Behring and E. Wernicke, *Z. Hyg.* **12**, 10, 45 (1892).

10. P. Ehrlich, *Klin. Jahrb.*, **6**, 299 (1897).

11. J. Bordet, *Ann. Inst. Pasteur* **12**, 688 (1899). Some years earlier, Richard Pfeiffer had shown that cholera vibrios are similarly destroyed by specific antibody and complement within the immunized host (*Z. Hyg.* **18**, 1 (1895)).

12. *Ann. Inst. Pasteur* **14** (1900).
13. It was Karl Landsteiner's observation of isoantibodies in the blood of most humans, specific for the erythrocytes of other individuals (*Centralbl. Bakteriol. Orig.* **27**, 357 (1900)), which opened up the field of blood groups, eventually of great importance in the areas of blood transfusion, immunogenetics, forensics and anthropology.
14. Thus, the finding of experimental spermicidal autoantibodies by S. Metalnikoff (*Ann. Inst. Pasteur* **14**, 577 (1900)) and antierythrocyte antibodies in the human disease paroxysmal cold haemoglobinuria by J. Donath and K. Landsteiner (*Münch. Med. Wochenschr.* **51**, 1590 (1904)).
15. E. Weil and H. Braun (*Wien. Klin. Wochenschr.* **22**, 372 (1909)) proposed that an autoimmune response to the tissue breakdown products in the syphilitic lesion exacerbates the disease; ophthalmologists S. Santucci (*Riv. Ital. Ottal. Roma* **2**, 213 (1906)) and S. Golowin (*Klin. Monatsbl. Augenheilk.* **47**, 150 (1909)) suggested that sympathetic ophthalmia might be caused by autoantibodies to damaged ocular tissues.
16. I have discussed elsewhere the full measure of the value of Bordet's observation on immune haemolysis: A. M. Silverstein, 'The heuristic value of experimental systems: the case of immune hemolysis', *J. Hist. Biol.* **27**, 437 (1994).
17. J. Bordet and O. Gengou, *Ann. Inst. Pasteur* **15**, 289 (1901).
18. A. von Wassermann, A. Neisser, C. Bruck and A. Schucht, *Z. Hyg.* **55**, 451 (1906).
19. P. Portier and C. Richet, *C.R. Soc. Biol.* **54**, 170 (1902).
20. M. Arthus, *C.R. Soc. Biol.* **55**, 817 (1903).
21. C. von Pirquet and B. Schick, *Die Serumkrankheit*, Deuticke, Vienna (1906).
22. A. Wolff-Eisner, *Das Heufieber*, Lehmann, Munich (1906).
23. S. J. Meltzer, *Trans. Assoc. Am. Phys.* **25**, 66 (1910); *J. Am. Med. Assoc.* **55**, 1021 (1910).
24. The efforts to come to grips with this paradox are reviewed in *A History of Immunology*, note 1, pp. 214–251.
25. To fix a specific date to the admission of a research area into the ranks of 'scientific discipline' is difficult. If we accept as adequate criteria the existence of a group of individuals who: (1) share the same research interests and methodologies; (2) share a special language peculiar to that area; and (3) utilize and debate one anothers' results to advance their research programme, then clearly immunology had become a discipline during the first decade of this century.
26. We owe this term to Robert Boyle in the 1640s. It describes informal groups of scientists established for the exchange of information and the advancement of learning. See also D. Crane, *Invisible Colleges: Diffusion of Knowledge in Scientific Communities*, University of Chicago Press, Chicago, IL (1972).
27. See A. M. Silverstein, 'The development of immunology in America', *Fed. Proc.* **46**, 240 (1987).
28. These studies are summarized in A. M. Silverstein, 'Ocular Immunology: on the birth of a new subdiscipline', *Cell. Immunol.* **136**, 504 (1991).
29. A. R. Rich, *The Pathogenesis of Tuberculosis*, 2nd edn, Chas. Thomas, Springfield, IL (1951).
30. T. M. Rivers, F. F. Schwentker and G. P. Berry, *J. Exp. Med.* **58**, 39 (1933); T. M. Rivers and F. F. Schwentker, *J. Exp. Med.* **61**, 689 (1935).
31. Many aspects of the history of allergy are covered in the fiftieth anniversary issue of *J. Allergy Appl. Immunol.*, **64**, 306–474 (1979).
32. H. H. Dale, *J. Pharmacol. Exp. Ther.* **4**, 167 (1913); H. H. Dale and P. P. Laidlaw, *J. Physiol. (London)* **52**, 355 (1919).
33. S. Arrhenius, *Immunochemistry*, Macmillan, New York (1907).
34. F. Obermeyer and E. P. Pick, *Wien. Klin. Wochenschr.* **19**, 327 (1906).
35. E. P. Pick, in *Handbuch der Pathogenen Mikroorganismen* (W. Kolle and A. von Wassermann, eds), 2nd edn, Fischer, Jena (1912), vol. 1, pp. 685–868.
36. K. Landsteiner and H. Lampl, *Z. Immunitätsforsch.* **26**, 258, 293 (1917).
37. K. Landsteiner, *The Specificity of Serological Reactions*, Thomas, Springfield, IL (1936).

38. M. Heidelberger, *Physiol. Rev.* 7, 107 (1927). This work owes much to the support of Oswald T. Avery, with whom Heidelberger published the initial papers (*J. Exp. Med.* 38, 81 (1923); 42, 367, 709 (1925)).

39. Heidelberger's contributions were celebrated in a book by his students E. A. Kabat and M. M. Mayer, *Quantitative Immunochemistry*, Chas. Thomas, Springfield, IL (1949).

40. F. Breinl and F. Haurowitz, *Z. Physiol. Chem.* 192, 45 (1930). There were other Lamarckian theories prior to this one, but they did not enjoy as great an influence.

41. L. Pauling, *J. Am. Chem. Soc.* 62, 2643 (1940); *Science* 92, 77 (1940).

42. F. M. Burnet, *The Production of Antibodies*, Macmillan, New York (1941); F. M. Burnet and F. Fenner, *The Production of Antibodies*, 2nd edn, Macmillan, New York (1949).

43. Two books typify this chemical approach to immunology, and summarize well its contributions: E. A. Kabat, *Structural Concepts in Immunology and Immunochemistry*, Holt, Rinehart & Winston, New York (1968); D. Pressman and A. Grossberg, *The Structural Basis of Antibody Specificity*, Benjamin, New York (1968).

44. A. Tiselius and E. A. Kabat, *J. Exp. Med.* 69, 119 (1939).

45. H. G. Wells, *The Chemical Aspects of Immunity*, Chem. Catalog Co., New York (1924); J. R. Marrack, *The Chemistry of Antigens and Antibodies*, HMSO, London (1934); K. Landsteiner, *The Specificity of Serological Reactions*, see note 37; Kabat and Mayer's *Quantitative Immunochemistry*, see note 39; W. C. Boyd, *Fundamentals of Immunology*, Wiley Interscience, New York (1943). Only in 1963 was a text written by and specifically for biologists: J. H. Humphrey and R. G. White, *Immunology for Students of Medicine*, Davis, Philadelphia (1963).

46. G. Lemaine, R. Macleod, M. Mulkay and P. Weingard (eds), *Perspectives on the Emergence of Scientific Disciplines*, Aldine, Chicago, IL (1976), p. 7.

47. H. Zinsser, *Bull. NY Acad. Med.* 4, 351 (1928).

48. Rich, see note 29.

49. L. Dienes and E. W. Schoenheit, *Am. Rev. Tuberc.* 20, 92 (1929).

50. F. A. Simon and F. M. Rackemann, *J. Allergy* 5, 439 (1934).

51. Rivers *et al.*, see note 30.

52. *The Production of Antibodies*, 1941 and 1949, see note 42.

53. P. B. Medawar, *J. Anat.* 78, 176 (1944); 79, 157 (1945). See also Medawar's *Harvey Lecture*, 52, 144 (1956–1957).

54. R. D. Owen, *Science* 102, 400 (1945).

55. *The Production of Antibodies*, 2nd edn, see note 42.

56. P. B Billingham, L. Brent and P. B. Medawar, *Nature (London)* 172, 603 (1953).

57. The first case of agammaglobulinaemia was described by O. C. Bruton, *Pediatrics*, 9, 722 (1952); the first case of a defect in T cells by A. M. DiGeorge, *J. Pediatr. (St Louis)* 67, 907 (1965); and the first case of severe combined immunodeficiency (so-called 'Swiss type') by E. Glanzmann and P. Riniker, *Ann. Pediatr. (Basel)* 175, 1 (1950).

58. N. R. Rose and I. R. Mackay (eds), *The Autoimmune Diseases*, Academic Press, New York (1985).

59. Kuhn, see note 4.

60. A. S. Coons, E. H. Leduc and J. M. Connolly, *J. Exp. Med.* 102, 49 (1955).

61. D. P. Pressman and G. Keighley, *J. Immunol.* 59, 141 (1948).

62. N. K. Jerne and A. A. Nordin, *Science* 140, 405 (1963).

63. K. Landsteiner and M. W. Chase, *Proc. Soc. Exp. Biol. Med.* 49, 688 (1942); N. A. Mitchison, *Proc. R. Soc. London, Ser. B* 142, 72 (1954); R. E. Billingham, L. Brent and P. B. Medawar, *Proc. R. Soc. London, Ser. B* 143, 43 (1954). See also H. N. Claman, E. A. Chaperon and R. F. Triplett, *Proc. Soc. Exp. Biol. Med.* 122, 1167 (1966).

64. R. I. Mishell and R. W. Dutton, *J. Exp. Med.* 126, 423 (1967); R. W. Dutton, *Adv. Immunol.* 6, 253 (1967).

65. N. K. Jerne, *Proc. Natl Acad. Sci. USA* 41, 849 (1955).

66. F. M. Burnet, *Aust. J. Sci.* 20, 67 (1957).

67. F. M. Burnet, *The Clonal Selection Theory of Acquired Immunity*, Cambridge University Press, London (1959).

68. D. W. Talmage, *Science* **129**, 1643 (1959); J. Lederberg, *Science* **129**, 1649 (1959).

69. See, for example, P. Galison, 'The trading zone: coordinating action and belief', in *Image and Logic: The Material Culture of Modern Physics*, chap. 9 (in press).

70. In 1964, in Prague, Burnet rose to declare the victory of his clonal selection theory, and few biologists in the audience disagreed (J. Sterzl (ed.), 'Molecular and Cellular Basis of Antibody Formation', Czech Academy of Science, Prague (1964)). The more chemically oriented immunologists converted only more slowly, and a few (for example, the late Felix Haurowitz and Alain Bussard) never conceded. Some identify the 1967 Cold Spring Harbor meeting (*Cold Spring Harbor Symp. Quant. Biol.* **32** (1967)) as the turning point.

71. There were, in fact, some interdisciplinary relationships. The study of antibodies and their specificity throughout this period was intimately connected with physical chemistry, and with developments in the understanding of protein and enzyme structure and function. Indeed, L. E. Kay (*Hist. Life Sci.* **11**, 211 (1989); and *The Molecular Vision of Life*, Oxford University Press, New York (1993)) suggests that immunology contributed much to the early development of molecular biology.

72. This coming together of chemically and biologically oriented immunologists is discussed in greater detail by A. M. Silverstein, 'The immunological synthesis: the unification of *cis* and *trans* science' (in press). It is reminiscent of the so-called 'evolutionary synthesis' (see E. Mayr and W. B. Provine, *The Evolutionary Synthesis: Perspectives on the Unification of Biology*, Harvard University Press, Cambridge, MA (1980)). In that case, it was the Mendelian geneticists working forward from the genome and the palaeontologists working backward from the whole organism and populations who melded their disparate languages and approaches to attack the problems of evolution.

73. A.-M. Moulin, *Rev. Hist. Sci.* **36**, 49 (1983); *Hist. Phil. Life Sci.* **11**, 221 (1989). See also her book *Le Dernier Langage de la Médecine: Histoire de l'Immunologie de Pasteur au Sida*, Presse Universitaire, Paris (1991).

Theories of Immunity

Origins of the Cell Selection Theories of Antibody Formation

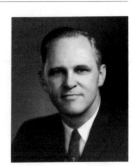

DAVID W. TALMAGE

Department of Immunology and the Webb–Waring Lung Institute,
Health Sciences Center, University of Colorado, Denver,
CO 80262, USA

The concept of cell selection is based on the rather simple notion that adaptation of the individual to environmental antigens requires selection of the individual's diverse components (differentiated cells) in the same way that adaptation of the species requires selection of its diverse components. This basic concept of cell selection was developed independently at the University of Chicago in 1956 and at the Hall Institute in Melbourne in 1957 (1–3). That this should happen almost simultaneously in two places so far apart indicates that the time was right for this development and that the concept was based logically on preceding knowledge and ideas.

The following attempt to describe and explain the origins of the cell selection theories will be divided into three parts. The first part is a brief description of developments in immunology that preceded the concept of cell selection and made its proposal possible and even inevitable. The second part discusses the events in the broader fields of science and scientific philosophy that led to the explosion of immunological knowledge that began around 1880. The last part is a more personal statement of the factors that led me to advance the concept of cell selection in 1956.

The Immunological Ideas that Preceded Cell Selection

The most important basic concepts on which cell selection draws are those of immunological memory and specificity. The idea of immunological memory has been around for a long time. It was known during the Middle Ages that those who had survived an attack of smallpox were immune to a second attack. The deliberate inoculation of a susceptible person with pustular material from a relatively mild case (known as 'variolation') was practised in the Near East for

IMMUNOLOGY: THE MAKING OF A MODERN SCIENCE
ISBN 0-12-274020-3

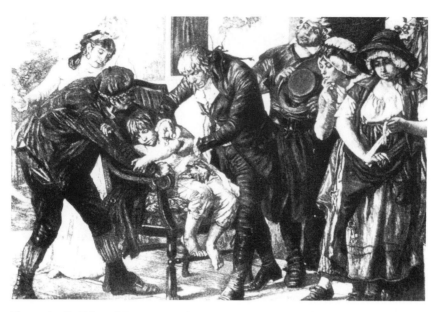

Figure 1 Dr Edward Jenner inoculating pus from the hand of Sarah Nelmes into the arm of James Phipps (4).

several centuries before it was introduced into Western Europe in 1718 by Lady Mary Montague, wife of the British Ambassador to Turkey. It was almost 80 years later, near the end of the eighteenth century, that Edward Jenner, a private practitioner of medicine in Berkeley, England, took note of a common local belief that dairy maids who had caught cowpox (a local infection of their hands) were immune to smallpox. In perhaps the most courageous and far-reaching clinical experiment of all times, Jenner took pus from the hand of Sarah Nelmes, and injected it into the arm of James Phipps, a healthy eight-year-old boy (4) (Fig. 1); six weeks later he injected the boy with pus from a smallpox patient without ill effect. As a direct consequence of this experiment, smallpox has been eliminated from the earth, although it took 180 years to complete the job.

From the point of view of immunological theory, Jenner's success had immense consequences. He had demonstrated that the specificity of immunological memory was not absolute. It was not necessary to inject a disease-producing organism to develop effective immunity. A related, less virulent organism would work equally well. But, surprisingly, it was 80 years before Pasteur generalized this concept to other diseases: chicken cholera, anthrax, swine erysipelas and rabies.

Although Pasteur understood the practical implications of Jenner's work, initially he did not have a clear idea of how the immune system worked. He proposed (5) that each organism had unique nutritional requirements and that

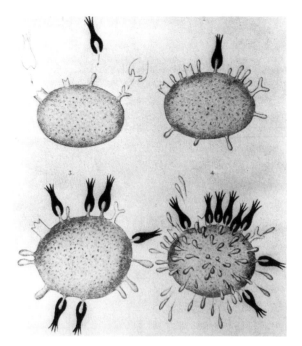

Figure 2 Ehrlich's side-chain theory. Cellular receptors are designed to bring nutrients into the cell. When a foreign substance (solid black) binds too many of these receptors, the cell makes an oversupply of them and some of them fall off and become antibodies (8).

the first attack of a particular organism consumed some of these, leaving the individual immune to the growth of that organism in the future. Thus, Pasteur's success with a rabies vaccine derived from heated spinal cord was important in the development of the idea that non-living components of the organism (antigens) could induce an immune response. The isolation of the first antigen (diphtheria toxin) by Roux and Yersin (6) and the demonstration of the first serum antibody by Nuttall (7), both in 1888, were important steps in establishing immunology as a separate field of science.

It was Paul Ehrlich (8) who first introduced an acceptable theory of immunity in 1900, the side-chain theory (Fig. 2). Ehrlich had an excellent concept of the interaction between antigen and antibody molecules, and the relation between cells, cellular receptors and humoral antibodies. His theory was the logical synthesis of existing theories of cellular and humoral immunity. It should have launched the beginnings of cellular immunology. But immunological science was not ready for Ehrlich. In fact the word 'immunology' was not introduced for another 11 years. Ehrlich was also somewhat rigid about his theory and insisted that the cellular receptors (side-chains) were physiologically important to the acquisition of nutrients by the cells.

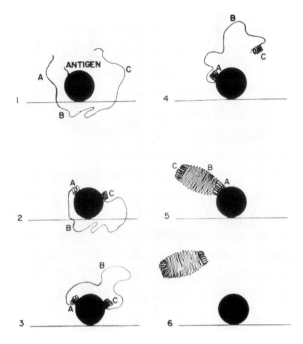

Figure 3   Pauling's variable folding theory of antibody formation (*11*).

When Landsteiner (*9*) showed that antibodies could be made to newly syn-thesized chemicals, the side-chain theory and the study of cells were dropped and forgotten for more than 30 years. This was the period of serology (1910–1940). Landsteiner and then Kabat and Heidelberger were the dom-inant figures in the field. In 1930, Breinl and Haurowitz (*10*) published their template theory of antibody formation, which was made more explicit by Pauling (*11*) in 1940 (Fig. 3). The word 'lymphocyte' did not appear in the index of the *Journal of Immunology* until 1948, when Harris and Henle (*12*) published a study on lymphocytes in hepatitis. Still, great progress was made in understanding the nature of immunological specificity during this time. Landsteiner (*13*) came very close to our modern concept of specificity in his discussion of Malkoff's (*14*) findings (Table 1). Malkoff came to the conclu-sion that normal serum contained as many specific agglutinins as there were sorts of erythrocytes that could be agglutinated by the 'natural' antibody in that serum. Because of the large number of different substances that could be agglutinated by normal serum and because each antibody amounted to several micrograms per millilitre of serum, Landsteiner rejected Malkoff's hypothesis. He was able to purify the agglutinins by absorption and elution, and to show that the purified agglutinins acted most strongly on the red cells used for absorption, but also agglutinated other sorts of cells. Landsteiner concluded that:

Table 1 Malkoff's results (from (*14*))

Blood	Unabsorbed serum	Goat serum absorbed with				
		Pigeon blood	Rabbit blood	Human blood	Pigeon and rabbit blood	Pigeon and human blood
Pigeon blood	+	0	+	+	0	0
Rabbit blood	+	+	0	+	0	+
Human blood	+	+	+	0	+	0

If one assumes that normal serum contains a sufficient number of agglutinins, each reacting with a certain proportion of all bloods, a given sort of blood will absorb from a serum all those agglutinins for which it has affinity and there will remain after absorption some that react with freshly added blood of other species . . . One may conjecture that there exists a much greater variety of globulin molecules in serum than would appear from physicochemical examination, some of which by virtue of accidental affinity to certain substrates are picked out as antibodies.

The preceding statement of Landsteiner had two of the essential ingredients of a selective theory: natural diversity and accidental affinity. He correctly attributed the specificity of natural antibodies to unique combinations of natural globulins. An extension of this concept to include immune antibodies might have seemed likely because of the similarity of Landsteiner's own results with synthetic haptens (*15*) (Table 2). Landsteiner rejected this concept as an explanation for the specificity of immune antibodies, apparently because of a firm conviction that immune antibodies were different from natural antibodies.

However, it was Landsteiner and Chase who started the trend back to cellular studies. Landsteiner had proposed that allergic reactions such as contact hypersensitivity were due to the same type of antibodies that could be measured in serum. This idea has been attacked by two allergists, Straus and Coca (*16*), and Landsteiner and Chase set out to determine if contact sensitivity could be due to humoral antibodies. This culminated in the classical report in 1942 (*17*) which showed that delayed hypersensitivity could be transferred only with cells. Thus Landsteiner, who had effectively buried Ehrlich's approach to cellular immunity, played a large role in its rebirth 30 years later.

Also in 1942, Coons, Creech, Jones and Berliner (*18*) described a new technique, using fluorescent antibody, that stained and localized antigens in tissue sections. This technique made possible the demonstration that antigens were missing from the highly specialized cell, the plasma cell, that made antibodies. The demonstration that plasma cells were the antibody producing cells was made by Fagraeus (*19*) in 1948. One year after Fagraeus' report, Burnet and Fenner (*20*) published the first edition of a small book called *Production of Antibodies*. In it they strongly attacked the then current chemical approach to immunology and the isolation of immunology from the

Table 2 Results obtained by Landsteiner and van der Scheer (15)*

Immune sera for m-aminobenzene sulphonic acid after absorption with	Azoproteins made from chicken serum and			
	o-Aminobenzene sulphonic acid	m-Aminobenzene sulphonic acid	m-Aminobenzene arsenic acid	m-Aminobenzoic acid
o-Aminobenzene sulphonic acid†	0	++±	±	+
o-Aminobenzene sulphonic acid‡	0	+++±	±	+
m-Aminobenzene arsenic acid†	+±	+++	0	+
m-Aminobenzene arsenic acid‡	++	++++	0	+±
m-Aminobenzoic acid†	+±	+++	±	0
m-Aminobenzoic acid‡	++	++++	±	±
Unabsorbed immune serum†	++	+++±	+	+±
Unabsorbed immune serum‡	+++	++++	++	++±

* Since the test antigens contained the same proteins, unrelated to the horse serum used for immunization, the protein component could not be responsible for the differential reactions.
† After standing for 1 hour at room temperature.
‡ After standing overnight in the icebox.

Antibody production

I   Adaptation phase – radiosensitive
(duration < 12 h)

Antigen + γ-globulin generator ⟶ Modified γ-globulin generator

II   Production phase – radioresistant
Modified
Antigen + γ-globulin ⟶ Antibody
generator

Figure 4   A modification of Burnet's and Fenner's globulin synthesizing unit was adopted as an explanation of the radiosensitive and radioresistant phases of antibody production (21).

mainstream of biology. They proposed a model of antibody formation that was based on the then current concept of adaptive enzyme formation in bacteria. They proposed that antigen modified the globulin synthesizing units in plasma cells, which were then able to replicate. In 1952, there were two reports, one by Dixon, Talmage and Maurer (21) and one by Taliaferro, Taliaferro and Janssen (22), that demonstrated radiosensitive and radioresistant phases in the antibody response. Dixon's group adopted Burnet and Fenner's modification of the globulin synthesizing unit to explain their findings (Fig. 4).

In 1953, Billingham, Brent and Medawar (23) extended Owen's earlier report (24) of red cell chimeras in cattle twins, by producing bone marrow chimeras in inbred mice. The injection of bone marrow cells into embryos and newborn mice produced a tolerance of subsequent skin grafts from the donor strain. This was a demonstration that immunological memory could be negative as well as positive. In 1955, Taliaferro and Talmage (25) and Roberts and Dixon (26) both reported the transfer of immunological memory with cells. This was the same year that Jerne proposed his natural-selection theory of antibody formation (27). But Jerne's theory did not involve cell selection. He proposed that the production of γ-globulins was randomized by some unspecified process, perhaps in the thymus. Once produced they could be replicated by antibody forming cells. The role of antigen was to select those random globulins with which they had a chance affinity and introduce them into the antibody producing cells, where they served as a model for further production of the same globulin. Jerne effectively reviewed the arguments against the direct and indirect template theories and focused immunological theory on the possibility of selection. By 1956 the field was ready for cell selection.

The Origin of Western Science and an Immunological Worldview

Many reasons have been given for the dramatic rise of Western science in the sixteenth century until the present. There was the introduction of Aristotelian philosophy and logic following the recapture of Spain from the Moors. There was the universal acceptance of a decimal numbering system following the invention of the zero in India around AD 600. Modern science could not exist without decimals, and decimals are impossible without the zero.

An important factor in opening people's mind to change was the conflict between the dogmatic, deductive logic of Aristotelian philosophy and the revealed knowledge of Christian orthodoxy (28). This may have opened minds to the possibility of settling arguments through observation rather than reason or revelation. The disastrous plague of 1348–1352 wiped out a quarter of the population of Europe and at the same time destroyed confidence in traditional ways of looking at nature and the cause of disease. Along with the plague, commerce with China brought three important and interdependent technological inventions: paper, reading glasses and the printing press. Movable type, which would not have been practical with China's more than 50 000 characters, was invented in Mainz, Germany, by Johannes Gutenberg around 1440.

A single event that marked the beginnings of Western science was the work of Nicolaus Copernicus, a Polish Catholic prelate who became interested in astronomical observations about the same time that Columbus discovered the New World and convinced the sceptics that the world was round. It was also clear from its circumnavigation that the Earth was unattached and free in space. Although Copernicus did not make any new discoveries or derive any famous equations, he made observations with crude instruments that convinced him that the stars were infinitely far away. Because of their distance they could not possibly travel all the way around the Earth in 24 hours. From this he reasoned that it must be the Earth that rotated. If the Earth rotated it could also move and Copernicus proposed that many of the peculiar motions of the planets could be explained if the Earth and the planets all revolved around the Sun.

Copernicus made a very important contribution to scientific philosophy by distinguishing between appearance and reality. With regard to whether it was the Earth or the sky that was moving, he said, 'The appearance belongs to the heavens but the reality belongs to the earth' (29). This distinction between appearance and reality was applied to medicine by Giralamo Fracastoro (30), a physician contemporary to Copernicus, who wrote in 1546, 'Contagion is an infection that passes from one thing to another'. Fracastoro also noted the similarity of symptoms in the donor and recipient of an infection and proposed that the infection originated in very small 'imperceptible particles'. Fracastoro's ideas were based on a careful balancing of observation, reason and causality and the postulation of an objective reality behind the perceptible. The germ theory of disease did not make much progress over the next two centuries partly because of the absence of good microscopes and partly because the science of physics went off in a different direction.

Beginning with Kepler and then with Galileo and Newton, physics became a science of absolute mathematical laws (31). The reality and the causes behind the laws became irrelevant or even meaningless. Newton, who showed that the inverse-square law of gravitation could explain the motion of the planets, said 'I frame no hypotheses' (32). Newton's distaste for speculation led some philosophers of science to downgrade the usefulness of all hypotheses. The word developed a bad connotation to the point that Thomas Reid, a Scottish mathematician and common sense philosopher discounted the value of all hypotheses. But Newton had made a causal hypothesis when he proposed that the force that held the Moon in its orbit was the same as the force that made the apple drop to the Earth. Among the reasons given by Reid for avoiding hypotheses were that it would prejudice the impartiality of the scientist and would assume that the mind of man was capable of understanding the works of God.

In the nineteenth century, causal hypotheses came under attack from another direction, the logical positivism of Comte and the Vienna school led by Ernst Mach. Comte was a French philosopher who claimed that human understanding had advanced through three states: theological, metaphysical and positive. Comte viewed positivism as the most advanced state in which one accepts only the objective evidence of the five senses. In retrospect, Comte's views seem to be a reaction to the claims of the Church that every cause had an earlier cause and God was the first cause. By eliminating causal hypotheses altogether, Comte freed himself from the dominance of the Church. Thus, the concept of God first prevented the use of causal hypotheses for fear of intruding on His domain, and then the revolt from God prevented its use for fear of giving Him too much credit.

Fortunately, medical science remained separate from these philosophical ruminations. Forced to deal with diseases that could not be predicted with mathematical equations, physicians framed causal hypotheses to explain what they observed. Then they did experiments to test, modify or reject these hypotheses. In Jenner's time it was assumed that smallpox was a contagious disease that produced immunity to subsequent attacks. Jenner was a country physician who demonstrated that immunity to smallpox could be produced by an attack of cowpox. Yet neither bacteria nor viruses were known at the time. Nor was there any idea of the mechanism of immunity.

Pasteur devised a dramatic test of a causal hypothesis. By his time it was known that bacteria growing in broth could be killed by boiling but would return again in a few days if the container were left open to the air. The current theory was that bacteria were spontaneously generated from the ingredients in the broth and the oxygen in the air, because if the container was kept closed no contamination occurred. Pasteur proposed an alternative cause of the contamination, namely that the bacteria came with the dust in the air. The controversy became heated and the French Academy of Sciences proposed a test of Pasteur's hypothesis in the Academy chambers. Pasteur built glass flasks that were sealed except for a long curved tube that let in the oxygen but not the dust. The broth in the flasks was sterilized and left at the Academy for months without becoming contaminated (*33*). This ended the controversy and the theory of spontaneous generation.

But Pasteur's demonstration did a great deal more. It established the value of the causal hypothesis in the biomedical sciences. Thus, while the physical sciences have grown more and more dependent on pure mathematics, biology has exploited the pragmatic value of causation. The purposes of this research are: (1) to understand the causes of natural phenomena, and (2) to control natural phenomena for the benefit of mankind. This differs from the purposes of physical science which are: (1) to describe natural phenomena with mathematical equations, and (2) to predict past and future events.

In addition to its dependence on the development of a biomedical worldview, which I have called 'causal realism' (*34*), immunology has benefited greatly from numerous technological inventions and support from related scientific fields. No technological advance has been more important to immunology than the perfection of the microscope. The fields from which immunology has drawn the most support are microbiology and, more recently, molecular biology.

Reading glasses were probably introduced to Europe in the fourteenth century (Fig. 5) and the first telescope was built in 1608 (Fig. 6). Within a year of that date, Galileo had discovered the moons of Jupiter and observed the phases of Venus as it travelled around the Sun. But the microscope was not perfected for more than two centuries (Fig. 7). Almost immediately there was a

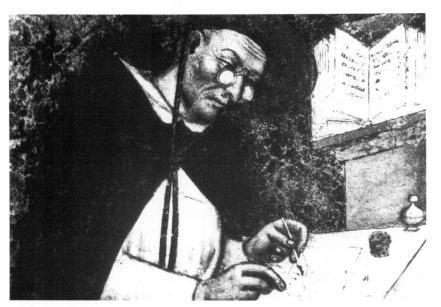

Figure 5   The earliest known painting showing the use of spectacles, according to Burke, dates from 1352 (*40*).

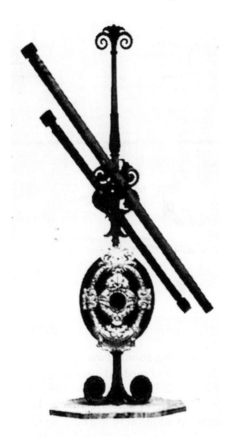

Figure 6 Two of Galileo's telescopes (from the Museo di Fisica e Storia Naturale, Florence, Italy). A lens from the telescope Galileo used when he discovered Jupiter's moons is on the plaque (*41*).

burst of activity. In 1850, Davaine saw anthrax bacilli in the blood of sheep suffering from anthrax and later was able to prove that the bacilli caused the disease. Both Koch and Pasteur were able to transmit anthrax to animals from isolated cultures in 1876. The first bacterium pathogenic for humans, the *gonococcus*, was isolated by Neisser in 1879. Within eight years ten more human pathogens had been isolated (*35*). The world was ready for the introduction of immunology with the isolation of antigens and antibodies in 1888.

A Personal Recollection of the Events of 1956

I graduated from medical school during World War II and took a rotating internship in Atlanta where I learned to sew up cuts in the emergency room and

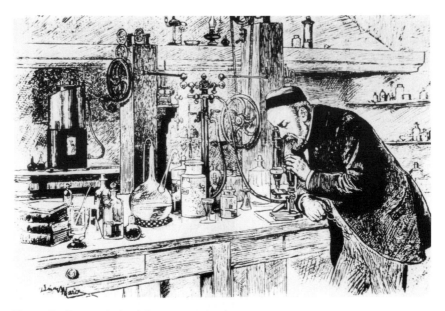

Figure 7 Pasteur in his laboratory. Note his microscope (42).

hold retractors in the operating room. Two years of active military service in Korea were followed by a year of medical internship and a year of medical residency at Barnes Hospital in St Louis. I was then fortunate to spend two years with Frank Dixon doing research on the immune response of rabbits to radioactively labelled proteins. In addition to learning how to handle radioisotopes, I learned how to design large experiments and became interested in the mechanism of antibody formation as indicated by our attempts in this direction shown in Fig. 4.

I moved to the University of Chicago in 1952 and began working closely with William Taliaferro. Tolly was a man with a great sense of humour and historical perspective who had lots of ideas about differentiation of lymphocytes and macrophages. Together we designed an experiment to determine whether the transfer of immunological memory with cells from an immunized to an unimmunized rabbit involved the synthesis of new protein or the release of old protein (25). The key to the experiment was to give ^{35}S labelled amino acids to either the donor or the recipient of the immune cells. When the radioactive label was given to the donor before transfer, the antibody made in the donor but not in the recipient was labelled. When the radioactive label was given to the recipient, the reverse was true. This was clear evidence that the transferred cells contained the machinery for making new antibody and not a store of already synthesized antibody. This was 1955, the year that Jerne published his natural selection theory.

By 1955 I had become firmly convinced that antibodies were just natural globulins that just happened to have affinity for antigen. Perhaps the most important experiment that led to this belief was the attempt to purify labelled antibodies by absorption and elution from solid antigen columns (36). There was always some antibody that came off the column spontaneously in the saline wash. Other antibody could be eluted by washing the column with unlabelled antiserum; and other antibody was attached so firmly that it could only be removed with acid solution. There seemed to be such a wide spectrum of avidities that the boundary between antibody and non-antibody globulin was a matter of arbitrary definition. This fitted with Jerne's previously published Ph.D. thesis describing the varying avidities of antidiphtheria toxin (37). It is probably not a coincidence that both of us, after studying the phenomenon of avidity, became convinced that antibodies were natural globulins selected by antigen.

But Jerne's proposed mechanism was not compatible with the new information on protein synthesis. When I arrived at the University of Chicago in 1952, I was impressed with the intense interest of the biochemists in the nucleic acids, and the evidence that the 'configuration of a protein molecule is determined solely by information contained in the hereditary units of the cell, the nucleic acids' (1). Recall that Watson and Crick's model of the DNA molecule was presented in 1953 (38).

Positive evidence that the cell was the site of immunological memory and selection was found in the experiments that cells but not antiserum could transfer memory to an unimmunized animal, in the long time required for sensitization, in the long persistence of memory in the absence of antigen and in the homogeneity of globulin produced by the plasma cells of multiple myeloma (39).

In summary, by 1956, there were a large number of objective signs pointing to cell selection. For me the most important were the following:

(1) The evidence that immunological memory was both positive and negative.
(2) The tremendous diversity of antibody molecules both in avidity and physicochemical properties.
(3) The increasing avidity of antibody during the immune response.
(4) The exponential increase in antibody titres during the immune response.
(5) The transfer of immunological memory with cells but not with antiserum.
(6) The very rapid rate of antibody production during the height of the immune response and its continued production for long periods.
(7) The evidence that protein structure was determined by information in the nucleic acids.

In addition, I was strongly influenced by the work of three people (Fig. 8): Landsteiner's evidence that the cross-reactivity of immune antibodies was similar to that of natural antibodies and his concept that the specificity of natural antibodies was based on random overlapping reactivities; Burnet's plea that immunology return to the mainstream of biology; and Taliaferro's concept of the differentiated cell.

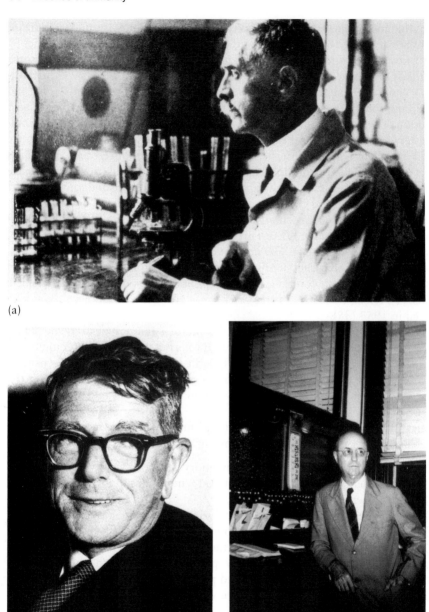

(a)

(b)   (c)

Figure 8   (a) Karl Landsteiner (from P. Speiser and F. G. Smekal, *Karl Landsteiner* (R. Rickett, trans.), Verlag Bruder Hollinek, Vienna (1975)). (b) Sir MacFarlane Burnet (from D. W. Talmage, Obituary: Frank MacFarlane Burnet 1899–1985. *J. Immunol.* **136**, 1528 (1986)). (c) William H. Taliaferro.

Finally, I believe that my training in medical science, which is based on the philosophy of causal realism, played an important role in preparing me to ask the right questions.

Notes and References

1. D. W. Talmage, *Ann. Rev. Med.* **8**, 239 (1957).
2. F. M. Burnet, *Aust. J. Sci.* **20**, 67 (1957).
3. D. W. Talmage, *Science* **129**, 1643 (1959).
4. G. Rosen and W. Jenner, in *The World Book Encyclopedia*, vol. 11, Field Enterprises Educational Corp., Chicago, IL (1971), pp. 73–74.
5. L. Pasteur, *C.R. Acad. Sci. (Paris)* **90**, 1033 (1880).
6. E. Roux and A. Yersin, *Ann. Inst. Pasteur* **ii**, 629 (1888).
7. G. Nuttall, *Z. Hyg. Leipzig* **iv**, 353 (1888).
8. P. Ehrlich, *Proc. R. Soc. (Biol.)* **66**, 424 (1900).
9. K. Landsteiner, *The Specificity of Serological Reactions*, Harvard University Press, Cambridge, MA (1936).
10. F. Breinl and F. Haurowitz, *Z. Physiol. Chem.* **192**, 45 (1930).
11. L. Pauling, *J. Am. Chem. Soc.* **62**, 2643 (1940).
12. S. Harris and W. Henle, *J. Immunol.* **59**, 9 (1948).
13. K. Landsteiner, *The Specificity of Serological Reactions*, Harvard University Press, Cambridge, MA (1945).
14. G. Malkoff, *Dtsch. Med. Wschr.* **26**, 229 (1900).
15. K. Landsteiner and J. van der Scheer, *J. Exp. Med.* **63**, 325 (1936).
16. H. Straus and A. Coca, *J. Immunol.* **33**, 215 (1937).
17. K. Landsteiner and M. Chase, *Proc. Soc. Exp. Biol. Med.* **49**, 688 (1942).
18. A. Coons, H. Creech, R. Jones and E. Berliner, *J. Immunol.* **58**, 1 (1942).
19. A. Fagraeus, *J. Immunol.* **58**, 1 (1948).
20. F. M. Burnet and F. Fenner, *Production of Antibodies*, Macmillan, Melbourne (1949), p. 133.
21. F. Dixon, D. Talmage and P. Maurer, *J. Immunol.* **68**, 693 (1952).
22. W. Taliaferro, L. Taliaferro and E. Janssen, *J. Infect. Dis.* **91**, 105 (1952).
23. R. Billingham, I. Brent and P. Medawar, *Nature (London)* **172**, 603 (1953).
24. R. Owen, *Science* **102**, 400 (1945).
25. W. Taliaferro and D. Talmage, *J. Infect. Dis.* **97**, 88 (1955).
26. J. Roberts and F. Dixon, *J. Exp. Med.* **102**, 379 (1955).
27. N. Jerne, *Proc. Natl Acad. Sci. USA* **41**, 849 (1955).
28. D. Lindberg, *The Beginnings of Western Science*, University of Chicago Press, Chicago, IL (1992), pp. 235–244.
29. N. Copernicus, in *Great Books of the Western World* (R. M. Hutchins, ed.), Encyclopedia Britannica, Chicago, IL (1952), p. 519.
30. H. A. Lechevalier and M. Solorovsky, *Three Centuries of Microbiology*, McGraw-Hill, New York (1965).
31. I. Newton, in *Great Books of the Western World* (R. M. Hutchins, ed.), vol. 34, Encyclopedia Britannica, Chicago, IL (1952), p. 270.
32. I. Newton, note 31, p. 371.
33. L. Pasteur, *Ann. Sci. Naturelles, Ser. 4* **16**, (1861). (Translated into English in *Milestones in Microbiology* (T. D. Brock, ed.), Prentice Hall, Englewood Cliffs, NJ (1961).)
34. D. Talmage, In *Immunologic Revolution: Facts and Witnesses* (A. Szentivanyi and H. Friedman, eds), CRC Press, Boca Raton, FL (1994), pp. 13–21.
35. H. J. Parrish, *Victory with Vaccines*, E. & S. Livingstone, Edinburgh (1968), p. 29.

36. D. Talmage, H. Baker and W. Akeson, *J. Infect. Dis.* **94**, 199 (1954).
37. N. K. Jerne, *Acta Pathol. Microbiol., Scand.* **87** (Suppl.), (1952).
38. J. Watson and F. Crick, *Nature* **171**, 737 (1953).
39. F. Putnam and B. Udin, *J. Biol. Chem.*, **202**, 727 (1953).
40. J. Burke, *The Day the Universe Changed*, Little Brown and Co., Boston, MA (1985).
41. C. T. Chase, Galileo, in *The World Book Encyclopedia*, vol. 8, Fred Enterprises Education Corp., Chicago, IL (1971), pp. 11–12.
42. H. Parish, *A History of Immunization*, E. & S., Livingston, Edinburgh (1965).

One Cell – One Antibody

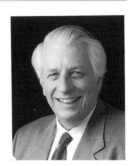

G. J. V. NOSSAL
The Walter and Eliza Hall Institute of Medical Research,
Post Office, Royal Melbourne Hospital, Victoria 3050, Australia

In 1957, when I had the good fortune to start in Sir Macfarlane Burnet's laboratory, cellular immunology was not yet a clearly demarcated specialty. In the nearly 40 years since then, it has made enormous progress. As Director of a medical research institute largely devoted to immunology, I have had the rare privilege of participating in some small way in this huge chapter of modern biology. It is quite difficult to put oneself back into the mental framework of 1957, when the lymphocyte was a cell of unknown function and vague terms like 'mesenchymal cells' and the 'reticuloendothelial system' were used to disguise our ignorance of the cellular basis of antibody formation. It is interesting that the early giants of immunology (Pasteur, Ehrlich, Bordet, Roux, von Behring and Koch) devoted relatively little attention to the question of which particular cells made antibodies, although Metchnikoff, of course, realized that macrophages were very important cells in immunity. Let us first summarize what was known in the prehistory of cellular immunology.

The Cellular Basis of Antibody Formation – 1957

In 1898, Pfeiffer and Marx (1) first pointed to the spleen as a major organ of antibody production, with lymph nodes and bone marrow also contributing. McMaster and Hudack (2) showed that the lymph node draining the site of a subcutaneous injection of antigen was the first tissue to produce antibody, and if two different antigens were injected on opposite sides of the body, the ipsilateral node made predominantly the appropriate antibody. The lymph node response to antigens was studied extensively by Ehrich and Harris (3) who first drew attention to the possible role of lymphocytes in immune responses. On the other side of the Atlantic, Bing and Plum (4) and Bjorneboe and Gormsen (5) drew attention to plasma cells as possible antibody producers. An important study by Fagraeus (6) charted the sequential appearance of 'transitional' cells, immature plasma cells and mature plasma cells in the red pulp of the spleen following immunization. In short-term tissue culture, the red pulp formed far more antibody than the lymphocyte-rich white pulp, so Fagraeus concluded that plasma cells, not lymphocytes, were the antibody-forming cells. Thorbecke and Keuning (7), using differential centrifugation to separate the two cell types, supported this conclusion. Definitive proof had to await the 'sandwich' variant of the Coons' fluorescent antibody technique (8), which showed much antibody present in the plasma cells of the red pulp of the spleen and the medullary cords of lymph nodes. Many more antibody-containing (presumably antibody-forming) cells developed in the secondary, as compared with the primary, immune response. The work of Coons' group supported the cellular sequence described by Fagraeus (6), but neither group believed that the plasma cell series was actually derived from lymphocytes. Indeed, the predominant view was that plasma cells came from primitive mesenchymal cells or cells of the connective tissue reticulum. Furthermore, in the late 1950s, it was still not possible to initiate antibody formation *in vitro*, and maintenance of production initiated *in vivo* was possible for only a few days of tissue culture. Thus the search for the initiating cell had to rely on the relatively clumsy technique of adoptive transfer. Harris and Harris (9) were among the few to promote the view that lymphocytes were responsible.

Selective Theories of Antibody Formation

The chapters by Silverstein and Talmage in this volume have already dealt with theories of antibody formation and, in particular, the instructive theory involving antigens as a direct template versus selective theories that saw antibodies as natural products requiring amplification following the entry of antigen. The only perspective I wish to add is to reflect on the relative contributions of Talmage (10) and Burnet (11) to the development of the clonal selection theory. Both, I believe, were heavily influenced by Jerne (12) and both independently reached the conclusion that his ideas about how specific antibody was synthesized were seriously flawed. Jerne thought antigen, after injection, complexed with natural antibody. Then the complexes were taken up by macrophages, in which the antibody somehow acted as a template for the synthesis of more of itself. Though the Crick dogma had not been articulated in its final form in 1957, the informational primacy of DNA was already clear, rendering untenable the idea of protein as a template. Burnet, for example, was thoroughly familiar with the concept of transformation and transduction. Talmage certainly was first to claim that Jerne's hypothesis made more sense if the unit of selection was a cell bearing natural antibody on its surface.

It has not been sufficiently recognized that Burnet (11) actually cites the slightly earlier paper of Talmage (10) in his first articulation of clonal selection.

Equally, it is true that Burnet had been groping his way towards clonal selection for some time, since realizing the inadequacy of his own earlier speculations. It is possible that Talmage's paper was the triggering point that persuaded Burnet to put pen to paper. What makes Burnet's 1957 article so remarkable is its sweep into many of the key puzzles of immune regulation. Thus, he postulated very precisely a *unique* receptor for each cell. He noted the very large number of small lymphocytes in the body, permitting the existence of a large and diverse repertoire of individual elements. He saw that the theory could provide an elegant explanation of tolerance. While foreign antigens reaching the mature lymphoid system would stimulate a subset of lymphocytes with receptors preadapted to react with it, self-antigens would reach the immature immune system leading to the opposite result, namely clonal deletion of self-reactive lymphocytes. Should this purging of the repertoire break down for any reason, 'forbidden clones' of self-reactive lymphocytes could arise and cause autoimmune disease. Furthermore, Burnet saw how somatic mutation in antibody genes could promote affinity maturation. If somatic mutation occurred among the lymphocytes originally selected by an antigen, then it was easy to see that mutants with higher affinity for the antigen in question would be favoured on continuing or repeated antigenic exposure. Finally, the antigen-induced increase in specifically reactive lymphocytes gave a ready explanation for the secondary or 'booster' response to readministration of antigen.

It seems to me that all three men deserve great credit: Jerne for realizing that antibodies were preformed products, covering a vast diversity of specificities; Talmage for seeing that it had to be the cell that was the unit of selection; and Burnet for fleshing out what clonal selection meant for immunobiology as a whole.

One Cell, One Antibody

My youthful ambition had been to become a biochemically oriented virologist. I was surely influenced by my six-year-older brother, P. M. Nossal, a student of Hans Krebs and a successful biochemist in Adelaide. A seminal year for me was 1952, when I took a year off from my medical studies to work with a highly original virologist at the University of Sydney, P. M. de Burgh. Like many of my generation, I was enormously influenced by the writings of Luria and Delbrück, and was convinced that studying the biochemistry of the replication of the simplest forms of life, the viruses, would reveal all of life's most precious secrets. Fascination with bacteriophages was tempered by a local consideration. Macfarlane Burnet, then committed entirely to a study of animal viruses, was Australia's greatest scientist, and Frank Fenner, then also working in Melbourne, had gained deep insights into the *in vivo* replication of ectromelia (mousepox) virus (*13*). De Burgh (*14*) was investigating this model to determine how the virus perverted the host cell's metabolic machinery, but I was more interested in one-step growth curves within individual liver cells, reaching the then surprising finding (intracellular 'factories' had not yet been discovered) that as many as 20 independent virus-synthesizing centres could exist in a single liver cell (15). My mentor, de Burgh, took me down to Melbourne for a week in the winter of 1952 and meetings with both Burnet and Fenner seeded the idea of a fellowship within the Walter and Eliza Hall Institute. So, I finished my medical degree, did two years as a hospital resident, and journeyed down to Melbourne with my wife and our tiny baby in February 1957. However, to my considerable dismay, Burnet's interests were rapidly shifting from virology to immunology. I was indoctrinated into the mysteries of the growth of influenza virus in embryonated hen's eggs, but was urged to apply this knowledge to a study of immunological tolerance. I soon showed that tolerance induction to influenza virus was not possible (16) but, provided multiple injections were given, tolerance to foreign erythrocytes could readily be induced in newborn but not adult rats (17). However, I was still reading the virus literature, and remember being very impressed by the technology of growing viruses in single tissue-cultured cells to determine details of the growth curve (18).

When Burnet brought a draft of his brief clonal selection paper into the laboratory, most of us thought it was fairly 'way out'. In best Popperian tradition, I told Burnet that I thought I could disprove his hypothesis quite quickly, by showing that single cells grown in tissue culture might perhaps make two or three different antibodies simultaneously. To my surprise, Burnet became quite excited. He wondered (not very seriously, I imagine) whether he should cancel a planned overseas trip to help me get started. But fate had decreed a better solution. One of the great pioneers of microbial genetics, Joshua Lederberg, was soon to arrive at the Hall Institute for a short sabbatical leave. His purpose was to understand more completely Burnet's last major discovery in virology, namely recombination among influenza viruses. Of course, I pored over the great man's papers and found that he had done some work (19) necessitating micromanipulation of single bacteria. Who better to get me started in learning micromanipulation? The interaction with Lederberg, really my third great mentor, was sheer joy. He, too, was enthusiastic about my proposal. He was prepared to accept clonal selection as a substantial contribution to the debate about mammalian somatic genetics, then in its very early stages. He was generous with his time both within and outside the laboratory. Burnet was 32 years my senior, a stern and aloof figure of authority, demanding a certain respect. Lederberg was only 32, thus six years older than me, informal and friendly, with a lightning-fast brain and a bewildering variety of deep scientific interests. In fact, during his three brief months in Melbourne, he did very little on influenza and spent much of his time working with me.

Wally Spector, a visitor in the laboratory, persuaded me that the lymph nodes of mice would be much too small to work on, and that I should become a rat man like himself. We soon decided on foot-pad injections and the popliteal node as a relatively virginal responding organ. But what antigen to use, and what titration method for the tiny amounts of antibody that a single cell could make? We canvassed a number of alternatives and settled on two possibilities: different foreign red blood cells as antigens and complement-dependent lysis (I had been inducted into the wonders of complement fixation by Beverly Perry) as the antibody titration technique; or formalin-killed *Salmonella* bacteria as antigens and specific immobilization of the different serotypes by antiflagellar antibody to detect antibody synthesis. Both methods had the potential to be made into very sensitive assays, and I tried both, but soon discarded the erythrocyte alternative, as I encountered unacceptable degrees of non-specific lysis within microdroplets. So, our rats were immunized three times with two unrelated *Salmonella*, *S. typhi* and *S. adelaide*.

The popliteal lymph node cells were collected, washed and micromanipulated into hanging droplets under mineral oil, and incubated. After culture, about 10 highly motile bacteria (first of one strain, then of the other) were micromanipulated into each droplet. In the first set of experiments, which unfortunately took place after Lederberg had returned to the USA, 62 antibody-forming cells were identified, 33 active against *S. adelaide* and 29 against *S. typhi* (20). No cell produced antibody active against both bacteria. The results, as far as they went, supported the clonal selection theory, but we commented at the time: 'However, further studies will be needed to determine whether the assortment of antibody-forming phenotypes reflects a genotypic restriction or whether it is more akin to such phenotypic effects as interference between related viruses or diauxie and competition in enzyme formation.' A more extensive series of experiments, involving purified flagellar preparations as antigens, much improved ways of selecting, washing and culturing cells; the use of three simultaneous antigens and a wide variety of immunization protocols, and much more quantitative assessment of antibody yield, identified 347 antibody-producing cells with not a single double or triple producer (21). This study made me feel very secure about the 'one cell, one antibody' finding. Indeed, confirmation was not long in coming.

Albert Coons was an early supporter, as he never saw plasma cells appearing to contain two antibodies (22). A similar result was described by White (23). When the haemolytic plaque technique was developed (24) it soon became possible for many people to play the 'antibody formation by single cells' game, and the absence of double producers was extensively documented. However, different results were presented by Attardi *et al.* (25). Using bacteriophage neutralization as an antibody assay, they reached the conclusion that, while most cells form one antibody, up to 20% of cells can actually form two separate ones. The reasons for this discrepancy have never been explained. Using essentially similar methods, but with more extensive cellular washing, Mäkelä (26) failed to find double producers in the phage neutralization system and instead obtained very clean 'one cell, one antibody' results. Mäkelä (27) also examined antibody cross-reactivities in this system, using related phages. He noted that each single cell had its own unique cross-reactivity pattern, with occasional cells producing *heteroclitic* antibody, capable of neutralizing the cross-reactive phage even more extensively than the immunogen. It is this unique quality of the single cell's product that lends to monoclonal antibodies their special properties.

From Phenotypic Restriction to Genotypic Potential

The single-cell technique proved useful for other purposes. We were able to show that cells could switch from immunoglobulin M to immunoglobulin G synthesis without a change in specificity (*28*), a finding which preceded the later discovery of the molecular mechanisms of isotype switching. Through sensitive autoradiographic techniques, we showed that single antibody-forming cells taken from animals immunized with small amounts of highly radioactive antigen contained less (and probably much less) than four molecules of antigen (*29*). This was a strong argument against the direct template hypothesis of antibody formation. Nevertheless, the pathway towards formal proof of clonal selection was slow and tortuous. Knowledge about the immunoglobulin antigen receptors grew in the second half of the 1960s, and a pivotal contribution was that of Naor and Sulitzeanu (*30*), who showed that only a tiny minority of lymphocytes from an unimmunized animal could bind a given radiolabelled antigen, exactly as clonal selection would have predicted.

Gordon Ada and I kicked ourselves when we saw this paper. Clearly we should have made this discovery! We had been talking about clonal selection for a decade and working with ^{125}I labelled antigens and autoradiographic techniques for four years. Either we were simply not smart enough to have thought of this very simple experiment, or we had so convinced ourselves of the existence of the receptors and the diversified repertoire that we did not place sufficient priority on its direct demonstration. In any case, Ada soon made amends with his famous 'hot antigen suicide' experiment (*31*). In this, a population of lymphocytes was held for 24 hours with highly radioactive antigen. This delivered sufficient ionizing radiation to the lymphocytes which bound the antigen to prevent their later division. As a result, the population specifically lost the capacity to form the corresponding, but not an irrelevant, antibody. This proved that cells with receptors for an antigen were the ones capable of responding to it, but did not formally eliminate the possibility that such cells could also possess other receptors and form other antibodies. The experiments of Raff *et al.* (*32*) provided further important information. They induced 'capping' of the immunoglobulin receptors in antigen-binding B cells by incubating them at 37°C with a highly multivalent antigen bearing a fluorescent tag. They then subjected the cells to a second tagged antibody capable of detecting all surface immunoglobulin. This second step was at 4°C, that is, under non-capping conditions. The great majority of B cells now showed linear staining, that is, randomly distributed receptors, with the anti-immunoglobulin, but the few specific antigen-binding B cells showed all the membrane immunoglobulin to be in the cap, suggesting a receptor population of only a single specificity.

Isolation and study of the few antigen-binding B cells present in unimmunized animals proved difficult. Some early results using flow cytometry were helpful to the clonal selection cause (33). We thought it important to press on to formal proof at the single cell level. We set out to purify antigen-binding B cells from unimmunized mice, to stimulate the single cells into clonal proliferation in microcultures, and to show that the resulting clone made only the expected single antibody and no other. When all the demanding elements for this formal experiment fell into place (34), with the anticipated result, the immunological community was not particularly impressed. In fact, clonal selection had been the almost universally accepted paradigm since the late 1960s. The brilliant molecular biological analysis of somatic assembly of immunoglobulin genes added a further dimension to the prior cellular work and firmly cemented clonal selection, first for B and later for T cells. A recent extension of the single-cell approach may be worth noting in passing. It is now possible (35) to take single antigen-specific B cells by six-parameter flow cytometry and to analyse their immunoglobulin V genes by polymerase-chain-reaction technology. This has shown, among other things, that *in vitro* expansion of single B cells into a clone of antibody-forming cells is not accompanied by somatic V gene hypermutation. That process occurs in germinal centres during the creation of memory B cells (reviewed in Nossal (36)).

Another good thing to come out of an obsession with cloning single antigen-binding B cells was the use of the technology in the analysis of immunological tolerance. It turns out that Burnet was only partially right in ascribing tolerance to clonal deletion of self-reactive cells during ontogeny. As far as B cells are concerned, concentrations of antigen far lower than those needed for deletion can cause tolerance. The relevant B cells can be isolated and subjected to analysis in single-cell culture. They fail to develop into antibody-forming cells, clearly having registered and stored some negative signal which, however, did not kill them. We described this state as 'clonal anergy' (37), a phenomenon that has since been confirmed for both B (38) and T (39) cells.

Conclusions

The cellular basis of antibody production was only one of a linked series of discoveries that had their origins in the 1950s. As Silverstein noted in his chapter, this decade saw the rise of a whole series of endeavours that looked at immune processes in a new way. Transplantation biology was fused into immunology. The autoimmune diseases began to be defined into a coherent group. Tumour immunology emerged from the shadows and became a substantial discipline. Understanding of the thymus and the separation of T and B cells came just a little later, during the 1960s. Gradually cellular immunology spread its web, entering embryology, cell biology, haematology, pathology and clinical medicine. Quite naturally, cellular immunology both informed and learnt from the great revolutions of the 1960s (antibody structure) and the 1970s (immunoglobulin gene structure and organization). Through this fusion, a huge edifice of knowledge became the springboard for three revolutions of the 1980s (molecular basis of T cell recognition; cytokines; and transgenic studies of immunoregulation) and one already of the 1990s (gene targeting to dissect the molecular physiology of the immune response). Along the way, there has been a rich harvest of clinically useful information and products. The ship of state of world immunology is in remarkably good shape! We can afford the luxury of a little retrospection. If this helps some who are now 26, as I was in 1957, the effort of producing this volume will have been worthwhile.

Acknowledgements

This work was supported by the National Health and Medical Research Council, Canberra, Australia; by Grant AI-03958 from the National Institute of Allergy and Infectious Diseases, United States Public Health Service; and by a grant from the Human Frontier Science Program (Principal Investigator Professor K. Rajewsky).

Notes and References

1. R. Pfeiffer and Z. Marx, *Z. Hyg. Infektionskrankch.* **27**, 272 (1898).
2. P. D. McMaster and S. S. Hudack, *J. Exp. Med.* **61**, 783 (1935).
3. W. E. Ehrich and T. N. Harris, *J. Exp. Med.* **76**, 335 (1942).
4. J. Bing and P. Plum, *Acta Med. Scand.* **92**, 415 (1937).
5. M. Bjorneboe and H. Gormsen, *Acta Path. Microbiol. Scand.* **20**, 649 (1943).
6. A. Fagraeus, *J. Immunol.* **58**, 1 (1948).
7. G. J. Thorbecke and F. J. Keuning, *J. Immunol.* **70**, 129 (1953).
8. E. H. Leduc, A. H. Coons and J. M. Connolly, *J. Exp. Med.* **102**, 61 (1955).
9. S. Harris and T. N. Harris, *J. Immunol.* **80**, 318 (1958).
10. D. W. Talmage, *Ann. Rev. Med.* **8**, 239 (1957).
11. F. M. Burnet, *Austral. J. Sci.* **20**, 67 (1957).
12. N. K. Jerne, *Proc. Natl Acad. Sci. USA* **41**, 849 (1955).
13. F. Fenner, *J. Immunol.* **63**, 341 (1949).
14. P. M. de Burgh, *Aust. J. Exp. Biol. Med.* **28**, 213 (1950).
15. G. J. V. Nossal and P. M. de Burgh, *Nature*, **172**, 671 (1953).
16. G. J. V. Nossal, *Aust. J. Exp. Biol. Med.* **35**, 549 (1957).
17. G. J. V. Nossal, *Nature*, **180**, 1427 (1957).
18. A. Lwoff, R. Dulbecco, M. Vogt and M. Lwoff, *Virology* **1**, 128 (1955).
19. J. Lederberg, *J. Bacteriol.* **68**, 256 (1954).
20. G. J. V. Nossal and J. Lederberg, *Nature* **181**, 1419 (1958).
21. G. J. V. Nossal, *Br. J. Exp. Pathol.* **41**, 89 (1960).
22. A. H. Coons, *J. Cell. Comp. Physiol.* **52** (Suppl. 1), 55 (1958).
23. R. G. White, *Nature* **182**, 1383 (1958).

24. N. K. Jerne and A. A. Nordin, *Science* **140**, 404 (1963).
25. G. Attardi, M. Cohn, K. Horibata and E. S. Lennox, *Bacteriol. Rev.* **23**, 213 (1959).
26. O. Mäkelä, *Cold Spring Harbor Symp. Quant. Biol.* **32**, 423 (1967).
27. O. Mäkelä, *J. Immunol.* **87**, 477 (1965).
28. G. J. V. Nossal, A. Szenberg, G. L. Ada and C. M. Austin, *J. Exp. Med.* **119**, 485 (1964).
29. G. J. V. Nossal, G. L. Ada and C. M. Austin, *J. Exp. Med.* **121**, 945 (1965).
30. D. Naor and D. Sulitzeanu, *Nature* **214**, 687 (1967).
31. G. L. Ada and P. Byrt, *Nature* **222**, 1291 (1969).
32. M. Raff, M. Feldmann and S. de Petris, *J. Exp. Med.* **137**, 1024 (1973).
33. M. H. Julius, T. Masuda and L. A. Herzenberg, *Proc. Natl Acad. Sci. USA* **69**, 1934 (1972).
34. G. J. V. Nossal and B. L. Pike, *Immunology* **30**, 189 (1976).
35. M. G. McHeyzer-Williams, M. McLean, P. A. Lalor and G. J. V. Nossal, *J. Exp. Med.* **178**, 295 (1993).
36. G. J. V. Nossal, Cell **68**, 1 (1992).
37. G. J. V. Nossal and B. L. Pike, *Proc. Natl Acad. Sci. USA* **77**, 1602 (1980).
38. C. C. Goodnow, J. Crosbie and S. Adelstein *et al.*, *Nature* **334**, 676 (1988).
39. M. R. Jenkins and R. H. Schwartz, *J. Exp. Med.* **167**, 302 (1989).

Roots of and Routes to Autoimmunity

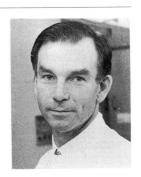

IAN R. MACKAY
Centre for Molecular Biology and Medicine, Monash University,
Clayton 3168, Victoria, Australia

Not one, but two, eras could be nominated for the 'discovery' of autoimmunity as a cause of disease, *c.*1900 and *c.*1950.

The First Era of Autoimmunity

In 1900, a recognized science of immunology did not exist, although serology was beginning to evolve from the science of bacteriology, based on procedures such as immunoprecipitation, haemogglutination, haemolysis and complement fixation. Thus, in 1898, Bordet described the haemolytic effects of sera of animals that had been injected with erythrocytes of other species, recognizing that the sera of such animals contained a thermostable moiety, 'antibody' in later usage, and a thermolabile moiety, 'complement' in later usage. In 1900, Ehrlich and Morgenroth (*1*) extended Bordet's observations in experiments on goats, and found that erythrocytotoxic sera were not generated by immunizing an animal with its own erythrocytes, and only rather weakly so with cells of animals of the same species. This resistance to autoimmunity was regarded by Ehrlich as a natural physiological effect, 'tolerance' in later usage.

Soon after 1900, Ehrlich developed the first general theoretical concept of specific immunity and natural self-tolerance. His side-chain receptor theory, with its striking similarities to the current selection theory of acquired immunity, proposed that cells involved in immune responses produced sessile 'side-chain' receptors that were initially anchored to the cell. The attachment of an antigenic molecule to a receptor would stimulate the formation by the cell of new receptors, and there would be production of the same receptors by additional cells in the body, 'activated cells' and 'memory cells' in later usage. The production of a surplus of receptors resulted in these being shed as free particles – antibodies – that could bind antigen in the circulation. Ehrlich classified

IMMUNOLOGY: THE MAKING OF A MODERN SCIENCE
ISBN 0-12-274020-3

receptors with one binding group (haptophore) as first order; with two binding groups (haptophore and zymophore), which as free antibodies could agglutinate antigens, as second order; and complement fixing as third order.

As mentioned, this process in animals could not be set in train by immunization with autologous cells (erythrocytes), leading Ehrlich to surmise that the production of cytotoxic antibodies to autologous molecules would be 'dysteleologic in the extreme' and further, according to Silverstein (2), that autoreactive antibody would not be found because either the appropriate receptors did not exist in the individual or, more probably, that such antibodies may be formed but are inhibited in their cytotoxic action. Thus Ehrlich (3) stated:

> The organism possesses certain contrivances by means of which the immunity reaction, so easily produced by all kinds of cells, is prevented from acting against the organism's own elements and so giving rise to autotoxins – so that we might be justified in speaking of a 'horror autotoxicus' of the organism. These contrivances are naturally of the highest importance for the individual.

This statement, interpretable as the first enunciation of natural immune tolerance as a requirement for health, sadly succumbed to misinterpretations, as recorded by various historians (2,4), and came to have a 'mind-closing' effect on the existence of a state of pathological autoimmunity.

However, it was only a few years later, in 1904, that Donath and Landsteiner (5) described their three patients with a cold-induced haemoglobinuria, which they attributed to the presence in the blood of an autohaemolysin. The discussion to their 1904 paper contains the following statements: 'Die Erscheinung entspricht der Absorption eines Hämolysins durch die empfindlichen zellen' and, further, 'Die Auflösung erfolgt mit Hilfe der als Komplement (Alexin, Cytase, etc.) bezeichneten Agentien des Serums'. The haemolysin described by Donath and Landsteiner was reactive in the cold with the erythrocytes of the patient, and of other individuals, but the lytic effects depended on warming and on the presence of the thermolabile moiety (complement) described earlier by Bordet. Silverstein's (6) view was that Donath as the clinical partner interpreted the disease in his earlier writings in terms of antibody and complement but, in the collaborative paper with Landsteiner as the scientific partner, such terms were used more guardedly. Nevertheless, this seminal paper led to an acceptance that haemolytic disease could be attributed to the spontaneous development of an autocytotoxic antibody to erythrocytes, as judged by the publications of Chauffard (7) and Widal et al. (8) in France in the years 1907–1909, Dameshek et al. (9) in the USA in 1938, and Gear (10) in South Africa in 1946 in the context of malaria and blackwater fever.

There were various other indications in the post-1900 era that pointed to the possibility of pathological autoimmune responses. These included anti-spermatozoal cytotoxicity (11), anaphylaxis and serum sickness as examples of harmful, as opposed to protective, effects of antibodies (3), and the capacity to raise cytotoxic antisera against various tissues (heart, liver, kidney, etc.), noting that, even by 1903, Sachs could cite 104 references to experiments with such cytotoxic antisera, although these were not shown to arise spontaneously. Of more direct relevance is the use in 1903 by Uhlenhuth (*12*) of ocular antigens since, in contrast to Ehrlich's attempts with erythrocytes, immunization within the same species proved successful, and the procedure was later adapted by Krusius (*13*) to induce an experimental autoimmune disease. He reported in 1910 that guinea-pigs could become immunized to lens protein by rupture of the lens capsule and that, in a presensitized animal, release in this way of lens protein could induce ocular disease. This led Römer and Gebb (*14*) to specu-late that autologous lens protein was actually seen as 'foreign' and, therefore, excluded from the dogma of *horror autotoxicus*; even so, these authors recog-nized that Ehrlich's proposed 'contrivances' against autocytotoxicity could be circumvented – 'failure of immunoregulation' in later usage. These observa-tions led to proposals in 1910 (*15*) and 1922 (*16*) that uveitis in humans, phaco-genic or lens-induced uveitis, is due to an autoantibody-mediated inflammatory response to leakage of lens substance into the eye.

Also among the early observations (1900–1910) was the recognition that an effective Wassermann antigen could just as readily be derived from normal as from syphilitic tissue. This raised the idea (*17*) that the serum antibody could have anti-tissue as well as antispirochaetal reactivity; in fact the antibody could be provoked by damaged cells, and could react with normal cells to liberate more antigen and so perpetuate disease. This 'vicious circle' concept for auto-immune damage was subsequently reinvoked many years later in considera-tions on autoimmunity (*18*).

Autoimmunity in Limbo

However, notwithstanding all these observations, it is difficult to discern whether any general concept of autoimmune disease had emerged in this 1900–1910 era. Certainly there is a lack of general texts or reviews on 'auto-immunity and disease' of the type that proliferated in the 1960s. In any event, autoimmunity became dormant after 1910. The reasons attributed for this included the interruption of European science by World War I and the shift thereafter of scientific leadership to the USA. Also, there were other preoccupa-tions of the new science of immunology in the 1920–1930 period, including explanations for the specificity of antibody, particularly in the light of Landsteiner's studies on the capacity of simple chemicals to elicit specific anti-body responses. These led to the template theories of antibody specificity which were not adaptable to the failure, normally, of autologous molecules to elicit antibody responses in the host animal. Of relevance also, clinical scientists in the post-war period had perceptions of immunology in the context of allergic diseases in which the antigenic culprits were extrinsically derived molecules. However, the most potent reason for the failure of an autoimmunity paradigm to develop was that the 'denkkollectiv', using Silverstein's term (2), had transliterated *horror autotoxicus* from a condition of health to a condition of life. This can be selectively illustrated by the writings of three influential immunologists of the post-war era, Karl Landsteiner, F. Macfarlane Burnet and Ernest Witebsky.

Karl Landsteiner enjoyed an eminent and authoritative position as an immunologist and serologist through to the 1940s. Despite being the coreporter, in 1904, of the first autoimmune disease, the discussions in his well-known monograph, *The Specificity of Serological Reactions*, of which the final 1943 revision was republished in 1962 (19), contain only a few brief references to autoimmunity, indicative of his indifference to the subject. For example, the index to the 1943 edition contains only one pertinent listing, this being to autohaemolysin under which the 1904 paper on cold haemoglobinuria is mentioned, although the entry is actually made in the context of the diagnostic reaction for syphilis described by Wassermann in 1906. Landsteiner noted that the sera of syphilitic patients reacted with extracts of various organs that contained spirochaetes, and also with extracts of practically any normal organ, and recalled that the haemolysin of cold haemoglobinuria developed almost exclusively in syphilitic patients. The monograph cites the opinion expressed by Sachs and coworkers that the Wassermann antibodies are produced in consequence of an 'autoimmunization' (Landsteiner's quotation marks), with consideration of two possibilities. First, the Wassermann reagins are engendered by spirochaetes but have a capacity for overlapping reactivity with organ extracts, by reason of these containing chemically similar substances. Alternatively, the Wassermann reagins could be explained by an observation that foreign proteins could have an enhancing effect on the capacity of animals to respond to isologous erythrocytes, and here Landsteiner cites data reported by Fischer who stimulated the formation of autohaemolysins in rabbits in this manner. There are just a few other brief and non-indexed citations in the 1943 edition, to autoimmunization, autoantibodies and autoagglutinins, but with no comment on pathogenetic mechanisms.

Macfarlane Burnet's first treatise on immunology was *The Production of Antibodies* in 1941; it contains no references to autoantibodies or autoimmunity (20). The better-known second edition, published in 1949 with Fenner (21), introduces the concept of immune tolerance and its establishment in embryonic life, and there is a passing reference to autoimmunity in the context of experimental encephalomyelitis. Since Burnet at that time viewed tolerance in terms of a 'self-marker' hypothesis, he did not have an easy theoretical framework into which autoimmunity could be introduced. In fact, he conceded in this second edition that the self-marker concept 'must be left flexible enough to accommodate the results of future studies on pathological conditions which may be due to "autoantibody", foreshadowed by those of Kabat, Wolf and Bezer (1947) and Morgan (1947)'. However, although the Burnet and Fenner 1949 edition reflected the prevailing neglect of autoimmunity as a potential cause of disease, Burnet was in fact at this time beginning to engage this question, as discussed below.

Ernest Witebsky is of interest in being, as a student of Sachs, in a direct line of succession from Ehrlich; in addition, he had a major experimental interest in the immunogenicity of tissue extracts. It was he who took *horror autotoxicosis* to its terminal extreme, as described by Noel Rose in this volume. In fact, Witebsky was led by this mindset even to disbelieve the results of his own experiments (2)!

Renaissance

What, then, were the influences that allowed autoimmunity to emerge from its 'dark ages' and, eventually, to attain acceptance by immunologists and clinicians as an important general mechanism of disease? There were several contributions between the years 1940 and 1960. Remarkably, only a minority of these came directly from experimental or theoretical laboratory immunology, and the majority were made either accidentally or in the course of an enquiry quite unrelated to autoimmunity itself.

The first event in the renaissance was directed to responses of animals to deliberate immunization with tissue extracts, in this case brain. The studies were, to a degree, predicated on the neuroparalytic accidents that occasionally occurred after rabies vaccination using brain emulsions that contained killed rabies virus. The particular relevance for autoimmunity of immunization with brain was in the observable functional effects that accompany the specific serological and histopathological reactions. Interest in these studies developed from the 1930s when Rivers *et al.* (22) described an encephalitis in monkeys after repetitive injections with monkey neural tissue. In 1944, it was first proposed by Ferraro (23) that experimentally produced disseminated encephalomyelitis was the result of an antigen–antibody reaction. A key discovery was the adjuvant for immunization, an oil and water emulsion containing tubercle bacilli, introduced in the 1940s by Freund (24). Kabat *et al.* (25) and Morgan (26), among others, found that incorporation of the immunizing neural emulsion into Freund's adjuvant greatly accelerated the occurrence and increased the severity of disease after immunization with brain, and thereafter the idea of an immunological basis for the disease became quite popular, leading to terms such as experimental 'isoallergic' encephalomyelitis by Freund *et al.* (27), and allergic encephalomyelitis by Morgan (26). These terms became replaced in the 1960s by the term 'experimental autoimmune encephalomyelitis' (EAE).

Experimental allergic encephalomyelitis intrigued Burnet. He used the occasion of an invited address to allergists in 1947, subsequently published in 1948 (18), to discuss what he then called a 'dubious group of degenerative diseases, in which there are strong suggestions that the body is producing antibody against some of its own constituents' . . . 'an idea which has been current in speculative form for a good many years but has had very little experimental backing until recently'. He noted the possibility of producing acute degenerative and demyelinating changes in monkeys by immunizing with central nervous system substance, even from animals of the same species, and the impetus to this work from the use of 'certain adjuvants' attributed to Freund who 'popularized the idea in America'. Burnet regarded none of his interpretations as established, but felt 'reasonably certain that a large proportion of nephritic conditions and a number of demyelinating diseases of the central nervous system have in part at least a basis in some inappropriate immunological activity'. He said:

> It is simply that in certain individuals the normal scavenging process, by which damaged cells are eliminated, is switched into an inappropriately immunological process – an auto-antibody directed against some specific component of say, damaged nerve cells is produced. This causes damage presumably by interference with intracellular enzyme mechanisms when it reaches cells of appropriate type in the central nervous system. It may be that in this way further antigen is liberated, so that a vicious circle is developed. (18)

Burnet's selection in 1947 of diseases of possible autoimmune origin, 'nephritic conditions and demyelinating diseases', would have been from his particular perspective as an experimental scientist, since laboratory models of these diseases had been investigated: encephalomyelitis as noted above and nephritis which had been described in 1936 by Smadel (28). It is curious that Burnet made no reference at all to autoimmune haemolysis, for which human disease examples had long been recognized.

A particular problem with the encephalomyelitis models of autoimmunity of the 1940s was the lack of any relationship between neural disease and levels of circulating antibody to brain. At that time serum antibodies were the only indicator of immunological activity, since the understanding of cellular immunity was rudimentary, and based entirely on the cutaneous delayed-type hypersensitivity reaction and its adoptive transfer by lymphoid cells. In fact, it was not until 1951 that cellular immune processes became implicated in experimental encephalomyelitis, based on correlations between the occurrence of disease and cutaneous delayed-type hypersensitivity responses to the myelin extracts used for immunization, as described by Waksman and Morrison (29).

Advances in the Clinic

Then followed three clinically derived discoveries that were to prove really critical for the acceptance of a general concept of autoimmunity: the Hargraves' lupus erythematosus cell effect, the Coombs' antiglobulin test, and the

Waaler–Rose rheumatoid factor. None of these discoveries was made by an immunologist, and all were 'unpremeditated', at least in the context of auto-immunity. Two were described in 1948, a year described as an *annus mirabilis* for rheumatology, but equally applicable to autoimmunity.

The most influential of these unpremeditated observations was the lupus erythematosus (LE) cell effect, discovered by Malcolm Hargraves in Rochester, USA, in April 1943, although the actual report was delayed until five years later (*30*). Hargraves quaintly described the background on which the LE cell was discovered (*31*). It was created by his belief in the diagnostic utility of sternal bone marrow examination, despite a reluctance at the Mayo Clinic to include this procedure as 'accepted routine'. He engaged himself 'in a sales promotion venture in order to obtain enough patients to supply the needed material for bone marrow study. I was most happy in those days to do a bone marrow aspiration on any patient in whom the procedure seemed to offer any reasonable prospect of diagnostic help. Actually, as we shall see, this attitude was an important factor in the discovery of the LE cell'. The first description of the LE cell is his report on a bone marrow biopsy in 1943: 'some increase plasma cells – peculiar structureless globular bodies taking purple stain (artefact?). This is not diagnostic'. Cases in which the characteristic 'purple inclusion bodies' were seen had diagnostically obscure medical problems. With one such case in 1946, a discussion followed with a clinician whose diagnosis was that of 'one of the collagen diseases, most probably systemic lupus erythematosus', and this led to bone marrow material being obtained from two further patients with 'definite' disseminated lupus erythematosus. Hargraves (*31*) recalls: 'fate must have smiled and nodded her head; numerous LE cells were evident', and 'the more I looked, the more astonishing things I could see'. Although by 1947 the LE cell association with lupus erythematosus was well confirmed, Hargraves deferred publication, fearing that 'somewhere there were fallacies that I had not yet covered'. In 1948, he eventually published his 'small preliminary report' (*30*): 'the amount of investigative activity that was stimulated throughout this country and the world amazed me' (*31*).

Hargraves then took what was 'obviously, the next step', the incubation of blood plasma from patients with systemic LE with bone marrow material of patients who did not have this disease: typical LE cells were observed, leading in 1949 to his second paper (*32*), so 'rounding out my contribution'. He recognized that he had unearthed an immunological problem that 'had become an unexpected bonus to immunopathology', but 'as a physician primarily involved in the clinical practice of medicine and getting into the laboratory only a few specific hours each week, my ability to make further contributions to the LE cell phenomenon was exhausted' (*31*). Next followed the identification of the LE cell-inducing factor in serum as a 7S γ-globulin (*33*) and then, within a few years (1954–1960), beginning with the removal of LE serum factor activity by absorption of serum with cell nuclei (*34*), it became clearly established that the LE serum factor was an autoantibody to nucleoproteins.

The antiglobulin reaction, like the LE cell effect, came to have a profound influence on the emerging concept of autoimmunity, although it was developed in rather a different setting. Despite the occasional descriptions between 1903 and 1938 of haemolytic anaemia attributable to circulating haemolysins, cases of haemolytic anaemia were simply divided into the acquired or idiopathic type in contrast to the congenital spherocytic type in which haemolysins in the blood were not demonstrable. In 1945, Robin Coombs and colleagues (35) reported on a test applicable to the detection in maternal serum of antibodies to rhesus antigens in instances of fetal–maternal erythrocyte incompatibility. In such cases the rhesus-positive cells of the fetus crossed the placenta and stimulated the production by the mother of antibodies to rhesus antigens that became transferred to the fetus. Such antibodies that could adhere to erythrocytes but did not cause agglutination or lysis were regarded as 'weak' or 'incomplete'. Coombs' procedure to detect these was to immunize a rabbit with human globulins to yield an antiserum capable of agglutinating erythrocytes coated with a 'weak' (non-agglutinating) rhesus antibody. A similar test had in fact been devised by Moreschi as early as 1908 (see Silverstein (2), reference 53).

This antiglobulin reaction, subsequently known universally as the 'Coombs test', was applied soon after to cases of idiopathic acquired haemolytic anaemia, with positive results (36), so pointing to a pathogenesis due to attachment *in vivo* of serum globulin to the erythrocyte surface. Thus, haemolytic anaemia became the first disease for which there was a simple and specific laboratory test for an autoimmune origin, and the first disease to acquire the adjectival prefix of 'autoimmune', in 1951 (37). However, autoimmunity in the early 1950s was a far from accepted concept, and the original non-committal term of 'acquired' haemolytic anaemia persisted well into the 1950s (38). The Coombs' reaction subsequently was to reveal the first spontaneously occurring animal model of autoimmune disease, haemolytic anaemia in New Zealand black (NZB) mice, as described below.

The third of the unpremeditated observations on autoimmunity was the capacity of serum from rheumatoid arthritis patients to agglutinate sheep erythrocytes, first reported in 1940 by Erik Waaler (39) in Oslo, Norway. Waaler was responsible for supervision of the Wassermann tests at the Oslo City Hospital, and in 1937 there was brought to his attention an unusual Wassermann result in which there was agglutination of the sheep cells rather than the expected complement fixation. The 'agglutinating activating factor', as Waaler termed it, was present in high titre, 1:5120, and the serum donor was found to have rheumatoid arthritis. Waaler succeeded in establishing that the reaction required globulin coating on erythrocytes, that it was not directed to sheep cells, and that a globulin fraction of serum contained the agglutinating factor. Waaler sought other cases of rheumatoid arthritis to establish the specificity of the reaction. Unfortunately, only about one-third of the sera referred to him were reactive, perhaps reflecting the selection of cases by the local clinicians, and so there was no evident clinical utility for the procedure.

This, together with difficulties in pursuing his research in wartime Norway, led to a long-delayed recognition of his findings.

The agglutination reaction using antibody-coated sheep erythrocytes was independently rediscovered several years later in New York, in an equally fortuitous way, in the laboratory of Harry Rose (40). A complement fixation test was being used in the diagnosis of a rickettsial illness and, when a laboratory technician, who happened to be a sufferer from rheumatoid arthritis, contracted the infection she tested her own serum among a batch of others. However, feeling unwell, she left the tubes overnight instead of for the usual one hour and, next morning, she noted that her serum had agglutinated the indicator sheep red cells. Accordingly, further rheumatoid arthritis sera were tested, and the specificity of the agglutinating reaction for rheumatoid arthritis was established. There was recognition of the agglutinating factor as an immunoglobulin M type autoantibody to immunoglobulin G during 1954–1956, this being nearly 20 years after the initial discovery by Waaler, and several years after its rediscovery by Rose. Fraser (41) records Waaler's comment that 'new findings may be somewhat premature, the fruit needs some years to hibernate before it can be fully appreciated', as well as interesting biographical details on Waaler and Rose. For example, despite their names being linked eponymously for over 30 years with the world-wide use of an important diagnostic assay, they were never to meet – the disinclination apparently was on the part of Rose.

An observation in 1951 which has received relatively little comment in the modern history of autoimmunity was made by Harrington (42). This study involved the infusion intravenously into healthy volunteers of serum from persons with the disease then called 'idiopathic thrombocytopenic purpura' (now 'immune thrombycytopenic purpura' (ITP)). The resulting immediate and dramatic decrease in levels of circulating blood platelets was proof of a passive transfer of a serum agent presumed to be an autoantibody capable of reacting with platelets in the circulating blood and facilitating their destruction. This experiment is of historic interest for two reasons. First, it provided direct proof of the pathogenic potency of a putative circulating autoantibody, as a forerunner to observations on pathogenic effects of maternal autoantibodies after transfer to the foetus *in utero* (43). Second, it is an interesting marker of differences in attitudes to the ethics of human experimentation in the mid-century and later.

Advances in the Laboratory

The next contributions to autoimmunity came in the mid-1950s, with a swing in interest in yet another direction, towards the thyroid gland, in the laboratory of Ernest Witebsky in Buffalo, New York. Witebsky, who is described by Rose in this volume as the inheritor of the Paul Ehrlich mantle and a vigorous champion of the 'law' of horror autotoxicus, had developed a profound sceptism with respect to the autoimmune aetiology of human disease. Rose recalls how he joined Witebsky's laboratory in 1951 and was given the task of investigating the organ and species specificity of mammalian thyroglobulins, and the degree to which denaturation of the molecule might explain the then unexpected positive response (at least to Witebsky) to an autoantigen within the same species, the rabbit. To conserve the laboratory preparations of rabbit thyroglobulin antigen, a decision was made to use Freund's adjuvant for the immunizations. The rabbits were allocated experimentally into three groups: one thyroidectomized to exclude any natural thyroglobulin in the circulation overriding the effects of immunization; one hemi-thyroidectomized; and the third group was thyroid intact. There were two surprises: rabbits in all groups produced antibodies to rabbit thyroglobulin; and a mononuclear infiltration was evident in the thyroid tissue of the immunized rabbits. This prompted a surgical collaborator to remark on histological similarities with human Hashimoto's thyroiditis, a chronic inflammatory thyroid disease of then unknown cause, and therefore sera from patients with this disease were tested and, like the immunized rabbits, these contained antibodies to thyroglobulin. The unfolding of thyroid autoimmunity was portrayed in detail in the 1957 paper of Witebsky and colleagues (44), which included the traditional (albeit not always fulfilled) postulates for specifying a disease as autoimmune in origin.

At much the same time, thyroid disease caught the attention of Roitt and Doniach in London who collaborated to examine sera from patients with Hashimoto's thyroiditis (45). They recall how their discovery of very high levels of antithyroglobulin enabled Hashimoto's thyroiditis to be identified as the prototype of the group of organ-specific autoimmune diseases (46); Bayliss in his 1983 Harveian Oration of the Royal College of Physicians of London gives further background to their discovery, including the earlier observations by Fromm et al. in Argentina in 1953. However, harking back to the first era, Papazolu (47) in 1911 described complement fixation reactions with sera and autologous thyroid in 26 of 34 cases of thyrotoxicosis.

The discovery of thyroid autoimmunity in the mid-1950s prompts comment on yet another fortuitous observation, first reported in 1956 but only finally understood some 10 years later. The endocrinologists Adams and Purves in Dunedin, New Zealand, developed a bioassay based on release in vitro of thyroxin from thyroid gland tissue, to examine whether thyrotoxicosis sera contained a pituitary hormone that could stimulate the release of thyroxin (48). The bioassay refuted this idea, but showed that thyrotoxicosis sera did have a stimulatory effect albeit in a delayed and prolonged manner. The responsible agent in serum, called 'long-acting thyroid stimulator' was subsequently identified as an immunoglobulin, and became the prototype of an interesting group of autoantibodies that react with cell surface receptors, with functional effects (49).

Another pointer to autoimmunity and disease in the mid-1950s, in Melbourne, Australia, was derived from yet another fortuitous observation which, as for the rheumatoid factor, was based on an unexpected result in the complement fixation test. D. Carleton Gajdusek, a recent arrival in the laboratory of Burnet at the Walter and Eliza Hall Institute, decided to develop an assay for antibody to hepatitis virus using a complement fixation test. The source of antigen was liver tissue obtained at autopsy from a fatal case of infectious (viral) hepatitis, presuming this to be rich in viral antigen. At the same time, interest had developed at the Hall Institute in an unusual form of chronic hepatitis in which the lupus erythematosus cell effect had been demonstrable in the blood (50,51), prompting the idea of autoimmunity in such cases. Sera from cases of infectious hepatitis reacted weakly, if at all, with the virus-containing liver tissue in the complement fixation test, but when the test was applied to cases of lupoid (autoimmune) hepatitis, lupus erythematosus, and certain other diseases of autoimmune nature, very strong reactions were obtained (52). There was no requirement in the complement fixation test for virus-infected liver, since various normal tissues were equally reactive. Again returning to the past, it was noted (46) that a similar reaction in liver disease had been reported by Fiessinger in 1908. The identification of antigenic reactants in the complement fixation reaction as constituents of normal mammalian tissues led to the designation 'autoimmune complement fixation' (AICF) reaction, and further experience with this reaction encouraged my idea that autoimmunity would explain many hitherto obscure diseases (53).

Next came the NZB mouse. By the mid-1950s there were well-characterized autoimmune models in animals, including encephalomyelitis, thyroiditis and orchitis, but these did not entirely relate to human disease by reason of the unphysiological inductive procedures with adjuvants. The background, according to Casey (54) and Warner (55), was that W. H. Hall of the Animal Department of the University of Otago Medical School, Dunedin, New Zealand, brought some mice to New Zealand in 1930 from the Imperial Cancer Research Fund laboratories, Mill Hill, London. In 1948 Marianne and Felix Bielschowsky selected a pair of mice with agouti coats from the maintained mixed colony for inbreeding. Various separate strains were established according to coat colour, including one with a black coat and one with an agouti coat that developed obesity. A pair of black littermates was used to generate a black strain of mice, later known as NZB/BL, which were seen after 11 generations to die with hepatosplenomegaly and jaundice, later characterized as haemolytic jaundice by reason of a positive Coombs' reaction of the type seen in human autoimmune haemolytic anaemia. This observation was modestly reported by Bielschowsky, Helyer and Howie (56) in the *Proceedings of the University of Otago Medical School*. Hybrids with other strains, NZY/BL and NZW/BL, were derived from the original mixed colony from England, yielding mice that gave positive LE cell tests and had renal lesions typically seen in human lupus erythematosus (57).

The NZB/BL strain was quickly acquired in 1959 by Burnet who, with various collaborators (Holmes, Hicks, Russell and others), characterized the autoimmune haematological, renal and thymic expressions in these 'New Zealand mice' (58–60). This discovery of a spontaneously occurring murine model of autoimmunity had a profound if not clinching influence on the acceptance of the human autoimmunity paradigm, given the existence of a spontaneous murine model susceptible to experimental analysis at the laboratory bench.

The concept of autoimmunity in the late 1950s gained a potent impetus from the application of fluorescence microscopy. A microscopy procedure for detecting the binding of an antibody to cells had been described in 1950 by Coons and Kaplan (61). This technique initially applied to the recognition of antinuclear antibodies (62,63), and later in the early 1960s was coupled with the development by Pearse, at the Postgraduate Medical School in London, of the cryostat for preparing unfixed sections of frozen tissue as an antigen substrate for detecting autoantibody in serum. Indirect immunofluorescence provided a 'workhorse' technology for detection of serum autoantibodies that soon brought a widely diverse range of additional diseases into the autoimmune arena: the gastric lesion of pernicious anaemia, the adrenalitis of Addison's disease, myasthenia gravis, Sjögren's syndrome, and others.

Final Recognition

By 1960–1961, it seemed time to pull the story together, and I began work with Burnet on a monograph, *Autoimmune Diseases: Pathogenesis, Chemistry and Therapy* (64). However, notwithstanding the convincing experimental and clinical evidence, there was still widespread scepticism about a role for autoimmunity in disease. Nairn (65) recalls that soon after the Roitt–Doniach report from London on Hashimoto's disease (45), MRC grants were freely awarded to any proponent of a research project aimed at rejecting 'so-called autoimmunity' as a cause of human disease. The use of the term 'autoimmunity' remained current throughout the 1960s.

Autoimmune Diseases was published as a theoretical and clinical science description of autoimmunity and disease, as of 1963. The theoretical basis comprised Burnet's clonal selection theory of acquired immunity (66) which included deletion in embryonic life of any potential self-reactive immunocytes. Accordingly, the occurrence in postnatal life of a clone of cells with autoimmune potential would be 'forbidden' – Burnet (67) describes the curious origin of this term in his autobiography – and clones with such potential would be 'forbidden clones'. Given the proliferative requirement of cells in immune responses and the ensuing inevitability of somatic mutations, forbidden autoimmune responses among B cells in postnatal life could be expected, requiring the postulate of a 'homoeostatic control' over such reactions – 'peripheral tolerance' in later usage. The forbidden clone theory had the virtue of simplicity and fitted comfortably into the knowledge base of immunology of the early 1960s. This of course was before the discovery of T cells, T and B cell collaboration, major histocompatibility complex restriction, and generation of repertoires, all of which have complicated rather than simplified the understanding of natural immune tolerance. From the clinical standpoint, our 1963 mono-graph accommodated all the major autoimmune diseases recognized at that time, with just one exception: insulin-dependent diabetes mellitus. Despite some evidence, the climate of opinion on autoimmunity in 1963 seemed too inhibitory to consider the inclusion of that disease! However, diabetes became suspected shortly afterwards by reason of associated autoantibodies (68), and the more decisive evidence of autoantibody to pancreatic islet cells was obtained by means of immunofluorescence in 1974 (69).

The most appropriate end-piece to the 'modern' history of autoimmunity would be the two-volume report on the proceedings of the 1965 New York Academy of Sciences Conference on Autoimmunity – Experimental and Clinical Aspects (70). This 980-page compendium of 77 relevant publications established the reality of autoimmunity. I note that Witebsky in his Closing Remarks (p. 979) records the following: 'As a matter of fact, as Dr Mackay remarked today at luncheon, we are dealing here with a fascinating and most important problem which might actually revolutionize certain aspects of pathology and even the practice of medicine in general.'

Notes and References

1. P. Ehrlich and J. Morgenroth, *Berlin Klin. Wchnschr.* **37**, 453 (1900).
2. A. Silverstein, *A History of Immunology*, Academic Press, New York (1989), chap. 7.
3. P. Ehrlich and J. Morgenroth, *Berlin Klin. Wchnschr.* **38**, 251 (1901).
4. J. M. Cruse, D. Whitcomb and R. E. Lewis, Jr, *Concepts Immunopathol.* **1**, 32 (1985).
5. J. Donath and K. Landsteiner, *Münch Med. Wchnschr.* **51**, 1590 (1904).
6. A. M. Silverstein, *Cell. Immunol.* **97**, 173 (1986).
7. M. A. Chauffard, *Sem. Méd. Paris* **27**, 25 (1907).
8. F. Widal, P. Abrami and M. Brulé, *Arch. Mal. Coeur* **1**, 193 (1908).
9. W. Dameshek, S. O. Schwartz, and S. Gross. *Am. J. Med. Sci.* **196**, 769 (1938).
10. J. Gear, *Trans R. Soc. Trop. Med. Hygiene* **39**, 301 (1946).
11. S. Metalnikoff, *Ann. Inst. Pasteur* **14**, 577 (1900).
12. P. Uhlenhuth, in *Festschrift zur Sechigsten Geburtstag von Robert Koch* (P. Theodor, ed.), Fischer, Jena (1903), pp. 49–74.
13. F. F. Krusius, *Arch. Augenh.* **67**, 6, (1910).
14. P. Römer and H. Gebb, *Arch. Opthal.* **81**, 376 (1912).
15. A. Elschnig, *Arch. Opthal.* **75**, 3 (1910); **76**, 509 (1910).
16. F. H. Verhoeff and A. N. Lemoine, *Am. J. Ophthal.* **5**, 737 (1922).
17. E. Weil and H. Braun, *Wein. Klin. Wchnschr.* **11**, 372 (1909).
18. F. M. Burnet, *Med. J. Aust.* **1**, 29 (1948).
19. K. Landsteiner, *The Specificity of Serological Reactions*, Dover, New York (1962).
20. F. M. Burnet, *The Production of Antibodies*, Macmillan, Melbourne (1941).
21. F. M. Burnet and F. Fenner, *The Production of Antibodies*, 2nd edn, Macmillan, Melbourne (1949).
22. T. M. Rivers, D. H. Sprunt and G. P. Berry, *J. Exp. Med.* **58**, 39 (1933).
23. A. Ferraro, *Arch. Neurol. Psychiatr.* **52**, 443 (1944).
24. J. Freund, *Ann. Rev. Microbiol.* **1**, 291 (1947).
25. E. A. Kabat, A. Wolfe and A. E. Bezer, *J. Exp. Med.* **85**, 117 (1947).
26. I. M. Morgan, *J. Exp. Med.* **85**, 131 (1947).

27. J. Freund, E. R. Stern and T. M. Pisani, *J. Immunol.* **57**, 179 (1947).
28. J. E. Smadel, *J. Exp. Med.* **64**, 921 (1936); **65**, 541 (1937).
29. B. H. Waksman and L. R. Morrison, *J. Immunol.* **66**, 421 (1951).
30. M. D. Hargraves, H. Richmond and R. Morton, *Proc. Staff Meet. Mayo Clin.* **23**, 25 (1948).
31. M. M. Hargraves, *Mayo Clin. Proc.*, **44**, 579 (1969).
32. M. M. Hargraves, *Proc. Staff Meet. Mayo Clin.* **24**, 234 (1959).
33. J. R. Haserick, L. Lewis and D. W. Bortz, *Am. J. Med. Sci.* **219**, 660 (1950).
34. P. Miescher and M. Fauconnet, *Experimentia* **10**, 252 (1954).
35. R. R. A. Coombs, A. E. Mourant and R. R. Race, *Br. J. Exp. Pathol.* **6**, 255 (1945).
36. K. E. Boorman, B. E. Dodd and J. F. Loutit, *Lancet* i, 812 (1946).
37. L. E. Young, G. Miller and R. M. Christian, *Ann. Intern. Med.* **35**, 507 (1951).
38. J. V. Dacie, *Lectures Sci. Basis Med.* VII, 59 (1957–58).
39. E. Waaler, *Acta Pathol. Microbiol. Scand.* **17**, 172 (1940).
40. H. M. Rose, C. Ragan, E. Pearce and M. Lipman, *Proc. Soc. Exp. Biol. Med.* **68**, 1 (1948).
41. K. J. Fraser, *Sem. Arth. Rheumatol.* **18**, 61, (1988).
42. W. J. Harrington, V. Minnich, J. W. Hollingsworth and C. V. Moore, *J. Lab. Clin. Med.* **38**, 1, (1951).
43. J. S. Scott, *Lancet* i, 78 (1976).
44. E. Witebsky, N. R. Rose, K. Terplan, J. R. Paine and R. W. Egan, *J. Am. Med. Assoc.* **164**, 1439 (1957).
45. I. M. Roitt, D. Doniach, P. N. Campbell and R. V. Hudson, *Lancet* ii, 820 (1956).
46. D. Doniach and I. M. Roitt, *Autoimmunity* **1**, 11 (1988).
47. A. Papazolu, *CR Soc. Biol. Paris* **71**, 671 (1911).
48. D. D. Adams, *Autoimmunity* **1**, 3 (1988).
49. P. R. Carnegie and I. R. Mackay, *Lancet* ii, 684 (1975).
50. R. A. Joske and W. E. King, *Lancet* ii, 477 (1955).
51. I. R. Mackay, L. I. Taft and D. C. Cowling, *Lancet* ii, 12 (1956).
52. I. R. Mackay and D. C. Gajdusek, *Arch. Intern. Med.* **101**, 30, (1958).
53. I. R. Mackay and L. Larkin, *Aust. Ann. Med.* **7**, 251 (1958).
54. T. P. Casey, *NZ Med. J.* **65**, 105 (1966).
55. N. L. Warner, Genetic aspects of autoimmune disease in animals, in *Autoimmunity. Genetic Immunologic, Virologic and Clinical Aspects* (N. Talal, ed.), Academic Press, New York (1977), pp. 33–62.
56. M. Bielschowsky, B. J. Helyer and J. B. Howie, *Proc. Univ. Otago Med. Sch.* **37**, 9 (1959).
57. B. J. Helyer and J. B. Howie, *Nature* **197**, 197 (1963).
58. M. C. Holmes, J. Gorrie and F. M. Burnet, *Lancet* ii, 638 (1961).
59. M. C. Holmes and F. M. Burnet, *Ann. Intern. Med.* **59**, 265 (1963).
60. F. M. Burnet and M. C. Holmes, *Nature* **194**, 146 (1962).
61. A. H. Coons and M. H. Kaplan, *J. Exp. Med.* **91**, 1 (1950).
62. E. J. Holborow, D. M. Weir and G. D. Johnson, *Br. Med. J.* **5047**, 732 (1957).
63. G. J. Friou, *Ann. Intern. Med.* **49**, 866 (1958).
64. I. R. Mackay and F. M. Burnet, *Autoimmune Diseases: Pathogenesis, Chemistry and Therapy*, Thomas, Springfield, IL (1963).
65. R. C. Nairn, *Br. Soc. Immunol. Newsl.* **267**, 9 (1993).
66. F. M. Burnet, *The Clonal Selection Theory of Acquired Immunity*, Cambridge University Press, Cambridge (1959).
67. F. M. Burnet, *Changing Patterns. An Atypical Autobiography*, Heinemann, Melbourne (1968), p. 218.
68. B. Ungar, A. E. Stocks, F. I. R. Martin, S. Whittingham and I. R. Mackay, *Lancet* ii, 77 (1967).
69. G. F. Bottazzo, A. Florin-Christensen and D. Doniach, *Lancet* ii, 1279 (1974).
70. W. Dameshek, E. Witebsky and F. Milgrom, *Ann. NY Acad. Sci.* **124**, 1 (1965).

The Cellular Basis of Immunity

The Mysterious Lymphocyte

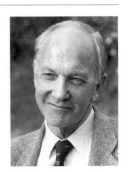

J. L. GOWANS
75 Cumnor Hill, Oxford OX2 9HX, UK

Those who accept an invitation to recall events that may have influenced their scientific work run the risk of confirming the old adage that autobiography makes bad history. In my own case the risk is all the greater because, in writing about experiments on lymphocytes which began 40 years ago, I realize the extent to which I shall have to depend upon memory, jogged along, I hope, by a collection of letters and reprints.

I have always thought that my start in research was due to a piece of extraordinary good luck and that, subsequently, I owed a great deal to two outstanding men. In 1947, I was a recently qualified house physician in London and not enjoying the deferential and hierarchical system we were expected to work under in those days. In this mood, I wrote a short note to the Secretary of the Medical Research Council, Sir Edward Mellanby, saying I wanted to do research, any openings? I had no idea what I wanted to do research on, although the idea of laboratory work had always attracted me. To my surprise, I received a personal note inviting me to see him. In a brisk interview, Mellanby painted a gloomy picture of my prospects but said that Howard Florey, in Oxford, was looking for medically qualified recruits and he was passing my letter to him. He was as good as his word and within a couple of weeks I was in Oxford being interviewed and accepted by Florey. I would like to conclude that it is a good rule always to write to the top man, but it was sheer luck that my letter to Mellanby arrived just after his conversation with Florey.

The interview with Florey was equally brisk and soon confirmed him in the view that I was ill prepared for a career in research. I was sent to learn physiology with the undergraduates before he would take me on as a D.Phil. student in his laboratory. Florey was himself a physiologist and had published his earliest work under the supervision of Sherrington in 1925 (1). Fifteen years later, in wartime Oxford, he was transforming an observation by Fleming into the most powerful agent for treating human infections hitherto available in medical prac-

IMMUNOLOGY: THE MAKING OF A MODERN SCIENCE
ISBN 0-12-274020-3

tice. He was a man of outstanding ability and greatly admired by those of us who trained under him, but he ran a somewhat austere regime. The currency, for him, was the simple, telling experiment with the minimum of speculative chatter. You would have a job as long as you continued to live successfully by your wits; if you were unsuccessful you could always go back to what he called 'the clinic'.

The Disappearing Lymphocytes

The work for a D.Phil. and a sabbatical at the Pasteur Institute had led to an interest in infection and immunity but, on returning to Oxford at the end of 1953, I had no clear idea what to do next. It was Florey who suggested that I should work on lymphocytes. The much-quoted indictment in those days was a ringing phrase by Arnold Rich (2) that 'the complete ignorance of the function of this cell is one of the most humiliating and disgraceful gaps in all medical knowledge'. Rich meant the 'small lymphocyte', the cell in the blood which was also a major component of lymphoid tissue and which accumulated, often in large numbers, in a variety of pathological lesions. Florey suggested I should look at a puzzling feature of its life history. In several species, lymphocytes had been shown to enter the blood from the major lymphatic vessels in numbers sufficient to replace all those in the blood many times each day. Thus, a large number of lymphocytes, numerically equal to those entering the blood, left it again for some unknown destination. The fate of these cells was the subject of much speculation. Maximov and his school regarded lymphocytes as haemopoietic stem cells capable of developing into all forms of circulating blood cells and into fibroblasts. This was the dominant view in 1953 and was based entirely on identifying the alleged transformations in histological preparations. A minor school regarded them as short-lived end cells, dying after performing their unknown function, possibly in the gut or the skin.

I was told to break with the tradition of morbid anatomy and do some experiments: if I could discover the fate of these disappearing lymphocytes I would also, no doubt, discover their function. Florey drew my attention to a method for collecting lymph from the thoracic duct of unanaesthetized rats and to an interesting finding by Mann and Higgins in 1950 (3) that the high, initial output of cells from the thoracic duct was not maintained if drainage from the fistula was continued for several days – the output fell progressively day by day to a low, relatively constant level. This observation launched my own studies and, from the beginning of 1954, I was on my own.

The observation of Mann and Higgins raised doubts about the true magnitude of the output of cells from the thoracic duct. Was the high output an artefact of cannulation or was it dependent, in some unknown way, on the input into the blood? This was solved by showing that the output of cells was indeed maintained at a high level if all the cells emerging from the fistula were pumped back into the blood. The rate of reinfusion was adjusted to the rate of lymph flow from the fistula and was continued for several days. This physiological design was important because the less tedious method of repeated injections of concentrated suspension of cells resulted in their large-scale arrest in the lungs. The experiments were tedious and required attention day and night to clear small clots from the pumping circuit.

The demonstration in 1957 that the lymphocytes which entered the blood were somehow responsible for maintaining their output from the thoracic duct (4) was most simply explained by a continuous recirculation of cells from blood to lymph. This was not a new idea; there was simply, at that time, no good evidence to support it. The next step was to see if the animals' own lymphocytes could, in fact, migrate from the blood into the lymph. A short intravenous infusion of lymphocytes which had been labelled *in vitro* with inorganic ^{32}P resulted in a wave of cell-associated radioactivity in the lymph which overlapped in time with an associated wave of increased cell output. This increase in output was not due to the generation of new small lymphocytes because a continuous infusion of tritiated thymidine failed to label them. Only the large lymphocytes, which normally make up about 5% of the cells in rat thoracic duct lymph, became labelled, thus providing a control for the labelling procedure.

I was confident enough about the results of these experiments to talk about them to the Physiological Society and to publish them in its journal in 1959 under the title 'The recirculation of lymphocytes from blood to lymph in the rat' (5). However, this confidence was not shared by a referee who recommended rejection on the grounds that the ^{32}P label had been exchanged during the destruction of the transfused cells. Objections to these experiments were also aired in 1959 at a conference in Utah organized by the Hematology Study Section of the National Institutes of Health (6). Some argued that, if recirculation occurred at all, it was probably on a small scale and did not explain the high turnover of the blood lymphocytes. Others recommended caution because new lymphocytes might be formed by incorporating the DNA from old lymphocytes so they might not have labelled with tritiated thymidine in my experiments. There was no biochemical evidence for this idea of DNA reutilization and I think it arose partly from an initial reluctance to accept the exceptionally long life span of blood lymphocytes which others had inferred from labelling data after giving tritiated thymidine *in vivo*. Looking again at the discussions at this meeting I wonder whether some of the hostility to the notion of a large-scale recirculation did not come from a feeling that it was a rather boring idea. One of my friends said it was not 'biologically illuminating'. At least, the classical haematological view gave a function to small lymphocytes; recirculation might give an answer to where they went but, at that time, it gave no clue about what they did.

It was clear from the Utah conference that we needed to trace the precise route taken by the traffic of cells as it passed from blood to lymph, if the critics were to be answered. This was achieved by an autoradiographic study on rats given intravenous infusions of lymphocytes which had been labelled *in vitro* with tritiated adenosine (7). The stability of the label in the RNA of small lymphocytes enabled them to be followed from the blood, into the lymph nodes and, thence, back into the thoracic duct lymph; they also entered and left the spleen via the blood. The large, dividing lymphocytes, in which the DNA could be labelled, did not recirculate but migrated from the blood into the lamina propria of the small intestine where they developed into plasma cells. This last observation led later to studies on local immunity in the gut.

The location of the labelled small lymphocytes within the lymph nodes was particularly interesting. At first, we simply noted a bulk transfer of cells from the blood into the cortex of the nodes, that is, into areas normally occupied by small lymphocytes. However, when the nodes were examined at short intervals after intravenous infusion, the labelled cells could be seen passing through an unusual set of blood vessels in the cortex – the so-called postcapillary venules or, as I believe they are now called, high endothelial venules. The vessels were ringed with labelled cells which had accumulated under the endothelium, prior to their migration into the cortex and on into the lymph sinuses. Vincent Marchesi, a medical student from Yale, had been doing an electron microscopic study with Florey on the migration of leucocytes in acutely inflamed tissues. He had produced some striking pictures of polymorphonuclear leucocytes (PML) with slim waists and bulbous ends passing through gaps between the endothelial cells of inflamed vessels. These photographs appeared in the 1962 edition of Florey's textbook of general pathology. Marchesi carried out a similar study on serial sections through the lymph nodes of normal rats (8). We were pleased to see lymphocytes caught in the act of migrating from the blood and arranging themselves under the endothelium, exactly as had been seen in the experiments with labelled cells. Marchesi was familiar with the appearance of leucocytes passing between enthothelial cells, but the appearance in the nodes was quite different. A detailed study of serial sections led to the conclusion that lymphocytes were passing not between, but through, the endothelial cells. This unorthodox view was subsequently challenged, but the matter has not, to my knowledge, been resolved.

Postcapillary venules are highly selective and will normally permit the migration of lymphocytes, but no other kind of leucocyte. However, Marchesi found that if the nodes were artificially inflamed, PML migrated from the blood by way of gaps between the endothelial cells – the PML remained orthodox. The contrast between the orthodox and unorthodox appearances gave us some confidence in concluding that there was something odd about the migratory behaviour of lymphocytes. There is currently some interest in identifying the molecular features of the cell surface which mediate the normal traffic of lymphocytes into lymphoid tissue: clearly, the repertoire of ligands on lymphocytes must be different from that on other leucocytes.

The two papers describing this work in 1964 appear to have convinced most people that we had solved the problem of lymphocyte turnover in the blood: the cells in the blood simply recirculated into the lymph by way of the lymph nodes and the Peyer's patches; we found no migration through the thymus. It is no longer held that lymphocytes are haemopoietic stem cells nor, incidentally, that they transform into macrophages (9). In 1959, I had been disappointed that Florey's prediction – find out where they go and you will find out what they do – was looking distinctly overoptimistic; but by 1964 we were well into other studies for which the audience had changed once more: from physiology and haematology to immunology. The change was quite rapid.

Immunology I

In 1959, the year of the Utah conference, Burnet wrote in his *The Clonal Selection Theory of Acquired Immunity* that 'there was no evidence of immunological activity in small lymphocytes' (10). Certainly, it was accepted that lymph nodes made antibody and, from the use of adoptive immunization, that they were the seat of delayed hypersensitivity and of the reaction to allografts; but the major cell within them was still without a function. Albert Coons (11) in a classic paper in 1955, had confirmed Fragraeus's claim that it was plasma cells within lymphoid tissue that made antibody but, again, lymphocytes had no place in his scheme; the elusive precursor of plasma cells was a 'primitive reticular cell'.

I owe my own entry into immunology to Peter Medawar, the second of the outstanding men I referred to at the outset (12). He had carried out some of his earliest work under Florey in Oxford and his wife, Jean, had published a paper on lymphocytes from the same department in 1940 (13). It must have been in 1955 that I first met Medawar at University College London because I see that I had started a correspondence with him in 1954. He sent a long reply in answer to my query about raising immunological tolerance in rats. All the initial experiments on recirculation had involved reinfusing an animal with its own cells and I wanted to transfuse lymphocytes between animals, which would be equivalent to performing an allograft. He said raising tolerance would be extremely tedious and that, instead, I should raise inbred strains of rats. We followed his advice and most of our later experiments were carried out on inbred donor–recipient pairs. I see also from correspondence that we did a strange experiment together in Oxford in 1957 to see if a nucleoprotein fraction, prepared from lymphocytes, could substitute for living lymphocytes in maintaining the output of cells from the thoracic duct. This experiment, the results of which were completely negative, was in the context of the arguments for the re-utilization of nucleic acids, mentioned earlier; it also arose because, for a while, it was believed that histocompatibility antigens might be associated with such a fraction.

This new connection with the field of transplantation immunology led to a much wider circle of ideas and scientific contacts, largely through the generosity of Peter Medawar. I already knew Avrion Mitchison, who was an early contemporary in Oxford, and I soon met Morten Simonsen and the members of Medawar's group in London. The common interest was in the cells involved in the reactions to alloantigens.

It was already known that cells in the peripheral blood could cause graft-versus-host (GVH) reactions in neonatal recipients and suspicion was falling on some kind of lymphocyte as being responsible. The injection of cells from the thoracic duct would be a cleaner test of this idea because the inocula would consist exclusively of lymphocytes. I discussed this experiment with Medawar in 1958 and he wrote to say it rather appealed to him; others, I knew, were also interested, so I provided the usual instruction in cannulating the rat thoracic duct. I decided instead to do the same experiment by injecting parental strain lymphocytes into adult F_1 hybrid rats. This was partly because it was technically easier than working with neonates and because, in a large recipient, I could more easily follow the fate of the injected cells – something for which I was anyway developing techniques in concurrent experiments on recirculation. The upshot of this flurry of activity was the report from several laboratories in 1960–1961 that lymphocytes from the thoracic duct could, indeed, cause GVH reactions in both neonatal and F_1 hybrid rats. There remained one problem. Thoracic duct lymph in the rat contains a minority population of large, dividing lymphocytes; the rest, about 95%, are small lymphocytes. It was a guess as to which was causing GVH reactions. We suspected that the small lymphocyte was responsible because we knew that the large cells migrated preferentially into the gut and not into the lymph nodes and spleen which were the first targets of the immunological attack. We were able to show that it was small lymphocytes and not large lymphocytes that caused the reactions by enriching the inocula for the two classes, respectively. The most striking and unexpected finding came from studying the fate of inocula of small lymphocytes labelled independently with three different isotopic markers. An autoradiographic study showed that a proportion of the small cells started enlarging and dividing in the lymphoid tissue of the host within 24 hours of their injection. The donor origin of these dividing cells was also confirmed with a chromosome marker. The results of these experiments were published in 1961 and, more fully, in 1962 (14,15). They aroused no serious criticisms; indeed, they may have been received with some relief because, at last, small lymphocytes did something. These were interesting times. In 1960, Nowell (16) had shown that phytohaemagglutinin could induce mitoses in cultures of human leukocytes; that these dividing cells came from small lymphocytes was shown conclusively in 1963 by Marshall and Robert (17). The news that the thymus played a crucial role in the development of the immune system broke in 1961 with Jacques Miller's paper in the Lancet (18).

Still under the influence of the Medawar school, we continued to work for a while on GVH reactions and allografts. Our small lymphocytes performed in a predictable way: populations of them exhibited the property of specific immunological tolerance (19); and normal, syngeneic lymphocytes could destroy long-standing skin allografts borne by tolerant animals (20). All this confirmed the idea that small lymphocytes were endowed with alloreactivity, a field in which one of my first research students, the late Bill Ford, worked with great distinction. So far, I have hardly mentioned colleagues or research students. This is because, up to 1962, there was little space for expansion from the single room I occupied in the School of Pathology. Things changed for the better in 1963 when the Medical Research Council set up a research unit and provided a new building which we called the Cellular Immunology Unit. In it, I enjoyed the company of many excellent visitors and long-term colleagues, only a few of whom I can mention in this short account.

The Function of Lymphocytes

The experiments on the response to alloantigens and some preliminary studies with Douglas McGregor on the possible role of lymphocytes in antibody formation, led us to propose in 1962 a more general function for small lymphocytes which also incorporated the phenomenon of recirculation (21). We suggested that the potentiality of an animal to react to all antigens resided in its large population of small (non-dividing) lymphocytes; and that the small lymphocyte itself, following interaction with antigen, would be triggered to divide and differentiate to produce the cellular effectors of the various responses. What had been called an 'immunologically competent cell' could be regarded as an antigen-sensitive cell with developmental potentialities. The missing evidence in 1962 was a demonstration that small lymphocytes could develop into the plasma cells that made antibody. I thought this very likely, but there was still the lingering view at that time that lymphocytes were only involved in the so-called 'cellular immunities'. Lymphocyte recirculation fitted our general scheme because it provided a means of selecting cells with particular specificities from the large recirculating pool into regionally stimulated lymphoid tissue. A selection of this kind was later demonstrated in vivo both for histocompatibility antigens (22) and for antigens yielding conventional antibody responses (23,24). Thus, recirculating lymphocytes ideally fulfilled the requirements of Burnet's clonal selection theory. I first met Burnet when he visited our laboratory in Oxford. He exchanged a few words with Florey, but I was surprised to discover that these two great Australian scientists hardly knew one another.

Immunology II

'A well recognized procedure for discovering the function of an organ is the study of the effects of its operative removal in animals.' This statement needs some qualification because I suspect that, since Jacques Miller's experiments on the thymus, there are no longer any organs with unknown functions left to remove. The quotation is the first line in a paper by Sanders and Florey in 1940 (25) in which they recorded the consequences of trying to excise surgically as much lymphoid tissue as possible from rats and rabbits – unfortunately without illuminating the function of the lymphocyte which was their objective. It was in the same spirit that in the early 1960s we depleted rats of lymphocytes by prolonged drainage from a thoracic duct fistula and examined their ability to make antibody to sheep red blood cells (SRBC) and to tetanus toxoid (26). The responses were profoundly depressed, but could be restored by returning the lymphocytes intravenously. This was an indication that small lymphocytes might initiate the cellular changes that lead to antibody formation as well as reacting to alloantigens in the way previously described. We particularly wanted to find out, in such experiments, if the antibody-producing cells were the descendants of the restorative small lymphocytes; the demonstration that small lymphocytes could develop into plasma cells was a missing piece of evidence in the general scheme proposed in 1962.

Sublethally irradiated rats, which themselves cannot make antibody, are convenient hosts for testing the developmental potentiality of lymphocytes from normal donors; and by choosing suitable donor–recipient combinations, alloantisera can be used to distinguish donor from recipient cells in the irradiated hosts (27). With this technique Jonathan Howard showed that the cells making antibody to SRBC in the spleens of irradiated recipients had arisen from the restorative inocula of small lymphocytes (28). A similar strategy was used to show that recirculating lymphocytes carry the property of immunological memory. In this case, irradiated rats had received thoracic duct cells from immunized donors; they then gave large secondary responses when challenged with the immunizing antigen. This carriage of memory was shown with a bacteriophage antigen (29) during a sabbatical with Jonathan Uhr in New York in 1964 and to tetanus toxoid by Susan Roser (née Ellis) in Oxford (30). In the memory experiment with tetanus toxoid it was shown that the plasma cells making antibody in the red pulp of the spleen again arose from the injected small lymphocytes, using the design with alloantisera. I have to admit that demonstrating the potential of recirculating small lymphocytes to develop into plasma cells has become something of an obsession and the experiments extended into an era when cell collaboration in immune responses had become the major focus. But it is a key point in any explanation of the dynamics of immune responses *in vivo*. There was a suggestion in the 1960s that lymphocytes, already in cell division, might be the antigen-sensitive precursors of plasma cells in primary responses in mice. I do not know what the adherents of this view now feel; in any case, it does not affect the point about the potentiality of small lymphocytes to become plasma cells.

We were never sure what happens, in cellular terms, when an animal is primed and acquires immunological memory. Certainly, recirculating lymphocytes from our primed rats contained all the ingredients for mounting secondary responses, but we also found that animals depleted of recirculating cells by prolonged drainage from the thoracic duct still responded normally to challenge. Apparently, priming also established a population of resident cells, sufficient in number to generate a response. Part of this population may have been derived from germinal centres about which much more is now known; indeed, they may have also given rise to part of our recirculating memory pool. It would be interesting to know what controls the choice between residence and vagrancy among lymphocytes. Chronic drainage from the thoracic duct does not remove all small lymphocytes from the lymph nodes, but we do not know whether, among those that remain, there is a group which is normally sessile. We do know that a cell is not necessarily condemned to residence simply because it is already launched on its pathway of differentiation. We know this because there is a traffic of plasma cell precursors, from lymph into the blood, on its way to mediate local immunity, for example, in the gut. In the lymph and blood they would be identified as 'large lymphocytes', but some of them already contain immunoglobulin, which is easily identifiable by immunofluoresence (31); in the gut they complete their development into plasma cells.

It was no surprise that the picture which emerged from our immunological work turned out to be an oversimplification. A major problem was the nature of what we had called 'the functional heterogeneity' of our populations of small lymphocytes – the ability of a single cell-type (small, recirculating, not yet dividing) to initiate all classes of immune response. The first answer to this problem that I found convincing came in 1968 from experiments by Mitchell and Miller in which the ability of irradiated mice to make antibody was restored by mixtures of cells from the thymus and bone marrow (32). They found that the antibody-forming cells in the irradiated host were derived from the marrow, but that restoration only occurred if thymus cells were simultaneously present. The era of cell collaboration between B and T cells had begun. I shall not attempt to interpret our old experiments in terms of T and B small lymphocytes and their dividing progeny, although this would not be difficult; it is simply that we did not make the important discovery that now makes it necessary.

I left experimental work in 1977 for a different career and handed over the Cellular Immunology Unit to Alan Williams whose premature death in 1992 was a great national and international loss to science. Many molecular structures involved in the interaction of lymphocytes with antigen and with each other have now been characterized and we now know the answer to the major problem that puzzled workers in the early days – the mechanism by which antibody diversity is generated. However, there is still a gap to be filled. The recirculation of lymphocytes through lymphoid tissue and the migration of differentiating lineages within it tell us that, despite contributing to an apparently stable architecture, the cells in lymphoid tissue are in a highly dynamic state. This cellular traffic no doubt favours cellular interactions but, to my knowledge, it is not yet possible adequately to describe the initiation and evolution of any immune response in terms of the structure and cellular dynamics of a lymphoid organ *in vivo*.

Notes and References

1. E. A. P. Abraham, Howard Walter Florey, in *Biographical Memoirs R. Soc.* **17**, 255 (1971).
2. A. R. Rich, *Arch. Pathol.* **22**, 228 (1936).
3. J. D. Mann and G. M. Higgins, *Blood* 5, 177 (1950).
4. J. L. Gowans, *Br. J. Exp. Pathol.* **38**, 67 (1957).
5. J. L. Gowans, *J. Physiol.* **146**, 54 (1959).
6. J. L. Gowans, in *The Kinetics of Cellular Proliferation* (F. Stohlman, ed.), Grune & Stratton, New York (1959), p. 64.
7. J. L. Gowans and E. J. Knight, *Proc. R. Soc., Ser. B* **159**, 257 (1964).
8. V. T. Marchesi and J. L. Gowans, *Proc. R. Soc., Ser. B* **159**, 283 (1964).
9. A. Volkman and J. L. Gowans *Br. J. Exp. Pathol.* **46**, 62 (1965).
10. F. M. Burnet, in *The Colonal Section Theory of Acquired Immunity*, Cambridge University Press, Cambridge (1959), p. 110.
11. E. H. Leduc, A. H. Coons and J. M. Connolly, *J. Exp. Med.* **102**, 61 (1955).
12. N. A. Michison, Peter Brian Medawar in *Biographical Memoirs R. Soc.* **35**, 281 (1990).
13. J. Medawar, *Br. J. Exp. Pathol.* **21**, 205 (1940).
14. J. L. Gowans, B. M. Gesner and D. D. McGregor, in *Biological Activity of the Leucocyte* (G. E. W. Wolstenholme and M. O'Connor, eds), Churchill, London (1961), p. 32.
15. J. L. Gowans, *Ann. NY Acad. Sci.* **99**, 432 (1962).
16. P. C. Nowell, *Cancer Res.* **20**, 462 (1960).
17. W. H. Marshall and K. B. Robert, *Q. J. Exp. Physiol.* **48**, 146 (1963).
18. J. F. A. P. Miller, *Lancet* ii, 748 (1961).
19. P. J. McCullagh and J. L. Gowans, in *The Lymphocyte in Immunology and Haemopoiesis*, Edward Arnold, London (1966), p. 234.
20. J. L. Gowans and D. D. McGregor, *Prog. Allergy* **9**, 1 (1965).
21. J. L. Gowans, D. D. McGregor, D. M. Cowen and C. E. Ford, *Nature* **196**, 651 (1962).
22. W. L. Ford and R. C. Atkins, *Nature New Biol.* **234**, 178 (1971).
23. J. Sprent, J. F. A. P. Miller and G. F. Mitchell, *Cell. Immunol.* **2**, 171 (1971).
24. D. A. Rowley, J. L. Gowans, W. L. Ford, R. C. Atkins and M. E. Smith, *J. Exp. Med.* **136**, 499 (1972).
25. A. G. Sanders and H. W. Florey, *Br. J. Exp. Path.* **21**, 275 (1940).
26. D. D. McGregor and J. L. Gowans, *J. Exp. Med.* **117**, 303 (1963).
27. S. T. Ellis, J. L. Gowans and J. C. Howard, *Antibiot. Chemother.* **15**, 40 (1969).
28. J. C. Howard and J. L. Gowans, *Proc. R. Soc. London, Ser. B* **182** 193 (1972).
29. J. L. Gowans and J. W. Uhr, *J. Exp. Med.* **124**, 1017 (1966).
30. S. T. Ellis and J. L. Gowans, *Proc R. Soc. London, Ser. B* **183**, 125 (1973).
31. A. F. Williams and J. L. Gowans, *J. Exp. Med.* **141**, 335 (1975).
32. G. F. Mitchell and J. F. A. P. Miller, *J. Exp. Med.* **128**, 821 (1968).

The Discovery of Thymus Function

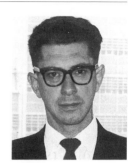

JACQUES F. A. P. MILLER
The Walter and Eliza Hall Institute of Medical Research,
Post Office, Royal Melbourne Hospital, Victoria 3050, Australia

To my mind one of the most important advances in immunology that we may look forward to in the next 5 or 10 years is an explanation of the mechanisms of the 'cellular' immunities. (Medawar, 1958 (1).)

The outstanding feature of the development of immunology in the last 10 years has been the recognition of the function of the lymphocyte and of the importance of the thymus in the immune process. (Burnet, 1966 (2).)

Prior to 1960, the functions of the thymus and its lymphocytes were unknown. By contrast, the circulating small lymphocytes found in blood, lymph and lymphoid tissues, had been shown to be immunologically competent by Gowans (3). Yet, although the thymus was known to be a lymphocyte-producing organ, immunologists were not willing to attribute to it any immunological function. There were at least three reasons for this. First, the cytological hallmarks of an immune response, such as the occurrence of plasma cells and germinal centres, were never seen in the thymus of normal immunized animals. Second, thymus lymphocytes, unlike cells from other lymphoid tissues, could not mount any immune response to antigen on transfer to appropriate recipients. Third, animals thymectomized in adult life could produce both cellular and humoral responses as efficiently as intact animals. This was even taken as 'evidence that the thymus gland does *not* participate in the control of the immune response' (4).

Early Studies

In 1958, after graduating in Medicine from the University of Sydney, I obtained from the University of Queensland a 'Gaggin' Fellowship which paid for me to go to London and spend two years in a suitable Cancer Research Institute. I

IMMUNOLOGY: THE MAKING OF A MODERN SCIENCE
ISBN 0-12-274020-3

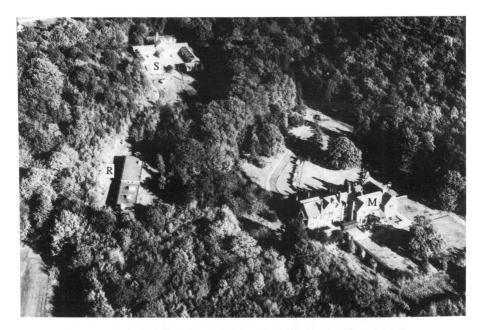

Figure 1   Aerial view of Pollards Wood Research Station at Chalfont St Giles, Buckinghamshire, England. It previously belonged to Bertram Mills, the circus owner, and was later purchased by the Chester Beatty Research Institute. The rooms in the mansion (M) were transformed into well-equipped laboratories. A modern building was added for work with radioisotopes (R). Converted stables (S) housed additional laboratories and mouse colonies.

approached several laboratories and was finally granted permission to work at the Chester Beatty Institute of Cancer Research. Having performed some experiments on virus multiplication during my undergraduate studies (5), I was pleased to learn that Dr R. J. C. Harris was interested in the Rous sarcoma virus of chickens. His laboratory was not in the main building of the Institute in South Kensington, but at a place called Pollards Wood (Fig. 1) near Amersham which, at that time, belonged to the Institute. It was a magnificent Tudor-style mansion and some of the laboratories and mouse colonies were situated in converted horse stables. Harris suggested that I might use my time at Pollards Wood to work on the pathogenesis of mouse leukaemia, as a leukaemogenic virus had recently been discovered by Ludwik Gross (6). I took up this challenge with great enthusiasm and began numerous experiments to find out why the thymus was so intimately involved in the leukaemogenic process. This required large numbers of mice of different inbred strains and hence considerable mouse space which, unfortunately, was not available. Six months after my arrival, Harris was offered the directorship of the Division of Virology of the Imperial Cancer Research Funds at Mill Hill, London, and I

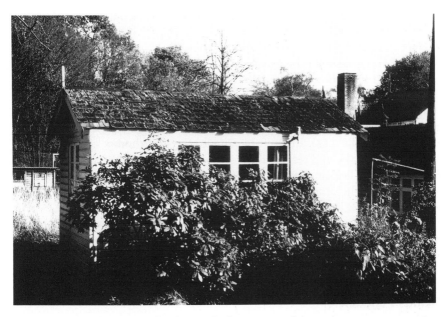

Figure 2   The 'shack' at Pollards Wood where many of the early experiments with neonatally thymectomized mice were done.

was left without a supervisor, but lucky to inherit some of his animal space and to acquire a small shack (Fig. 2).

I prepared extracts from leukaemic tissues and filtered them according to the method of Gross. They had to be inoculated into newborn mice, otherwise leukaemia would not develop. As adult thymectomy had been shown to prevent spontaneous mouse leukaemia developing in high leukaemic strains and leukaemia induced in low-leukaemic strains by ionizing radiation and chemical carcinogens, my first plan was to find out whether it would also prevent the disease in virus-infected mice. It did so even though the virus had been inoculated at birth (7). Thymus implantation six months after thymectomy (which was performed at one month of age) restored the potential for leukaemogenesis in neonatally inoculated mice (8). Hence the virus must have remained latent, and the next experiment showed that it could be recovered from the non-leukaemic tissues of thymectomized mice (9). I wondered, therefore, whether the virus could multiply outside thymus tissue. Since, however, it had to be given at birth, this could be resolved only by thymectomizing the mice before the virus was inoculated. I therefore decided to thymectomize baby mice and then inject them with virus. The experiment met with some difficulty because the neonatally thymectomized mice died prematurely whether inoculated with virus or not. This suggested 'that the thymus at birth may be essential to life' (10). Further investigations showed clearly that mice thymectomized at one day of age, but not later than a few days, were highly susceptible to infections, showed a marked deficiency of lymphocytes in the circulation and in the lymphoid tissues and were unable to reject foreign skin grafts. As extrathymic lymphocytes were known to be immunologically competent and skin-graft rejection had been shown by Medawar and colleagues (1) to be the result of a cell-mediated immune response, my results led me to postulate that 'during embryogenesis the thymus would produce the originators of immunologically competent cells many of which would have migrated to other sites at about the time of birth. This would suggest that lymphocytes leaving the thymus are specially selected cells' (11). I therefore came to the unorthodox conclusion that the thymus was the site responsible for the development of immunologically competent cells. It is interesting to note with hindsight that, had not my mice been housed in the non-pathogen-free conditions which prevailed at Pollards Wood at the time, the neonatally thymectomized mice would not have died of 'wasting disease' as a result of intercurrent infections (as I showed later with germ-free mice (12)) and I probably would not have been alerted to their immune deficiencies.

Thymus Function

Prior to their first publication, I sent my results to a number of well-known immunologists. They were considered with interest, but the conclusion was regarded with scepticism. For example, Medawar did not seem convinced, as shown in a letter he sent to me dated four days before the publication date of my *Lancet* paper (11) (Fig. 3). He remained in doubt even as late as 1963 when he stated 'we shall come to regard the presence of lymphocytes in the thymus as an evolutionary accident of no very great significance' (13). Other immunologists, with the notable exception of Burnet, also expressed doubts and incredulity when I presented my results, prior to their publication, at various meetings during 1961. For example, at the Ciba Foundation Symposium on Tumour Viruses of Murine Origin held in Perugia in June 1961, my former mentor, R. J. C. Harris, claimed the following: 'Dr Delphine Parrott in our laboratory has been thymectomizing day-old mice and there is at present no evidence that these animals are immunologically weaker than normal animals. They do not retain skin grafts, they are living and breeding quite normally. They do not die of laboratory infections' (14). At the New York Academy of Sciences meeting in February 1962, I gave my results in great detail and emphasized that mice thymectomized at birth failed to reject skin both from MHC-incompatible strains and from other species such as rats (15). During the discussion, Martinez (from Good's group) stated without showing data that they also had shown that neonatally thymectomized mice were somewhat immunodeficient but, in contrast to my findings, they observed prolonged skin graft survival *only* in strains of mice isogenic at the H-2 histocompatibility locus but homologous with respect to other weaker histocompatibility genes. They later published this

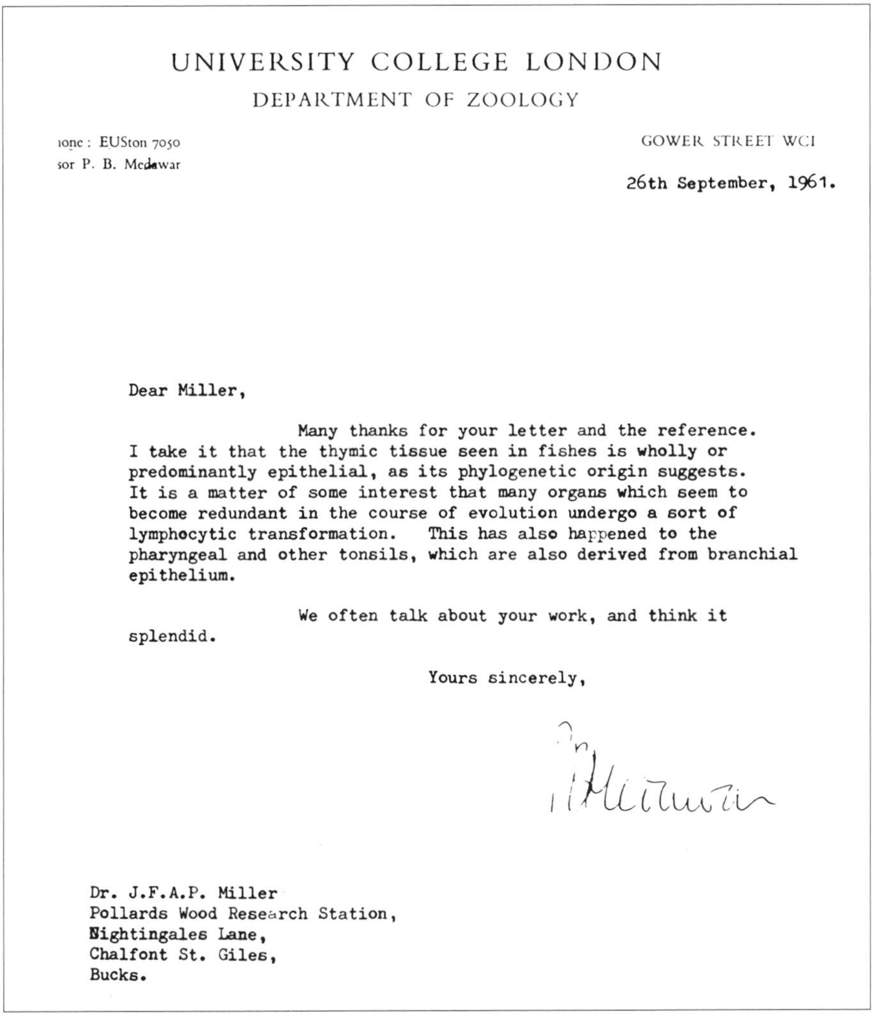

UNIVERSITY COLLEGE LONDON

DEPARTMENT OF ZOOLOGY

ione : EUSton 7050
sor P. B. Medawar

GOWER STREET WC1

26th September, 1961.

Dear Miller,

Many thanks for your letter and the reference. I take it that the thymic tissue seen in fishes is wholly or predominantly epithelial, as its phylogenetic origin suggests. It is a matter of some interest that many organs which seem to become redundant in the course of evolution undergo a sort of lymphocytic transformation. This has also happened to the pharyngeal and other tonsils, which are also derived from branchial epithelium.

We often talk about your work, and think it splendid.

Yours sincerely,

Dr. J.F.A.P. Miller
Pollards Wood Research Station,
Nightingales Lane,
Chalfont St. Giles,
Bucks.

Figure 3   Peter Medawar's letter in reply to one in which I had briefly summarized the effects of neonatal thymectomy. The letter is dated four days prior to the publication of my 1961 *Lancet* paper *(11)* documenting the immunological function of the thymus.

finding and statement *(16)*. Subsequently, Good offered an explanation for the discrepancy between these results and mine: 'Careful autopsies performed in the thymectomized animals often revealed minute amounts of residual thymic tissue in these animals. With perfection of our technique a large proportion of neonatally thymectomized mice accepted H-2 incompatible grafts in contrast to partially thymectomized mice' *(17)*. In my experience, however, partial thymectomy was never associated with any immune defects, an observation in keeping with the well-documented fact that the thymus is composed of multiple autonomous subunits, each of which is independent of the other and not subject to external feedback mechanisms (18).

Independent investigations using rats, performed by Waksman's group and published in 1962, confirmed the immune deficiencies associated with neonatal thymectomy (19).

In adult mice, thymectomy had for long been known *not* to have any untoward effects, and it was partly this fact that had led many to claim that the thymus did not have an immune function. Since total body irradiation destroyed lymphoid tissues, I wondered if recovery of immune function following irradiation might be thymus dependent. I showed this to be true in late 1961 and the results were accepted for publication in *Nature* (20). As expected, implanting thymus tissue into neonatally thymectomized or adult thymectomized and irradiated mice allowed a normal immune system to develop. When the thymus tissue came from a foreign strain, the neonatally thymectomized recipients became specifically immunologically tolerant of the histocompatibility antigens of the donor. This led to the suggestion that 'when one is inducing a state of immunological tolerance in a newly born animal', for example by the classical technique of injecting allogeneic bone marrow cells at birth, 'one is in effect performing a selective or immunological thymectomy' (21). In other words, lymphocytes developing in the thymus in the presence of foreign cells would be deleted, implying that the thymus should be the site where self-tolerance is imposed. Sir Alexander Haddow, FRS, the director of the Chester Beatty Research Institute, urged me to send these and other results for publication and he communicated them on my behalf to the *Proceedings of the Royal Society London, Series B* in late December 1961 (received by the journal on 5 January 1962, and published later that year (21)). In view of what I had suggested about tolerance in that paper, I was most interested to hear Burnet's lecture given at the University of London in June 1962 when he stated: 'If, as I believe, the thymus is the site where proliferation and differentiation of lymphocytes into clones with definable immunological functions occurs, we must also endow it with another function – the elimination or inhibition of self-reactive clones' (22).

T Cells and B Cells

In the late 1950s and early 1960s, there was no reason to believe that mammalian small lymphocytes could be divided into entirely distinct subsets. In birds, on the other hand, it was known that the bursa of Fabricius was involved in antibody production (23). Szenberg and Warner (24) were the first to show a division of labour among chicken lymphocytes, early bursectomy being associated with defects in antibody formation and early thymectomy with defects in

cellular responses. Since mice do not have a bursa and since neonatal thymectomy in mice prevented both cellular immune responses and normal antibody
production (21,25), it was widely held that the mammalian thymus fulfilled the
functions of both the avian thymus and bursa. For example, Burnet stated in
1962 that in 'mammals it is highly probable that the thymus also carries out
the function performed by the bursa of Fabricius in the chicken, which is to feed
into the body the cells whose descendants will produce antibody' (26).
Nevertheless, a hint that two subsets of lymphocytes may be involved in antibody formation in mice came from the experiments of Claman and colleagues
in 1966 (27): irradiated mice receiving a mixed population of marrow and
thymus cells produced far more antibody than when given either cell source
alone. The investigators could not, however, determine the origin of the
antibody-forming cells in their model for lack of genetic markers.

Davies and his collaborators (28) were investigating the response of adult
thymectomized irradiated mice given bone marrow and thymus grafts from
donors which differed slightly immunogenetically. When spleen cells from these
mice were injected soon after challenge with sheep erythrocytes into irradiated
recipients presensitized against either the thymus or the marrow donor, mice
capable of rejecting cells of thymus-donor type produced antibody. Those
immunized against marrow donors made much less. These transfer experiments
were, however, performed 30 days after irradiation and thymus grafting. At this
time, my colleagues and I had already shown that the lymphoid cell population
of the thymus graft had been entirely replaced by cells of marrow origin (29).
Thus, the haemolysins detected in Davies's irradiated recipients presensitized
against the thymus donor might well have been produced by marrow-derived
cells that had repopulated and migrated from the thymus graft. The cells producing antibody could, therefore, have had the immunogenetic characteristics
of the marrow donor and yet be thymus derived. Davies, himself, admitted this
when stating: 'it may be that thymus-derived cells can produce antibody, but
only in the presence of cells of bone marrow origin. Equally, cells of bone
marrow origin may be the cells whose immunological potential is enhanced by
association with cells of thymic origin. These are not problems which the
present analysis can resolve' (30).

In independent studies performed with Graham Mitchell immediately after
my return to Australia in 1966, we investigated the ability of various cell types
to restore immune functions to thymectomized mice. By introducing genetically
marked cells into neonatally thymectomized or thymectomized irradiated
hosts, we established beyond doubt and for the first time that antibody-forming
cell precursors (B cells) were derived from bone marrow, and that thymus-
derived cells were essential to allow B cells to respond to antigen by producing
antibody (31–33). The immunological community regarded the existence of
two distinct lymphocyte subsets with surprise and scepticism. Gowans (34),
who had proven that the recirculating small lymphocyte could initiate both cellular and humoral immune responses stated: 'Had it not been for Dr Miller's

experiments I would have assumed that a single variety of small lymphocyte was involved in each of our experiments.' Good (*35*) was 'concerned at separating thymus-derived from marrow-derived cells', since the former 'are in fact, marrow-derived cells'. It was undoubtedly the use of genetically marked cells and of adult thymectomized, irradiated and bone marrow-protected ('AT×XBM') mice, which I first developed in late 1961 (*20,36*), that proved the existence of the two major types of lymphocytes, T and B cells, with their distinct functions. Yet some expressed doubts 'about the significance of results obtained in such biological monstrosities as pure line mice thymectomized, lethally irradiated, and salvaged by injection of bone marrow from another mouse' (*37*). But it was only by using such 'monstrosities' that Zinkernagel *et al.* (*38*) were subsequently able to demonstrate that restriction is imposed by the major histocompatibility complex intrathymically on developing T cells and, even today, in experiments relying on sophisticated transgenic technology, one still has to use AT×XBM mice to uncover basic facts about self-tolerance and autoimmunity (*39*)!

In the post-1960 decades, the immunological function of the thymus is being taken for granted and the term 'T cell' has become a household name. The immune deficiency associated with opportunistic infections in patients with AIDS is reminiscent of the postneonatal thymectomy syndrome I first observed in 1961. The existence of T and B cells was not only confirmed, but also led to a reinvestigation of numerous immunological phenomena, including the carrier effect (*40,41*), memory (*42*), tolerance (*43–45*), autoimmunity (*46*) and genetically determined unresponsive states (*47*). T cells were clearly responsible for the 'cellular' immunities, the mechanism of which Medawar (*1*) wished to elucidate, and even T cells themselves became subdivided into subsets based on function, cell surface markers and secreted products or interleukins. Hardly an issue of any immunological journal now appears without some reference to T lymphocytes.

Acknowledgements

I am most grateful to the University of Queensland for the award of the Fellowship which allowed me to pursue my early studies on thymus function in London. I thank many colleagues who encouraged me during these early years, in particular the late Sir Alexander Haddow, director of the Chester Beatty Research Institute, who gave me complete freedom in choosing whatever line of work I thought was essential, and also the late Sir Peter Medawar who gave me tremendous encouragement to continue what I was doing, work which, as he put it, led to a 'wholly new conception' (*48*). I am grateful to Professor R. A. Weiss, Director of the Chester Beatty Research Laboratories, Institute of Cancer Research, London, for permission to reproduce the aerial view of Pollards Wood Research Station.

Notes and References

1. P. B. Medawar, *Proc. R. Soc. London, Ser. B* **149**, 145 (1958).
2. F. M. Burnet, in *The Thymus: Experimental and Clinical Studies (Ciba Foundation Symposium)* (G. E. W. Wolstenholme and R. Porter, eds), Churchill, London (1966), pp. 1–2.
3. J. L. Gowans, in *Biological Activity of the Leucocyte (Ciba Foundation Study Group)* (G. E. W. Wolstenholme and M. O'Connor, eds), Churchill, London (1961), pp. 32–44.
4. L. D. MacLean, S. J. Zak, R. L. Varco and R. A. Good, *Transpl. Bull.* **41**, 21 (1957).
5. J. F. A. P. Miller and P. M. de Burgh, *Aust. J. Exp. Biol. Med. Sci.* **35**, 115 (1957).
6. L. Gross, *Proc. Soc. Exp. Biol. Med.* **78**, 342 (1951).
7. J. F. A. P. Miller, *Nature* **183**, 1069 (1959).
8. J. F. A. P. Miller, *Nature* **184**, 1809 (1959).
9. J. F. A. P. Miller, *Nature* **187**, 703 (1960).
10. J. F. A. P. Miller, *Nature* **191**, 248 (1961).
11. J. F. A. P. Miller, *Lancet* **ii**, 748 (1961).
12. K. R. McIntire, S. Sell and J. F. A. P. Miller, *Nature* **204**, 151 (1964).
13. P. B. Medawar, in *The Immunologically Competent Cell (Ciba Foundation Study Group)* (G. E. W. Wolstenholme and J. Knight, eds), Churchill, London (1963), p. 70.
14. R. J. C. Harris, in *Tumour Viruses of Murine Origin (Ciba Foundation Symposium)* (G. E. W. Wolstenholme and M. O'Connor, eds), Churchill, London (1962), p. 283.
15. J. F. A. P. Miller, *Ann. NY Acad. Sci.* **99**, 340 (1962).
16. C. Martinez, J. Kersey, B. W. Papermaster and R. A. Good, *Proc. Soc. Exp. Biol. Med.* **109**, 193 (1962).
17. C. Martinez, A. P. Dalmasso and R. A. Good, in *The Thymus in Immunobiology* (R. A. Good and A. E. Gabrielsen, eds), Harper & Row, New York (1964) pp. 465–477.
18. D. Metcalf, *The Thymus*, Springer-Verlag, Berlin (1966).
19. B. G. Arnason, B. D. Jankovic and B. H. Waksman, *Nature* **194**, 99 (1962).
20. J. F. A. P. Miller, *Nature* **195**, 1318 (1962).
21. J. F. A. P. Miller, *Proc. R. Soc. London, Ser. B* **156**, 410 (1962).
22. F. M. Burnet, *Br. Med. J.* **2**, 807 (1962).
23. B. Glick, T. S. Chang and R. G. Japp, *Poultry Sci.* **35**, 224 (1956).
24. A. Szenberg and N. L. Warner, *Nature* **194**, 146 (1962).
25. J. F. A. P. Miller, in *La Tolérance Acquise et la Tolérance Naturelle à l'égard de Substances Antigéniques Définies*, C.N.R.S. Colloque, Paris (1963), pp. 47–75.
26. F. M. Burnet, *Sci. Am.* **207**, 50 (1962).
27. H. N. Claman, E. A. Chaperon and R. F. Triplett, *Proc. Soc. Exp. Biol. Med.* **122**, 1167 (1966).
28. A. J. S. Davies, E. Leuchars, V. Wallis, R. Marchant and E. V. Elliott, *Transplantation* **5**, 222 (1967).
29. P. Dukor, J. F. A. P. Miller, W. House and V. Allman, *Transplantation* **3**, 639 (1965).
30. A. J. S. Davies, E. Leuchars, V. Wallis, N. R. St. C. Sinclair and E. V. Elliott, in *Advance in Transplantation* (J. Dausset, J. Hamburger and G. Mathé, eds), Munksgaard, Copenhagen (1968), pp. 97–100.
31. J. F. A. P. Miller and G. F. Mitchell, *Nature* **216**, 659 (1967).
32. J. F. A. P. Miller and G. F. Mitchell, *J. Exp. Med.* **128**, 801 (1968).
33. G. F. Mitchell and J. F. A. P. Miller, *J. Exp. Med.* **128**, 821 (1968).
34. J. L. Gowans, in *Immunological Tolerance. A Reassessment of Mechanisms of the Immune Response* (M. Landy and W. Braun, eds), Academic Press, New York (1969), p. 169.
35. R. A. Good, in *Immunological Tolerance. A Reassessment of Mechanisms of the Immune Response* (M. Landy and W. Braun, eds), Academic Press, New York (1969), p. 136.
36. J. F. A. P. Miller, S. M. A. Doak and A. M. Cross, *Proc. Soc. Exp. Biol. Med.* **112**, 785 (1963).
37. F. H. Burnet, *Auto-immunity and Auto-immune Disease*, MTP, Lancaster (1972), p. 45.
38. R. M. Zinkernagel, G. N. Callahan, A. Althage, S. Cooper, P. A. Klein and J. Klein, *J. Exp. Med.* **147**, 882 (1978).

39. J. F. A. P. Miller and W. R. Heath, *Immunol. Rev.* **133**, 131 (1993).
40. N. A. Mitchison, *Eur. J. Immunol.* **1**, 18 (1971).
41. K. Rajewsky, *Proc. R. Soc. London, Ser B* **176**, 385 (1971).
42. J. F. A. P. Miller and J. Sprent, *J. Exp. Med.* **134**, 66 (1971).
43. J. F. A. P. Miller and G. F. Mitchell, *J. Exp. Med.* **131**, 675 (1970).
44. G. J. V. Nossal, *Ann. Rev. Immunol.* **1**, 33 (1983).
45. A. Basten, *Proc. R. Soc. London, Ser. B* **238**, 1 (1989).
46. A. A. Sinha, M. T. Lopez and H. O. McDevitt, *Science* **248**, 1380 (1990).
47. G. F. Mitchell, F. C. Grumet and H. O. McDevitt, *J. Exp. Med.* **135**, 126 (1972).
48. P. B. Medawar, in *Transplantation (Ciba Foundation Symposium)* (G. E. W. Wolstenholme and M. P. Cameron, eds), Churchill, London (1962), p. 412.

About the Discovery of MHC-restricted T Cell Recognition

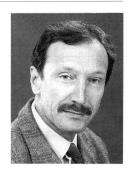

ROLF M. ZINKERNAGEL
Institute of Experimental Immunology, Department of Pathology,
University of Zurich, Zurich, Switzerland

After having finished a wonderful time at the Medical Schools of the Universities of Basle, Paris and Berlin in 1968, I originally wanted to become a surgeon. I had considered neurology first, because an externship at the Hôpital Salpétrère in Paris had attracted me to the clear diagnostics and had motivated me to write my thesis on a 'peripheral form of the Plexus brachialis neuritis' in Basle. But then, because I liked to work with my hands, I started out as assistant at a local surgical clinic and spent most of my time taking up patient's histories and confirming diagnoses that had already been confirmed several times before. I spent the rest of my time holding hooks and assisting at operations for hours. Somehow this did not seem the right thing for me to do and, therefore, with the support of the head surgeon, I looked around for an alternative job. Fortunately, the University of Zurich offered a postgraduate course in experimental medicine to ten young MDs to train them in basic sciences, so as to hopefully enrich clinical research efforts in Switzerland.

After six months of lectures and seminars, I spent the next two years in the laboratory of H. Isliker at the Institute of Biochemistry at the University of Lausanne, where I was introduced to biochemical and immunological techniques. My project was to attempt to establish a killer assay using ^{51}Cr labelled enteropathogenic *Escherichia coli* to evaluate their lysis by antibody and complement. This was part of a project where orally administered bovine colostral antibodies were to be evaluated for passive protective immunity in infants. This labelling method was at the time thought to be a logical extension of the classical ^{51}Cr release assay developed by T. Brunner (1) in Lausanne to monitor cytotoxic T cell activity against foreign transplantation antigens. Brunner's test became very popular because it permitted relatively easy definition of T cells and effector function of T cells *in vitro* (2). Of course, *E. coli* did

IMMUNOLOGY: THE MAKING OF A MODERN SCIENCE
ISBN 0-12-274020-3

not like ^{51}Cr as much as cells did, so the test never worked. But in Lausanne I learned my immunology the hard way in an excellent institution.

When I was looking around for a second postdoctoral position, my wife Kathrin, also an MD and planning to become an ophthalmologist, helped me to type some 50 letters of application to places all over the world to do immunological research in cancer, infectious disease or clinical immunology. I also applied in response to an advertisement in *Nature* by the Australian National University in Canberra. Classical studies on *Listeria* and *Salmonella* immunity had been performed there by G. Mackaness and R.V. Blanden, and by G. Ada on B cell responses to *Salmonella* flagellin in the Department of Microbiology at the John Curtin School of Medical Research, where I hoped to extend my fragmentary experience with intestinal pathogens.

All of the 50 applications, including the one to Canberra, failed. However, by chance, Lausanne and the Institute of Biochemistry also hosted the WHO training laboratory and reference laboratory for immunoglobulins. Each year this laboratory ran a training course in immunology for some 20–30 trainees from all over the world. I had applied to this course, was accepted and profited greatly from the lectures by eminent immunologists in 1970 and the following years. Since Ada knew Isliker through work at the International Union of Cancer in Lyon and through WHO, and since Blanden from Ada's department was teaching at one or two of the WHO courses in Lausanne, they interviewed me, despite the fact that my application had been declined. With the help of Isliker I received a fellowship from the Stiftung für Biologisch-Medizinische Grundlagenforschung, which helped to get me accepted in Canberra after all. My wife, courageous and willing to go to the other end of the world with two small children aged 1 and 3 years, packed things up into a few boxes, and we left for Canberra in January 1973.

Canberra, 1973

Upon arrival in Canberra (3), Blanden met us at the airport and talked about a series of experiments he and Gardner, his Ph.D. student, had done since he had returned from the last course in Lausanne. They found for mousepox virus (4) what Oldstone and Dixon (5), Cole (6) and Marker and Volkert (7) had found earlier for lymphocytic choriomeningitis virus (LCMV) infections; similar to cytotoxic T cells involved in transplant rejection, the Brunner–Cerottini assay could be used to measure cytotoxic T cell activity against virus infected target cells. Gardner and Blanden had worked out all the technical details and the assay worked very reliably (4). Since I had applied to Canberra to work on facultative intracellular bacteria, I started to work on *Listera monocytogenes* with Blanden. I thereby profited from his vast experience in the cellular immunology of mice and his understanding of disease.

The Department of Microbiology at the John Curtin School of Medical

Research consisted of some ten small laboratories, each including a cubicle for two people to write and a hot-air vent-hood for working with infectious agents (8). I was put into a laboratory with Peter C. Doherty who had moved in some six months earlier, on returning to Australia from Edinburgh, where he had written a Ph.D. thesis on antibody responses to virus infections in the brain of sheep. In Canberra he had started to analyse inflammatory processes in the brains of mice infected with various viruses including Semliki forest virus and LCMV. In addition to working on *Listeria*, I joined forces with Peter and we started to work on cell-mediated immunity to LCMV. I had come from the 'Mecca' of ^{51}Cr release assays (Lausanne) and therefore had some knowledge with which to establish the cytotoxicity assay against LCMV. Since most of the initial work on antiviral cytotoxic T cells that had been published was based on LCMV and now also had been done with mousepox in Canberra, these studies were not particularly encouraged by other members of the department, because it was thought to be too late to compete with the various laboratories doing research on LCMV. After some problems because of our inexperience with LCMV, we nevertheless managed to establish a reliable ^{51}Cr release assay much along the lines of Gardner and Blanden's assays (4).

This test was then applied to find out whether inflammatory cells in the cerebrospinal fluid of mice infected intracerebrally with LCMV and suffering from choriomeningitis were cytolytic *in vitro*. For this purpose, we miniaturized the ^{51}Cr release assay by adapting it to 96-well plates – this permitted assessment of cytotoxic T cell (CTL) activity of small numbers of cells. Peter Doherty was very good at harvesting cerebrospinal fluid from the cisterna magna of mice, using a method described by Carp (9). These experiments were successful and revealed potent antiviral cytotoxic T cells, suggesting that T cell mediated destruction of LCMV-infected meningeal and ependymal cells *in vivo* was the essential pathogenetic mechanism causing a breakdown of the blood–brain barrier (10). We postulated that the ensuing brain oedema caused death by compression of the brainstem. In fact, when Doherty injected Evans' blue, pathological extravasation was dramatically illustrated since the brains of mice with choriomeningitis turned blue (10).

In March 1973, a paper in the *Journal of Experimental Medicine* (11) by Oldstone, McDevitt and collaborators had appeared describing evidence that mice with different major histocompatibility gene complex (MHC) types exhibited distinct susceptibilities with respect to lethality and kinetics of disease after intracerebral LCMV infection. We therefore decided to check whether the notion that antiviral cytotoxic T cells were responsible for lethal choriomeningitis could be tested by correlating susceptibility to disease with the cytolytic T cell activity generated in different mouse strains. Six to eight mice of each of the inbred and cross-bred strains available at the School were infected intracerebrally with LCMV. Two of each were sacrificed on day 7 after infection when the first mice had become sick, to test antiviral cytotoxic T cell activities in spleens. The remaining mice were monitored for the development of lethal disease during the next ten days.

The first experiment, in August 1973, gave a very clear result that did not fit our predictions: only some strains of mice generated virus-specific cytotoxic T cell activities, but all mice died of LCMV, some on day 7, some a few days later, but by day 11 or 12 all had died. This meant that cytotoxic T cells had nothing to do with lethal choriomeningitis or, alternatively, that our test was somehow strange. It became quickly obvious that the test we used explained the findings. Remember, we were in a Department of Microbiology, where virologists dominated; plaquing of virus on tissue cultured cells was a standard procedure and, therefore, a central tissue culture facility provided us twice a week with single cell suspensions of monkey (Vero), hamster (BHK) and mouse (L929) cells. We all used L929 cells for cytotoxicity assays because they were of murine origin and were readily infected by LCMV. By chance, and fortunately, the mouse strain used most commonly in the Department was CBA; because CBAs were available in greatest numbers, all basic experiments were performed on these mice. Again by chance, L929 cells had been derived from C3H mice that possess the MHC H-2^k haplotype, as do CBA mice. All the LCMV-immune spleen cells from H-2^k mice, including the cross-breeds with H-2^k mice, that were tested in an attempt to understand susceptibility to LCMV, lysed infected L (H-2^k) cells. In contrast, spleen cells from all mice that were not of H-2^k type failed to do so.

Two additional experiments done within the next two weeks very convincingly confirmed these findings. It seemed important to us to confirm that LCMV immune lymphocytes from non-H-2^k strains of mice were able to lyse LCMV infected target cells of corresponding syngeneic origin. This proved not to be easy, because the other available mouse cell lines such as the H-2^d mastocytoma P815 or the H-2^b thymoma EL4 could not be infected with LCMV. Because of my work on *Listeria* – which infects macrophages and is essentially controlled by T cell mediated activation of macrophages, as had been shown by Mackaness (*12,13*) – we experimented with macrophages directly isolated from peritoneal washings of mice. These macrophages stuck well to plastic, were readily infected and could be labelled with ^{51}Cr. Proper criss-cross experiments done in October 1973 showed that LCMV immune T cell from H-2^b mice lysed LCMV infected macrophages of H-2^b but not of other H-2 types, and vice versa. The report was sent off via John Humphrey in early December as a letter to *Nature*; it was accepted in January 1974 and was published in April 1974 (*10,14*).

T cell immunology 1973–1974

The biological function and *raison d'être* of MHC and of transplantation antigens was unclear in the early 1970s. Obviously their function was not to frustrate transplantation surgeons and restorative medicine. Transplantation antigens had been defined by Gorer (*15*) and by Snell based on the work of Little, Strong and others who developed inbred strains of mice to be able to transplant tumours (reviewed by Klein (16)). Haematologists, particularly Dausset and, then, van Rood, defined lymphocyte antigens in humans (17,18). Once many patients had been typed for their transplantation antigens, it became apparent that some disease susceptibilities were linked to transplantation antigens (19). Studies by Benacerraf (20) and McDevitt (21) on antibody responses and by Lilly (22) on susceptibility to tumours revealed that inbred strains of guinea-pigs and mice differed in their responses; in mice this was readily mapped to the MHC.

In the early 1970s, transplantation antigens were proposed (reviewed in (16,23–25)) to prevent mutual parasitism or tumour cell transmission, or to cause rejection of thymus cells if they had mutated. Others postulated that MHC polymorphism either prevented viruses or other pathogens from mimicking transplantation antigens and, therefore, from eliminating the species, or that they functioned as enzymes or as generators of antibody specificity. A most fascinating proposal had been formulated by Lawrence in 1959 (26), that infectious agents complexed with transplantation antigens (self + x) and triggered lymphocytes to produce a soluble, specific receptor for this complex (transfer factor). I discovered this reference only in 1975 and was enormously struck by this prophetic view.

The series of experiments that were to reveal the essential role of MHC in T cell recognition and antigen presentation all depended upon the bases built by tumour and transplantation immunologists and the summarized studies. Without inbred and MHC–H-2 congenic or mutant mouse strains, this problem would not have been accessible and solvable. Once cloned, effector T cells and molecularly defined T cell receptors would have been available; MHC-restricted T cell recognition would certainly have been discovered, however, by a different approach and by others.

Our results were surprising and immediately gave us the feeling that we had possibly found a biological function of transplantation antigens. Our results fitted other observations that had appeared during the past 12 months. We went through the available literature and found that some data on cytotoxic T cell responses against leukaemia virus infected or transformed target cells revealed hints (27,28) that could be interpreted to signal H-2 restriction. Also, Kindred and Schreffler had reported that H-2 incompatible T helper cells transfused to T cell deprived nude mice were not able to help nude B cells to make antibodies (29). McCullagh (30) and Katz, Hamaoka and Benacerraf (31) had shown that histoincompatible B cells, when mixed with T cells and antigen *in vitro* or *in vivo*, generated antibodies without a need for specific T helper cells. This allogeneic effect suggested that alloreactive T helper cells reacting against foreign transplantation antigens on B cells could do 'non-physiologically' what conventional T helper cells did under physiological conditions, that is, antigen-specific contact-dependent triggering of B cells to make antibodies. In parallel experiments with inbred strains of guinea-pigs, Shevach and Rosenthal (32,33) analysed antigen-specific poliferative T cell responses and found them only if primed T cells and antigen pulsed macrophages were from guinea-pigs with the same MHC types. Because of the considerable alloresponses and allogeneic effects, non-specific signals interfered; therefore, these findings were only accepted with hesitation by the immunological community. This changed when our data appeared, although not immediately, because viral and infectious disease immunology had not yet gained back the ground it had lost to sheep red blood cells and small haptens.

Our results stirred up a tremendous amount of discussion in the department. We thought simply that virus somehow altered the normal self-transplantation antigens and that this virus-specific alteration was recognized by cytotoxic T cells similar to foreign transplantation antigens as we all had learnt and accepted from the results of Brunner and Cerottini. Vigorous debate stimulated the imagination and intellect of each of us to come up with a simpler, more general and more convincing explanation. Discussions in the department were very lively also because Lafferty and Cunningham had during that time developed their ideas on second signals (factors) necessary to induce responses against foreign transplantation antigens. The players in these games included: Ada, our leader and head of the Department; Blanden, the great expert in cell-mediated immunity against intracellular bacteria and immunity to pox virus (ectromelia); Cunningham, Pilarski and Bretscher, who studied B cells and antibody specificities against red blood cells (always looking out for sombreros (34)); and theoretical immunologists who thought about general rules and asked why should T cells kill. Parish, establishing cell separation techniques; Gardner, working on cytotoxic T cells against ectromelia; Ramshaw, Hapel, Kirov, Davidson, Dunlup and Rosenberg, working on B and T cell responses in various virus infections; and overpowering Lafferty, with his blooming vocabulary and down-to earth arguments; and Walker and McCullagh, members of the Department of Immunology next door.

The first public presentation outside Australia was at a Brooklodge Meeting attended by Ada and at the Keystone meeting in Squaw Valley attended by Cunningham in February and March 1974. A letter sent back to Canberra summarized data from Shearer showing that TNP-specific cytotoxic T cells lysed syngeneic TNP-lated targets better than allogeneic TNP-lated targets. These data were submitted to the *European Journal of Immunology* shortly after our report in *Nature* had appeared. Obviously the two findings had emerged completely independently. Because coupling of TNP to cells at that time seemed to modify chemically the transplantation antigens and to render targets foreign (an interpretation that now has been rendered less likely), the evidence from the TNP model helped to establish the concept of 'altered self'.

The allogeneic reactivities encountered in the various T–B and T–macrophage models tested by others were subject to many different interpretations. We interpreted our finding to mean that virus infections somehow altered transplantation antigens by complex formation with antigen or other structural alterations and that these alterations were recognized by T cells

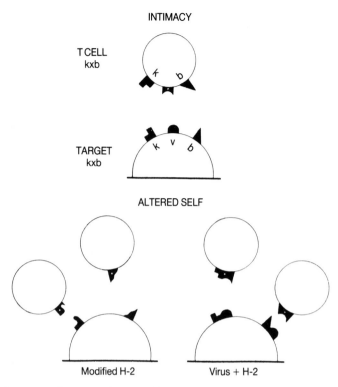

Figure 1   Capacity of sensitized F_1 (H-2$^{k/b}$) T cells to interact only with histocompatible virus-infected target cells may be considered to reflect any one of the models shown. The intimacy concept proposes a single immunologically specific T cell receptor for viral (v) antigen, additional to a requirement for physiological interaction coded for by the H-2 gene complex (mutuality between either H-2^k or H-2^b). The two models proposed for altered self postulate that, in each case, there are at least two T cell populations with receptors of different immunological specificities recognizing modified H-2, or virus +H-2 of either parent type.

(Fig. 1). Foreign transplantation antigens could then be viewed as genetically altered forms of self-transplantation antigens, and this explained why they were potent stimulators and targets for T cells. This view differed from the then favoured possibility that lymphocytes and target cells interacted mutually via transplantation antigens, that is, that H-2^k interacted best with H-2^k transplantation antigens in a like–like fashion (35). This intimacy model was soon excluded by experiments showing that virus-specific cytotoxic T lymphocytes from heterozygote H-2^k × H-2^b mice consisted of at least two subpopulations and that each was specific for either infected H-2^k or for infected H-2^b targets. Since MHC products were codominantly expressed on lymphocyte surfaces, H-2 restricted recognition signalled T cell receptor specificity rather than like–like or 'physiological' interactions. This was further confirmed in 1977–1978 by experiments with bone marrow chimeras (*36,37*) and with thymus transplants (*37*) which showed the crucial influence of the thymus in selecting specificity for the restricting MHC. These experiments showed that the H-2 of the thymus not the H-2 of the maturing thymocyte determined the 'learned' specificity of mature T cells.

Further experiments soon showed that the H-2D (and H-2K) regions were involved in virus specific cytotoxic T cell recognition. These findings submitted to the *Journal of Experimental Medicine* in June 1974 (*38,39*) separated MHC restriction of virus specific cytotoxic T cells from H-2I linked immune response phenomena. This was confirmed by formal genetic mapping of restriction in a letter to *Nature* in early 1975 (*40*), reflecting a common effort of the department to demonstrate for several viruses MHC-restriction of virus-specific cytotoxic T cells for H-2K or D. Studies demonstrating that restriction also applied to cytotoxic T cell interactions *in vivo* causing lethal immunopathology (*41*) or antiviral protection (*42*) and for T cells involved in protection against *Listeria monocytogenous* (*43*) confirmed that MHC restriction governed the specificity of T cells *in vivo*. All the data and our views on the biological role of transplantation antigens were finally summarized in a hypothesis in the *Lancet* in the summer of 1975 (*44*), where we attempted to compare class I and class II specific restriction and offered a unifying view that T helper and cytotoxic T cells were specific for altered class II or class I transplantation antigens, respectively.

Conclusions

Although some of the connections pointed out may be viewed in a distorted fashion in retrospect, they reflect my perception of my early years in science and immunology. A good portion of luck, a demanding but comfortable family and home, excellent schools, universities and postdoctoral training, stimulating scientific environments, a number of very intelligent and challenging, tough but fair colleagues, and excellent animal models of infectious disease have all contributed to these interesting results. Many chances and as many necessities have played crucial roles: what if I had stuck to surgery or if Isliker had not been involved in WHO or not known Ada, or if Kathrin had not been willing to move to Canberra of if I had not been put into the same laboratory with Doherty? This would probably not have happened; certainly not in the same way, and probably without me.

The story told above illustrates that a reasonable question, which can be addressed by good methods, opens up chances of finding something unexpectedly new, that was not planned for. It has certainly helped a lot that Doherty and I were both relatively new in the field, not yet fixed into doctrinaire views, and accepted results as they were. Probably most important was the fact that we worked with well-analysed viruses and excellently defined inbred strains of mice, providing us with some of the best genetics available in vertebrates. Probably the most important factors that contributed to the results we obtained were: that we compared an *in vitro* read-out, that is, cytotoxicity, with real and drastic disease *in vivo*, and that the model used was one of the best analysed immunologically and virologically *in vivo*; that we worked in the relative isolation of Canberra (45), thus permitting undisturbed consequential work; and, last but not least, that we had the privilege to work in a stimulating environment formed by an ideal mixture of virologists, immunologists and tinkerers in science assembled during 1973–1976 in the Department of Microbiology.

In April 1975 a wonderful period in Canberra ended for me. I left for the USA to take up a position at the Scripps with F. Dixon; Peter Doherty stayed another few months, and then moved to the Wistar Institute with H. Koprowsky.

Notes and References

1. K. T. Brunner, J. Mauel, J. C. Cerottini and B. Chapuis, *Immunology* **14**, 181 (1968).
2. J. C. Cerottini and K. T. Brunner, *Adv. Immunol.* **18**, 67 (1974).
3. Besides flies all over the place, two experiences struck us most: the friendly and easy way of life in Australia, and the enormous cost of everything except housing. In the early 1970s an Australian dollar was equivalent to more than 5 Swiss francs, and our stipend of SFR 32000 was worth Australian $6000. This was OK for buying meat because a pound of topside beef cost only 25 cents, but most other things were enormously expensive. This problem was offset by the fact that ANU provided excellent housing for postdoctoral workers and that Kathrin started work at the casualty department of the local hospital. It was further offset by the fact that ANU offered me a Ph.D scholarship, which not only improved our financial situation, but in addition provided me with a Ph.D to supplement the Dr.med. degree I had earned in Basle.
4. I. D. Gardner, N. A. Bowern and R. V. Blanden, *Eur. J. Immunol.* **4**, 63 (1974).
5. M. B. A. Oldstone and F. J. Dixon, *Virology* **42**, 805 (1970).
6. G. A. Cole, R. A. Prendergast and C. S. Henney, *Fed. Proc.* **32**, 964 (1973).
7. O. Marker and M. Volkert, *J. Exp. Med.* **137**, 1511 (1973).
8. The department ran on a budget virtually entirely provided by the Australian federal government. Only about Australian $3000–5000 per year per researcher was available in funds, but the infrastructure of the John Curtin School of Medical Research was tremendous and provided us with all necessities, except radioactivity, plastic materials and other exotic materials. Everything from mice, media, antisera, fetal calf serum to antibiotics, buffers, etc., was made in-house. This autarchy and the generosity of our chairman, G. Ada, made possible an open, dynamic, active atmosphere and enormous experimental efficiency.
9. R. I. Carp, A. I. Davidson and P. A. Merz, *Res. Vet. Sci.* **12**, 499 (1971).
10. P. C. Doherty and R. M. Zinkernagel, *Transplant Rev.* **19**, 89 (1974).
11. M. B. A. Oldstone, F. J. Dixon, G. F. Mitchell and H. O. McDevitt, *J. Exp. Med.* **137**, 1201 (1973).
12. G. B. Mackaness, *J. Exp. Med.* **129**, 973 (1969).
13. R. M. Zinkernagel and R. V. Blanden, *Experientia* **31**, 591 (1975).
14. R. M. Zinkernagel and P. C. Doherty, *Nature* **248**, 701 (1974).
15. P. A. Gorer, *J. Pathol. Bacteriol.* **44**, 691 (1937).
16. J. Klein, *Biology of the Mouse Histocompatibility-2 Complex*, Springer-Verlag, Berlin (1975).

17. J. Dausset, *Acta Haematol (Basel)* **20**, 156 (1958).

18. J. J. Van Rood and A. Van Leeuwen, *J. Clin. Invest.* **42**, 1382 (1963).

19. H. O. Sjögren and N. Ringertz, *J. Natl. Cancer Inst.* **28**, 859 (1961).

20. B. B. Levine, A. P. Ojeda and B. Benacerraf, *J. Exp. Med.* **118**, 953 (1963).

21. H. O. McDevitt and A. Chinitz, *Science* **163**, 1207 (1969).

22. F. Lilly, E. A. Boyse and L. J. Old, *Lancet* **ii**, 1207 (1964).

23. D. B. Amos, W. F. Bodmer, R. Ceppellini, P. G. Condliffe, J. Dausset, J. L. Fahey, H. C. Goodman, G. Klein, J. Klein, F. Lilly, D. L. Mann, H. McDevitt, S. Nathenson, J. Palm, R. A. Reisfeld, G. N. Rogentine, A. R. Sanderson, D. C. Shreffler, M. Simonsen and J. J. Van Rood, *Fed. Proc.* **31**, 1087 (1972).

24. F. M. Burnet, *Nature* **245**, 359 (1972).

25. W. F. Bodmer, *Nature* **237**, 139 (1972).

26. H. W. Lawrence, *Physiol. Rev.* **39**, 811 (1959).

27. J.-C. Leclerc, E. Gomard and J. P. Levy, *Int. J. Cancer* **10**, 589 (1972).

28. D. H. Lavrin, R. B. Herberman, M. Nunn and N. Soares, *J. Natl Cancer Inst*, **51**, 1497 (1973).

29. B. Kindred and D. C. Shreffler, *J. Immunol.* **109**, 940 (1972).

30. P. J. McCullagh, *Transplant. Rev.* **12**, 1180 (1972).

31. D. H. Katz, T. Hamaoka and B. Benacerraf, *J. Exp. Med.* **137**, 1405 (1973).

32. A. S. Rosenthal and E. M. Shevach, *J. Exp. Med.* **138**, 1194 (1973).

33. E. M. Shevach and A. S. Rosenthal, *J. Exp. Med* **138**, 1213 (1973).

34. A. J. Cunningham and S. A. Fordham, *Nature* **250**, 669 (1973).

35. R. M. Zinkernagel and P. C. Doherty, *Nature* **251**, 547 (1974).

36. M. J. Bevan, *Nature* **269**, 417 (1977).

37. R. M. Zinkernagel, G. N. Callahan, A. Althage, S. Cooper, P. A. Klein and J. Klein, *J. Exp. Med.* **147**, 882 (1978).

38. P. C. Doherty and R. M. Zinkernagel, *J. Exp. Med.* **141**, 502 (1975).

39. R. M. Zinkernagel and P. C. Doherty, *J. Exp. Med.* **141**, 1427 (1975).

40. R. V. Blanden, P. C. Doherty, M. B. C. Dunlop, I. D. Gardner, R. M. Zinkernagel and C. S. David, *Nature* **254**, 269 (1975).

41. P. C. Doherty and R. M. Zinkernagel, *J. Immunol.* **114**, 30 (1975).

42. I. D. Gardner, N. A. Bowern and R. V. Blanden, *Eur. J. Immunol.* **5**, 122 (1975).

43. R. M. Zinkernagel, *Nature* **251**, 230 (1974).

44. P. C. Doherty and R. M. Zinkernagel, *Lancet* **28**, 1406 (1975).

45. Two examples may illustrate this situation. First, the only phone call about science I had during the two and a half years was with Jacques Miller from the Hall Institute, when we discussed the possibilities of demonstrating MHC-restriction of T cells involved in DTH. Second, illustrating that Australia was still far away then, was when our new secretary mailed a manuscript describing MHC restriction of anti-*Listeria* protection to *Nature* and forgot to put the airmail sticker on. When we called *Nature* after three months to find out what they had decided about the manuscript, they told us it had just arrived by surface mail!

Two-signal Models of Lymphocyte Activation

RONALD H. SCHWARTZ
Laboratory of Cellular and Molecular Immunology,
National Institute of Allergy and Infectious Diseases,
National Institutes of Health, Bethesda, MD, USA

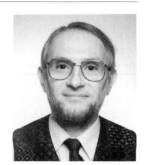

It was the summer of 1986 and suppressor T cells had just taken another damaging hit, this time from the DNA sequencing of the B10.A(3R) and (5R) recombinants (*1*). The *I–J* subregion did not appear to exist in the major histocompatibility complex (MHC), and molecular biologists were clamouring for the demise of suppressor cells. I thought to myself, 'I've seen this before – the macrophage in 1970, when I first came into the field: a body of science discarded in one fell swoop with the emergence of a set of new findings (in that case, it was T cell–B cell interactions) (*2*), but then a dramatic reemergence – like a phoenix from the ashes – when Shevach and Rosenthal demonstrated MHC restriction of T cell-macrophage interactions (*3*)'. It was time to follow my stockbroker grandfather's sage advice: buy low.

Initial Studies

Marc Jenkins had just finished his graduate work in Steve Miller's laboratory, cloning suppressor-inducer T cells specific for the random terpolymer GAT (*4*). My laboratory had just completed mapping out one of the first T cell peptide determinants (pigeon cytochrome *c*), defining residues that interact with the MHC molecule (agretopes) and residues that interact with the T cell receptor (epitopes) (*5*). I thought possibly we could combine Marc's knowledge of suppressor cells with our knowledge of pigeon cytochrome *c* to derive suppressor T cell clones specific for pigeon cytochrome *c*. In this way, we could determine the fine specificity of suppressor T cell recognition (supposedly capable of recognizing free antigen) (*6*) and compare it with that of the helper T cells we had already defined. Marc began by coupling pigeon cytochrome *c* to spleen cells and injecting them intravenously. This classic procedure of Battisto and Bloom (*7*) was the standard approach for eliciting suppression, and it did induce a

IMMUNOLOGY: THE MAKING OF A MODERN SCIENCE
ISBN 0-12-274020-3

70% reduction in the proliferative response subsequently elicited by priming the animals with cytochrome c in CFA and restimulating the T cells from draining lymph nodes *in vitro* seven days later (8). In working up the specificity of this suppression, however, we found that it had the same induction requirements (in terms of MHC and antigen specificity) as the priming for proliferation or the activation of CD4$^+$ T cell clones. Furthermore, if the cytochrome c was coupled to the spleen cells using a heterobifunctional cross-linker instead of the carbodiimide cross-linker ECDI, the mice were primed. This led us to explore the coupling reagent in *in vitro* assays and to the discovery that fixation of the cells, *per se*, was the critical component of the manipulation. This then allowed us to induce the proliferative unresponsive state in T cell clones and, thus, to set up an *in vitro* assay system which could be more easily dissected at a molecular level.

Our early ideas for what was going on were shaped by the experiments of another postdoctoral fellow in the laboratory, Helen Quill (9). She was exploring the question of why purified MHC class II molecules in planar membranes could not activate normal T cell clones to proliferate, whereas Tania Watts and Adrienne Bryan in Harden McConnell's laboratory had reported that such membranes could stimulate IL-2 production from T cell hybridomas (10). Helen was convinced that the normal clones were responding in some fashion because they appeared to enlarge. After quantitating this by flow cytometry, she went on to show that the cells were being induced into the same unresponsive state as that seen with the chemically fixed antigen-presenting cells (APC) and that this induction could be blocked by cycloheximide. This convincingly demonstrated that induction of the non-responsive state was an active process which only required occupancy of the antigen-specific receptor to achieve.

The Two-signal Model

At this point, we considered two possible mechanisms by which the unresponsive state was being induced. One was as a consequence of the way in which the T cell antigen receptor was cross-linked: planar membrane presentation and chemical fixation of the proteins on the APC surface could both be hindering the mobility of the MHC molecules and, thus, preventing the formation of a proper array of receptor aggregates for signal transduction. The second possibility was that something was missing. This additional signal would be required for activation, and its absence would result in non-responsiveness; presumably, the chemical fixation would have destroyed the ability of the APC to deliver this additional signal. We were attracted to the second idea for two reasons: it fitted nicely with the two-signal model for B cell activation first proposed by Bretscher and Cohn in 1968 (11), and it was easy to test.

We began by adding back molecules: cytokines, pharmacological agents such as phorbol esters, and antibodies against cell surface proteins such as anti-CD4. None of these resulted in activation, although anti-CD4 blocked the induction process (presumably by decreasing signalling through the T cell antigen receptor). The only thing that worked was adding live allogeneic APC (12). Because these cells expressed the wrong MHC molecule, they could not present the peptide antigen; however, they were capable of providing the additional signals (in *trans*) which both induced a proliferative response from the T cell clone and prevented the induction of the non-responsive state. Separating the allogeneic APC from the T cell by a semipermeable membrane prevented these effects, suggesting that a cell–cell interaction or a short-range soluble mediator was required. We thus concluded that T cell activation fit the general outline of the Bretscher and Cohn two-signal model in which signal one alone – through the antigen-specific receptor – was a negative signal to the cell, while signal one in conjunction with a second co-stimulatory T cell signal was activating (11). The non-responsive state in the T cell clones has since been termed 'anergy', in keeping with a tolerant state first described by Nossal and Pike (13) for B cells, in which the lymphocyte is not killed by the negative signalling, but only inactivated.

When I first presented these results to Mel Cohn at a symposium we both attended, he seemed reluctant to embrace our findings – or at least our interpretation of the findings. He sent me a long letter reinterpreting the results in his own framework of T cell recognition: the dual recognitive single-receptor model that he and Ron Langman had published in 1985 (14). I mistook his concerns at the time for a reluctance to abandon the T cell receptor model. It was not until several years later – after much harping by Polly Matzinger – that I appreciated that his real reluctance stemmed from his difficulty in accepting the non-antigen specificity of the second signal. Bretscher and Cohn's original model called for an antibody-mediated second signal specific for an independent determinant on the antigen (11). Its subsequent modification in the T cell era replaced this with signals provided by the antigen-specific T cell (15). In fact, as Polly also pointed out, our data were most consistent with the Lafferty and Cunningham model proposed to explain alloreactivity (16). In this model, T cell receptor engagement of the MHC molecule stimulates the APC to express a co-stimulatory molecule which, in turn, engages an independent receptor on the T cell to activate the second signal. Recent identification of the CD28 and B7 molecules and their interactions has provided a solid molecular foundation for this concept (17).

Two Signals in Context

When one reviews the literature on two-signal models of lymphocyte activation, one finds that the roots go quite far back. Felton spend his whole career studying the immune response to polysaccharides because of his medical interest in pneumococcal pneumonia. In 1949, he published his ideas on high-dose paralysis (18) where he concluded that too much antigen turns off the antibody-secreting cell. This idea was pursued by Dresser, who – in a classic paper in 1962 (19) – concluded that it was not necessarily the dose of antigen that was critical, but its form of presentation to the immune system. Dresser used proteins as antigens and found that removal of aggregates by spinning them in an ultracentrifuge produced a toleragen instead of an immunogen. Immunogenicity could be restored, however, if the soluble proteins were administered in Freund's complete adjuvant. Dresser coined the term 'adjuvanticity' to describe the property of an antigen or its method of administration that allows it to activate the immune system. It is quite stirring to read the discussion in his paper where he spells out clearly that antigen alone leads to paralysis, whereas antigen plus adjuvanticity leads to immunity.

The Bretscher and Cohn model also was initially an attempt to come to grips with the tolerance induction of high doses of antigen (11). How could antigen signalling through the same receptor give both on and off signals? Their thoughts were stimulated by a theoretical paper of Forsdyke (20), who proposed a scintillation counter model for cellular activation, that is a single signal detected by the cell is ignored, while detection of two coincident signals is perceived as an activating stimulus. They were also influenced by the hapten carrier experiments of Mitchison (21) and Rajewsky and colleagues (22) implying the need to recognize two determinants on the antigen in order to generate an immune response. Their model was an elegant synthesis of these thoughts and observations in which the signal received through the B cell antigen receptor always turned the cell off (tolerance), whereas a coincident second signal coming indirectly from another antigen-specific cell turned the cell on (immunity). This formulation allowed Bretscher and Cohn to explain the tolerance paradox caused by somatic hypermutation. In a simple, one-signal model such as that of Lederberg (23), where tolerance only occurs during development, mutation of a mature B cell antigen receptor could lead to an autoreactive cell. In contrast, in the Bretscher and Cohn two-signal model, such a mutational event would not cause a problem because engagement of the receptor by a self-antigen would turn the cell off in the absence of a second signal from the T cell.

Bretscher and Cohn insist to this day that application of their model to T cells requires a T cell–T cell interaction via an antigen bridge (15,24). This seems hard to fathom in light of what Mel Cohn calls 'the peptide revolution', where T cell receptors have been shown to visualize peptide–MHC molecule complexes on the surface of the APC (25). Furthermore, the T cell–T cell scenario of Bretscher and Cohn simply moves the problem to another level, because if one T cell provides the second signal for the other T cell to get primed, how does the first T cell get primed? This priming problem requires an ad hoc solution which, although conceivable, could just as easily be abandoned for a Lafferty and Cunningham type of model.

Lafferty and Cunningham were not concerned primarily with tolerance but rather with the nature of alloreactivity (16). Why did the immune system focus so much attention on MHC molecules? Their idea was that T cells could see all types of molecules, but that MHC molecules were located on special stimulatory cells which, when tickled through their MHC molecules, were induced to provide a second signal to the T cell to activate it. They coined the term 'co-stimulation' to describe this event. We now think that T cell receptors are evolutionarily selected to focus on MHC molecules because these molecules display the foreign peptides that the cells need to recognize. It has been argued by Charlie Janeway (26), however, that – early in their evolution – T cells recognized inflammatory signals displayed by phagocytic cells and that some of these signals may have been inflammatory self-peptides displayed by MHC molecules (for example for γδ T cells). The activation of these T cells may have involved current-day co-stimulatory molecules as well, and the eventual system evolved for αβ T cells may have converted the peptide presentation of MHC molecules for antigen specificity and maintained the co-stimulatory molecules for activation.

Some form of co-stimulation also appears to be involved in the activation of CD8$^+$ T cells. In the cytotoxic response of female B6 mice to the Qa1^b antigen, Keene and Forman showed that male cells were required for immunization (27). The male cells provided a helper stimulus in the form of a CD4$^+$ T cell response to the H-Y antigen. Both antigens, Qa1 and H-Y, had to be on the same immunizing cell in order to elicit cytotoxic T lymphocyte (CTL) responses. Subsequent experiments from the laboratories of Polly Matzinger (28) and Al Singer (29) demonstrated that prior administration of only the Qa1 antigen on female cells prevented the subsequent priming to Qa1 antigen on male cells. Thus, the activation of CD8$^+$ T cells appeared to follow the rules of Bretscher and Cohn, that signal one alone (Qa1) tolerizes the cell, whereas signal one plus signal two (the H-Y response) elicits an immune response. The nature of the second signal delivered by the antigen-specific CD4$^+$ cell is not clear. In the original idea of Cassell and Forman (30), the signal was IL-2. It was delivered by the CD4$^+$ T cell responding to the H-Y antigen in close proximity to the CD8$^+$ T cell responding to the Qa1 antigen on the same APC; however, the normal CTL responses recently described in IL-2 'knockout' mice (31) suggest that other molecules may also be involved.

Much current activity in this general area of immunology is focused on the molecular basis of co-stimulation and anergy. New co-stimulatory molecules and receptors are being discovered at a rapid pace (32–35). Our own work in collaboration with Mike Lenardo's laboratory has uncovered a block in anergic mouse T cells in IL-2 gene transcription at the level of the AP-1 transcription factor (36). Studies with human T cell clones suggest a block in early signal transduction through the antigen-specific receptor (37). What is most gratifying to see is the generation and use of new molecular tools for immunotherapy in transplantation, cancer, and autoimmunity (38–41) which have emerged out of this conceptual framework. My colleagues and I are glad to have played a small part in the historical development of this field. We hope some day our efforts will prove to be beneficial for humankind.

Notes and References

1. J. A. Kobori, E. Strauss, K. Minard and L. Hood, *Science* **234**, 173 (1986).
2. E. R. Unanue and D. H. Katz, *Eur. J. Immunol.* **3**, 559 (1973).
3. A. S. Rosenthal and E. M. Shevach, *J. Exp. Med.* **138**, 1194 (1973).
4. M. K. Jenkins and S. D. Miller, *J. Mol. Cell Immunol.* **2**, 1 (1985).
5. R. H. Schwartz, *Annu. Rev. Immunol.* **3**, 237 (1985).
6. M. Taniguchi and J. F. A. P. Miller, *J. Exp. Med.* **146**, 1450 (1977).
7. J. R. Battisto and B. R. Bloom, *Nature* **212**, 156 (1966).
8. M. K. Jenkins and R. H. Schwartz, *J. Exp. Med.* **165**, 302 (1987).
9. H. Quill and R. H. Schwartz, *J. Immunol.* **138**, 3704 (1987).
10. T. H. Watts, A. A. Brian, J. W. Kappler, P. Marrack and H. M. McConnell, *Proc. Natl Acad. Sci. USA* **81**, 7564 (1984).
11. P. Bretscher and M. Cohn, *Science* **169**, 1042 (1970).
12. M. J. Jenkins, J. D. Ashwell and R. H. Schwartz, *J. Immunol.* **140**, 3324 (1988).
13. G. J. V. Nossal and B. L. Pike, *Proc. Natl Acad. Sci. USA* **77**, 1602 (1980). |
14. R. E. Langman and M. Cohn, *Cell Immunol.* **94**, 598 (1985).
15. M. Cohn, *Annu. Rev. Immunol.* **12**, 1 (1994).
16. K. J. Lafferty and A. J. Cunningham, *Aust. J. Exp. Biol. Med. Sci.* **53**, 27 (1975).
17. P. S. Linsley and J. A. Ledbetter, *Annu. Rev. Immunol.* **11**, 191 (1993).
18. L. D. Felton, *J. Immunol.* **61**, 107 (1949).
19. D. W. Dresser, *Immunology* **5**, 378 (1962).
20. D. R. Forsdyke, *Lancet* **i**, 281 (1968).
21. N. A. Mitchison, *Eur. J. Immunol.* **1**, 18 (1971).
22. K. Rajewsky, V. Schirrmacher, S. Nase and N. K. Jerne, *J. Exp. Med.* **129**, 1131 (1969).
23. J. Lederberg, *Science* **129**, 1649 (1959).
24. P. Bretscher, *Immunol. Today* **13**, 74 (1992).
25. R. N. Germain, *Cell* **76**, 287 (1994).
26. C. A. Janeway, Jr, *Immunol. Today* **13**, 11 (1992).
27. J. Keene and J. Forman, *J. Exp. Med.* **155**, 768 (1982).
28. S. Guerder and P. Matzinger, *Cold Spring Harbor Symp. Quant. Biol.* **54**, 799 (1989).
29. M. A. Rees, A. S. Rosenberg, T. I. Munitz and A. Singer, *Proc. Natl Acad. Sci. USA* **87**, 2765 (1990).
30. D. Cassell and J. Forman, *Ann. NY Acad. Sci.* **532**, 51 (1988).
31. T. M. Kundig, H. Schorle, M. F. Bachmann, H. Hengartner, R. M. Zinkernagel and I. Horak, *Science* **262**, 1059 (1993).
32. K. S. Hathcock, G. Laszlo, H. B. Dickler, J. Bradshaw, P. Linsley and R. J. Hodes, *Science* **262**, 905 (1993).
33. D. J. Lenschow, G.H.-T. Su, L. A. Zuckerman, N. Nabavi, C. L. Jellis, G. S. Gray, J. Miller and J. A. Bluestone, *Proc. Natl Acad. Sci. USA* **90**, 11054 (1993).
34. V. A. Boussiotis, G. J. Freeman, J. G. Gribben, J. Daley, G. Gray and L. M. Nadler, *Proc. Natl Acad. Sci. USA* **90**, 11059 (1993).
35. M. Azuma, D. Ito, H. Yagita, K. Okumura, J. H. Phillips, L. L. Lanier and C. Somoza, *Nature* **366**, 76 (1993).
36. S.-M. Kang, B. Beverly, A.-C. Tran, K. Brorson, R. H. Schwartz and M. J. Lenardo, *Science* **257**, 1134 (1992).

37. J. M. LaSalle, P. J. Tolentino, G. J. Freeman, L. M. Nadler and D. A. Hafler, *J. Exp. Med.* **176**, 177 (1992).
38. D. J. Lenschow, Y. Zeng, J. R. Thistlewaite, A. Montag, W. Brady, M. G. Gibson, P. S. Linsley and J. A. Bluestone, *Science* **257**, 789 (1992).
39. L. A. Turka, P. S. Linsley, H. Lin, W. Brady, J. M. Leiden, R. Wei, M. L. Gibson, X. Zhen, S. Myrdal, D. Gordon, T. Bailey, S. F. Bolling and C. B. Thompson, *Proc. Natl Acad. Sci. USA* **89**, 11102 (1992).
40. L. Chen, S. Ashe, W. A. Brady, I. Hellström, K. E. Hellström, J. A. Ledbetter, P. McGowan and P. S. Linsley, *Cell* **71**, 1093 (1992).
41. S. E. Townsend and J. P. Allison, *Science* **259**, 368 (1993).

Ontogeny of the Immune Response

ARTHUR M. SILVERSTEIN
Institute of the History of Medicine, Johns Hopkins University
School of Medicine, Baltimore, MD 21205, USA

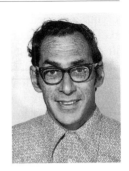

Among the many biomedical observations that challenged the chemically dominated immunology after World War II, perhaps none was so crucial as Ray
Owen's observation of blood cell chimeras in twin calves (*1*). It implied that something of profound immunological importance must occur in the fetus during
mammalian gestation. Macfarlane Burnet and Frank Fenner interpreted Owen's
finding to mean that the developing fetus is immunologically incompetent and
can somehow be rendered tolerant of self-antigens present during the transition
to full immunological competence (*2*). This suggestion was soon verified experimentally by Peter Medawar and colleagues (*3*). With the demonstration of the
incompetence of the fetus and neonate of many species to form antibodies (*4*) and
to manifest the morphologic characteristics of an immune response (germinal
centres and plasma cells) (*5*), it came to be assumed that all fetuses throughout
gestation are immature, and only attain maturity sometime after birth.

This was the situation in the late 1950s when a series of chance events caused
me to convert from chemistry to biology, and to spend the next two decades
studying fetal immunology. It happened, briefly, as follows: studying radio-
chemistry and nuclear physics in graduate school at Ohio State University, I
became disillusioned and left school in 1948 to return home to New York,
where I searched for a job. On the casual suggestion of a girlfriend, I applied at
the Sloan–Kettering Institute for Cancer Research, where I was hired as a technician in David Pressman's Immunochemistry Department. I had never even
heard of the word 'immunology' before this, but influenced by Pressman (and
by Fred Karush and Herman Eisen, who were fellows in the department at the
time), I did little work but read every book on Pressman's shelves. I quickly
became enthralled by the type of immunochemistry that Pressman and his
mentor Linus Pauling had pursued. During the next few years, I managed
to finish my Ph.D. in physical chemistry, and prepared myself to submit to a
fruitless two years of obligatory military service.

IMMUNOLOGY: THE MAKING OF A MODERN SCIENCE
ISBN 0-12-274020-3

Copyright © 1995 Academic Press Ltd
All rights of reproduction in any form reserved

Once again, the gods smiled upon me, for with typical military illogic I was, with no pertinent qualifications, assigned to the Armed Forces Institute of Pathology in Washington, DC, where Scientific Director Ernest Goodpasture took me under his protective and encouraging wing. Then, in 1958, two chance events occurred in quick succession. I happened to repeat to our paediatric pathologist the current dogma that fetuses are immunologically incompetent and cannot form plasma cells, whereupon he sent me several cases of human abortuses with congenital syphilis, each showing a luxuriant plasmacytosis. The second incident occurred in the Institute's lunchroom, when I overheard a veterinarian ask whether anyone could use six pregnant sheep he had just been given gratis. I asked whether he had ever worked on a fetus of any kind, and he replied, 'No, but I'm willing to give it a try. Let's learn together.'

It was while preparing to immunize these first fetal lambs that I wrote to my hero and that acknowledged leader in experimentation with young animals, Peter Medawar, to ask whether he thought there might be a future for me in fetal immunology. After some months, Medawar replied that it was common knowledge that fetuses are immunologically incompetent, and therefore I would do better to find a more productive outlet for my youthful ambitions (6). But by the time that I received this advice, we had already immunized the fetal lambs (gestation age unknown) and discovered that they had formed high titres of antiovalbumin and antiferritin antibodies when bled from the cord at birth. I had found my vocation! I had also found a series of superb collaborators who contributed not only useful technical approaches that I could never have developed alone, but also much good advice and an excellent postgraduate education. They included veterinary surgeons Keith Kraner and Charles Parshall, haematological pathologist Robert Lukes, immunologists Jonathan Uhr, Jeanette Thorbecke and Harvey Colten, and immunopathologist Robert A. Prendergast.

Human Fetal Immune Responses

The initial morphological studies of congenital diseases from the files of the Institute of Pathology proved quite rewarding. Not only were infections of the fetus with *Treponema pallidum* and *Toxoplasma gondii* accompanied by an impressive plasmacytosis in the lesions themselves, but plasma cells and a premature lymphofollicular maturation were also present in the draining lymph nodes and spleen in many cases (7). The human fetus is indeed immunologically mature *in utero*. But, more than this, it was also possible to obtain from these data an estimate of the gestational time of development of the capacity to mount an immune response, at least in the case of congenital syphilis. By analysis of a large series of cases of different gestational ages, it was possible to conclude that competence to respond to the antigen(s) of the treponemes appears at approximately the sixth month of gestation.

A subsequent study of the histopathology of congenital rubella infection suggested that the maturation of immunological capabilities in the human fetus had other interesting implications. It might lead to a modulation of the pathogenesis of certain congenital infectious diseases (8). Thus, fetuses infected with rubella virus during the first trimester show multiple disorders of development (ears, eyes, heart) with no signs of inflammation. The virus is known to affect mitotic rates, critical during organogenesis. However, some cases of congenital rubella, apparently infected late in gestation, show not developmental defects but rather multiple organ inflammatory changes (otitis, ophthalmitis, carditis). As with measles in the adult, where the pathology in the immunologically compromised patient is giant cell pneumonitis rather than dermal rash and fever, the presence or absence of a functioning immune system of the fetus may profoundly affect the pathological picture presented by the host–pathogen interaction.

Immune Responses in the Fetal Lamb

The initial crude, but successful, experiments on immunization of fetal lambs prompted us to continue the studies, arranging in succeeding years the procurement of large numbers of timed-gestation pregnant sheep. We learned as we went along, each year becoming increasingly more daring in our surgical procedures and working earlier and earlier in gestation (150 days in the ovine). It should be pointed out that the fetal lamb is an ideal subject for such studies, receiving no transfer of either proteins or cells across its syndesmochorial placenta. It is born agammaglobulinaemic and only receives its first passive transfer of maternal immunoglobulins in colostrum. In addition, it has a long (five months) gestation period and is large enough to be manipulated conveniently during the last two-thirds of gestation.

Immunization of large numbers of fetal lambs with many different antigens at different stages of gestation revealed a most curious situation. The ability to form antibody does not develop simultaneously for all antigens; rather, there appears to be a stepwise maturation of immunological competence for different antigens at different stages of gestation (9). Some antigens (for example, bacteriophage $\emptyset$X 174) can stimulate antibody formation as early as we could technically introduce it to the fetus, even prior to the maturation of organized lymphoid tissue in spleen or regional lymph nodes (10). Competence to respond to other antigens arises later in gestation, and to some (for example, diphtheria toxoid, *Salmonella typhosa*) only after birth, as summarized in Table 1. Moreover, this sequential attainment of competence to respond to the several antigens seemed not to vary from one animal to another within the species; it appeared as a carefully programmed maturational process like so many others during ontogeny. Curiously, even the ability to respond to allogeneic antigens with the rejection of skin grafts appears to be part of the timed maturation,

Table 1   The timing of acquisition of immunological competence to different antigens in the fetal lamb

Antigen	Days after conception
ØX 174 bacteriophage	<40
Ferritin	56
Q-fever	65
Allogeneic graft rejection	75
Haemocyanin	80
SV 40	90
T4 bacteriophage	105
Dinitrophenyl hapten	<110
Arsanilate hapten	<110
Ovalbumin	120
Bluetongue virus	122
LCM virus	140
- - - - - *Birth* - - - - -	150
Diphtheria toxoid	>190
Salmonella typhosa O antigen	>190
BCG vaccine	>190

graft rejection appearing at about 75 days' gestation in the fetal lamb (*11*). Equally interesting is the observation that T cell competence for a given antigen may arise earlier in gestation than B cell competence (*12*).

The finding of a precisely timed programme of immunological maturation in the fetal lamb had interesting theoretical implications as well as practical ones. It will be recalled that during the 1960s and 1970s, a lively dispute was taking place about the origin of the great diversity of antibody specificities. Some argued that the generation of immunological diversity depended upon the expansion of specificities from a few germline genes by somatic mutation and/or recombination – the paucigene model (*13*). Others argued a multigene model, wherein all specificities were encoded in the germline (*14*). The argument raged back and forth, with students of ontogeny like me generally taking the multigene side (*15*), since a carefully programmed maturational sequence seemed to argue against the chance occurrence that mutation implies.

Lymphoid Maturation in the Fetal Lamb

Comparison of the maturation of organized lymphoid tissues with the onset of immunological capabilities in the fetal lamb revealed several interesting facts. First, the earliest immune response (to bacteriophage ØX 174) took place before lymphocytes were found in spleen, regional nodes or thymus. Next, it was found that induction of precocious maturation of lymphoid tissues and lymphocyte numbers had no effect on the timing or order of appearance of competence to the several antigens (16). Finally, thymectomy of the fetal lamb at the end of the first third of gestation, while resulting in a marked lymphopenia that persisted into neonatal life, appeared to have little effect on the ability of the fetus or neonate to form antibodies or to reject skin allografts (17). This is in marked contrast to the profound immunosuppressive effect of thymectomy in mice and rats (18), and still remains unexplained.

One of the interesting consequences of the agammaglobulinaemic status of the fetal lamb *in utero* is the easy ability to suppress immunoglobulin formation using antiglobulin sera. It will be recalled that in the early 1960s it was still claimed by some that circulating antibody plays a role in allograft rejection (19). Studies of orthotopic skin allografts in fetal lambs treated with massive doses of rabbit antisheep immunoglobulins showed no diminution of their ability to reject these grafts (20).

Fetal Immune Responses in Other Species

In addition to the ability of the human fetus to mount an immune response to some pathogens, and of the fetal lamb to respond to many antigens as described above, experiments demonstrate that the fetus of many other species is similarly endowed. Thus, guinea-pig, Rhesus monkey, calf, opossum and other fetuses are able to form antibodies or to develop cellular immunity (21).

Modern Developments

All the studies described above are long since outdated. The maturation of lymphocyte lineages from the yolk sac onward has been well worked out, employing a variety of differentiation markers. The stepwise expansion of the B cell repertoire has been clarified for other species, and modern molecular biology has demonstrated that this is due to the preferential use of the most proximal V-region genes in early responses, subsequently expanded by somatic mechanisms. Thus, as so often happens in scientific disputes, both paucigene and multigene protagonists were partly right.

It is difficult in retrospect to assess the contributions of these early studies of fetal immune responses to modern developments. One can say, however, that at a time when so much of immunology depended upon findings in inbred mice and rats, results obtained in large animals such as primates and ungulates did perhaps temper certain overgeneralizations about the fine details of the immune system.

Notes and References

1. R. D. Owen, *Science* **102**, 400 (1945).
2. F. M. Burnet and F. Fenner, *The Production of Antibodies*, 2nd edn, Macmillan, Melbourne (1949).
3. R. E. Billingham, L. Brent and P. B. Medawar, *Nature* **172**, 603 (1953).
4. J. J. Osborn, J. Dancis and J. F. Julia, *Pediatrics* **9**, 736 (1952); R. T. Smith and R. A. Bridges, *J. Exp. Med.* **108**, 227 (1958).
5. R. A. Bridges, R. M. Condie, S. J. Zak and R. A. Good, *J. Lab. Clin. Med.* **53**, 331 (1959).
6. It was only later that we learned of the study, done as early as 1953, that the fetal lamb could reject tissue allografts (P. G. Schinkel and K. A. Ferguson, *Aust. J. Exp. Biol. Med. Sci.* **6**, 533 (1953)).
7. A. M. Silverstein, *Nature* **194**, 196 (1962); A. M. Silverstein and R. L. Lukes, *Lab. Invest.* **11**, 918 (1962).
8. A. M. Silverstein, *Science* **144**, 1423 (1964), in *Ontogeny of Acquired Immunity (Ciba Foundation Symposium*, No. 5), Elsevier, Amsterdam (1972).
9. A. M. Silverstein, J. W. Uhr, K. L. Kraner and R. J. Lukes, *J. Exp. Med.* **117**, 799 (1963); A. M. Silverstein, C. J. Parshall and J. W. Uhr, *Science* **154**, 1675 (1966).
10. A. M. Silverstein and R. A. Prendergast, in *Developmental Aspects of Antibody Formation and Structure*, Vol. 1 (J. Šterzl and I. Riha, eds), Czech Academy of Sciences, Prague (1970), in *Morphological and Functional Aspects of Immunity* (K. Lindahl-Kiessling, G. Alm and M. G. Hanna, eds), Plenum Press, New York (1971).
11. A. M. Silverstein, R. A. Prendergast and K. L. Kraner, *J. Exp. Med.* **119**, 955 (1964).
12. A. M. Silverstein and S. Segal, *J. Exp. Med.* **142**, 802 (1975).
13. See, for example, M. Cohn, *Progr. Immunol.* **2**, 261 (1974).
14. W. J. Dreyer and J. C. Bennet, *Proc. Natl Acad. Sci. USA*, **54**, 864 (1965); L. Hood and D. W. Talmage, *Science* **168**, 325 (1970). See also A. J. Cunningham, *The Generation of Antibody Diversity*, Academic Press, New York (1976).
15. A. M. Silverstein and R. A. Prendergast, in *Development Aspects*, see note 10; A. M. Silverstein, in *Phylogenic and Ontogenic Study of the Immune Response and its Contribution to the Immunological Theory* (P. Liacopoulos and J. Panijel, eds), INSERM, Paris (1973).
16. A. M. Silverstein and R. A. Prendergast, in *Morphological and Functional Aspects*, see note 10.
17. A. M. Silverstein and R. A. Prendergast, in *Developmental Aspects*, see note 10; G. J. Cole and B. Morris, *Aust. J. Exp. Biol. Med. Sci.* **49**, 33 (1971); A. M. Silverstein and R. A. Prendergast, in *Microenvironmental Aspects of Immunity* (B. D. Janković and K. Isaković, eds), Plenum Press, New York (1972).
18. See, for example, R. A. Good and A. E. Gabrielson (eds), *The Thymus in Immunobiology*, Hoeber, New York (1964); J. F. A. P. Miller and D. Osoba, *Physiol. Rev.* **47**, 437 (1967).
19. V. Hašková, J. Chutná and J. Hort, *Ann. NY Acad. Sci.* **99**, 602 (1962); C. A. Stetson, *Adv. Immunol.* **3**, 97 (1963).
20. A. M. Silverstein, R. A. Prendergast and K. L. Kraner, *Science* **142**, 1172 (1963); A. M. Silverstein and K. L. Kraner, *Transplantation* **3**, 535 (1965).
21. Guinea-pig: J. W. Uhr, *Nature* **187**, 957 (1960). Rhesus: A. M. Silverstein, R. A. Prendergast and C. J. Parshall, *J. Immunol.* **104**, 269 (1970). Calf: K. L. Fennestad and C. Borg-Petersen, *J. Infect. Dis.* **110**, 63 (1962). Opossum: S. E. Kalmutz, *Nature* **193**, 851 (1962).

The Molecular Basis of Immunity

The HLA Story

JEAN DAUSSET
Human Polymorphism Study Centre, C.E.P.H.,
27 rue Juliette Dodu, 75010 Paris, France

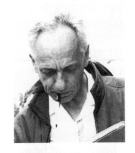

FELIX T. RAPAPORT
State University of New York at Stony Brook, Transplantation
Service, Department of Surgery, Health Sciences Center, T-19, 040,
Stony Brook, NY 11794–8192, USA

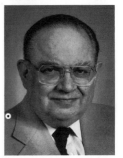

The development of our understanding of human leucocyte antigen (HLA) constitutes an adventure in biology that is possibly unique in all of science. Indeed, progress in this field, for the first time in scientific history, was the outcome of an exemplary and rigorous co-operative effort between all of the specialists involved in the discipline. This was necessary because of the extreme complexity of the problems involved, which were beyond the capacity of any one single laboratory. Only such a concerted and persistent collaborative effort over the years could have resolved the extraordinarily complex situation encountered with leucocyte groups, and the process of identifying them as tissue groups.

As an integral component of this process, biennial international workshops reuniting all workers in the field were begun in 1964 (*1–12*), initially including only ten or so teams, and eventually growing to more than 100 groups, representing all nationalities. At each workshop, one or more specific questions were asked, with all participating teams studying the same biological materials (antisera, cells, etc.), and then sharing the results. The central analysis of the thousands of reactions produced in this fashion then yielded new invaluable information and led, within a relatively few years, to a clear understanding of the genetics of the HLA system and its extreme polymorphism. The pre-eminent

IMMUNOLOGY: THE MAKING OF A MODERN SCIENCE
ISBN 0-12-274020-3

importance of HLA in transplantation was demonstrated, multiple associations with human disease were uncovered and, above all, the immunological role of the HLA determinants was discovered. This extraordinary progress was achieved in spite of (or possibly as a consequence of) a keen spirit of competition between the participating groups, which was tempered by full commitment to a collaborative effort, encouraged further by the rapid progress which this effort produced. During this exciting epoch, organ transplantation, that age-old dream of humanity, became a reality and a new kind of medicine, that is, predictive medicine, based on a growing knowledge of human predisposition to certain diseases, began to develop. Finally, the fundamental role of HLA molecules as the initiators of immune responses, opened the door to the entire panorama of immunological reactivity. This great progress has been the result of a joint effort by hundreds, if not thousands, of gifted investigators, all of whom cannot be named in this brief overview. It is only possible in the allowed space to allude to some key milestones of this great adventure. We refer the reader to the published volumes of the International Histocompatibility Workshops, from 1965 to date, for a more complete record of these events (1–12).

Discovery

As their name indicates, the HLA antigens were initially leucocyte groups. It was logical that, in the search for antileucocyte antibodies, the first three pioneers, all of whom were experts in red blood cell typing, utilized the basic technique of cell agglutination, which they had used routinely for erythrocyte studies. The point of departure was the observation of a strong leucoagglutination reaction, observed on a glass slide when serum from a polytransfused human was added to leucocytes obtained from another patient (13). The antibodies responsible for this reaction were not natural antibodies, such as those of the ABO system, but immune antibodies, produced in response to blood transfusions (14) or pregnancy (15,16). The demonstration of antigenic differences between various individuals provided further support for the existence of leucocyte groups. The first antibodies produced by planned transfusions obtained from the same donor were described in 1958, and were named Mac (17). Systematic study of leucocyte group reactions with various immune antisera, utilizing computer analysis for the first time, led Van Rood in 1962 (18) to describe the first leucocyte group 'system' (4A, 4B), shortly followed in 1964 by the description of a second system (LA1, LA2) by Payne and Bodmer (19). Simultaneously and independently, Rapaport et al. (1962) (20) had demonstrated for the first time the existence of 'tissue groups' in unrelated human subjects, on the basis of skin grafting experiments. The next logical step was to ascertain whether these 'tissue groups' were the same as the antigenic determinants recognized as 'leucocyte groups' by serological techniques. This central question triggered a long-term close collaborative transatlantic enterprise between the authors, which began in 1963.

It may be of interest that the first steps along the HLA highway were completely independent of the studies pursued since 1936 by Gorer and followed by Snell and many others, on the murine H2 system. In defence of the early HLA pioneers, it should be noted that an analogy between H2 and HLA was not clear at that time, since the H2 antigens were defined by erythrocyte agglutination techniques, while the HLA antibodies seemed to be recognized exclusively on leucocytes, although Amos, a student of Gorer, had already reported the presence of H2 antigens on murine leucocytes as early as 1953 (21). The role of co-ordinating the efforts of the international teams investigating HLA thus fell naturally to Amos, who initiated the International Histocompatibility Workshops, and was the Chairman and organizer of the first of these historic meetings in Durham, North Carolina, in 1964.

Development through Workshops

The early group of pioneers was soon joined by many other workers, representing a broad spectrum of disciplines, and including surgeons in particular. Indeed, renal transplantation was beginning to take its first faltering steps at this time, and one central motivating factor spurring on the HLA effort became the very urgent need to develop a method capable of providing the best possible and clinically relevant measurement of donor–recipient histocompatibility. By now, the principal techniques for histocompatibility studies with leucocytes had been defined, including lymphocytotoxicity (22) and mixed lymphocyte culture (MLC) (23–25). Other methods, such as platelet complement fixation (26), mixed cell agglutination (27), and indirect antiglobulin consumption (28) were also described, but were less popular. At the time of the first Workshop, clinicians also proposed *in vivo* compatibility tests, such as the third-man test by skin grafting (29) and the lymphocyte-transfer test, done by intradermal leucocyte injections (30). These remained experimental, however, and did not come into routine use. Subsequently, the key value of the experimental skin allograft studies (31–33) was in the definitive demonstration that the HLA antigens were indeed active as major transplantation antigens in man (34).

It is remarkable that, during the following 20 years, no additional techniques for the study of human histocompatibility were devised. The next phase had to await the advent of molecular biology. It is of interest, in retrospect, to note that the early pioneers remained undaunted by what appeared, at first, to be somewhat discouraging findings. At the time of the First International Workshop in 1964 (1), the available serological techniques failed to show a significant correlation between the observations of the various groups on the same cells. In one of his theatrical gestures, for which he was justly famous, Ceppellini publicly tore up the sheets bearing these results, which were thus never published.

In spite of this, however, the participants remained convinced that they were on an investigative path of great potential. A Second International Workshop was agreed upon, and was organized by Van Rood in Leiden, The Netherlands, only one year later (2). This was a crucial year, during which the early promise of leucocyte groups was fulfilled. With concurrent progress in the available techniques, very clear correlations appeared between the results of various groups on the same cell samples. Dausset's antigen Mac was found to be the same as the LA2 of Payne and Bodmer, the PLGrLyB1 of Shulman, and the 8A antigen of Van Rood. A number of other antigens were also defined, and the role of these antigens in transplantation was documented formally by skin graft studies in recipients who had undergone specific sensitization procedures with group-specific leucocytes (35,36).

There remained a strong disagreement at that time, however, between the proponents of a single genetic system (the Hu-1 system of Dausset and Ivanyi (37)) and those who favoured two systems (the LA1, LA2 system of Bodmer (38) and the 4a, 4b system of Van Rood (39)). Resolution of this issue required careful family studies. This was proposed by Ceppellini as the theme of the Third International Workshop, held under his aegis in Turin, Italy, in 1967 (4). Blood samples from members of local Italian families were distributed each morning in blind fashion, so that the results of the typing could be available that very same evening. Each participating team used its own technique, its own reagents and sera, and even some of their own equipment (unfortunately, a strike by Italian customs personnel prevented one of the teams from using the equipment which they had sent to Turin at great expense from the USA!). Analysis of the results of these family studies provided clear-cut evidence of the existence of a single major leucocyte antigen system. As our spokesman, Ceppellini presented a brilliant synthesis of the collective efforts of the group. He also described results of intrafamilial skin grafts which were in concordance with the serological results. The pre-eminent role of the ABO antigens in transplantation was also demonstrated, as ABO-incompatible skin grafts were rejected rapidly by the recipients, often without any vascularization (white graft reaction) (33,40). The principal biological laws of human transplantation had thus been uncovered:

(1) Natural anti-ABO antibodies (40) and immune antileucocyte antibodies (41) can cause acute allograft rejection;
(2) Kidney or skin grafts exchanged between HLA identical siblings exhibit highly favourable survival times; the results of similar transplants between unrelated or HLA different siblings yield mediocre results. Transplants between parents and children (that is, with 50% genetic identity) yield intermediate results between these two extremes.

It is difficult, in retrospect, to think of a more convincing demonstration of the key role of HLA antigens in transplantation than these data. This is particularly interesting in view of the fact that our knowledge was limited at this time to the antigens of the first two HLA series (that is, class I antigens). Unaware of this lacuna, but impatient to help patients who might benefit from transplantation, a number of organizations were created in order to promote organ exchanges, first in Europe (such as Eurotransplant in 1967 and France Transplant in 1969) and subsequently in the USA (UNOS). It is thus not too surprising that it was difficult to find a highly significant correlation between tissue compatibility and the survival of kidney grafts obtained from cadaver donors (that is, unrelated subjects). This produced a schism between the believers (largely immunologists) and the non-believers (largely clinical surgeons). This conflict still persists today, 30 years later!

The following years were marked by continuing efforts of immunologists to improve the precision of their techniques, and to search for as-yet undetected HLA antigens. The results were presented at the Fourth International Workshop, organized in Los Angeles in 1970 by Terasaki (5). Sandberg and Thorsby also suggested at this time the probable existence of a third allelic series in HLA (HLA-C). Two years later, Dausset organized the fifth workshop in Evian, France (6). The central theme of this workshop was a global anthropological effort, designed to study the distribution of HLA antigens in the various different world populations. Terasaki, who presided at this workshop, opened the meeting with a parable, featuring an Indian tribe, 'Hu-LA' (derived from Hu1 and LA), which held periodic pow-wows on both sides of the Atlantic, in a continuing search for weapons (antibodies) capable of destroying the enemy (cells) with ever-increasing efficiency (alluding to antibodies of ever-increasing specificity). This workshop was a culmination of a series of highly memorable expeditions by various tissue typing teams. Albert (Munich) identified HLA types in a tent in Nepal; Degos (Paris) went into the desert and lived with the Tuaregs for the same purpose. American Indians of the North and South (Walford), Pygmies, Polynesians, Eskimos, Tibetans and even a population of chimpanzees were studied and compared with each other. Although this study was only based upon sera recognizing class I antigens, it remains to this day a highly valuable source of information on the distribution of HLA antigens in these various different populations, and on their genetic relationships. It has even been possible to reconstitute the history of a number of human migrations with the help of this information.

It was also during this same period, limited by our knowledge of only the HLA class I antigens, that an association was discovered between certain HLA antigens and disease. Although several studies, begun as early as 1967 (42,43), had already touched on this issue, the first definitive correlation between HLA and psoriasis was published in 1972 by Terasaki (44), simultaneously with Bewerton's report on HLA and ankylosing spondylitis (45). All of the typing teams now began an intensive search for other associations between HLA and disease, with remarkable success. Today, one can identify at least 50 diseases which bear more or less strong associations with one or more antigens of the HLA system.

HLA Class II

It may be somewhat arbitrary to consider that the events described thus far constituted the first major chapter of the HLA adventure, where only the class I antigens were known. There is no question, however, that the formal demonstration of the existence of HLA class II antigens marked the beginning of a new era for HLA. As early as 1967, Amos and Bach (46) had observed an occasional disassociation between the results of intrafamilial serological determinations and *in vitro* lymphocyte proliferation reactions. Yunis and Amos (47) confirmed this finding in 1971. Another five years was required, however, for the full definition of the class II Dw series, on the basis of mixed lymphocyte cultures (MLC). This reached full fruition at the time of the sixth international workshop organized by Kissmeyer-Nielsen in Aarhus, Denmark, in 1975 (7). In the interim, Schreffler and Klein (48) had independently detected in mice a series of new H2 loci which governed antigens expressed only on B, but not T, lymphocytes. This provided a major stimulus to HLA immunogeneticists, who now sought evidence of a similar situation in man. The early publications on this topic emanated from the sixth workshop, and reached full fruition at the seventh international workshop organized by Walter and Julia Bodmer at Oxford University in 1977 (8). The new findings triggered yet another series of intensive world-wide studies, initiated with the same enthusiasm as that which had marked the early HLA days. The effort was considerable, since it was necessary to eliminate class I antibodies from reactive sera by first absorbing them with blood platelets (which only bear class I determinants). The number of new alleles of the DR series (class II antigens) grew rapidly. It also became evident within a relatively short time that there existed yet another series of class II antigens, located in close proximity to the determinants of the DR series on the sixth chromosome. This became fully accepted at the eighth international workshop, organized by Terasaki in Los Angeles in 1980 (9). The series described by Park as 'MB' became the DQ series; in addition, further MLC studies led to identification of a third series of class II antigens, named 'DP' (49,50). These advances seemed to support the concept that the arduous effort of identifying possible effects of these antigens in transplantation or in association with human disease would now have to be undertaken once again, from the beginning. New series of skin graft studies in normal volunteers (35) and of renal allograft results showed very soon that donor–recipient compatibility for the products of these new HLA loci greatly influenced the results of transplantation. With the help of now well-established methods of statistical analysis, new data were accumulated with great rapidity, and became directly applicable to the daily practice of clinical organ transplantation.

Matters were somewhat more complicated, however, in the search for associations between HLA antigens and human disease. These studies had to be started from the beginning once again because leucocytes from patients studied previously had not, as a general rule, been stored in the frozen state for

future reference. Even if such cells had been stored, the quantity of B lymphocytes required for the new studies would not have been sufficient. The effort
was worthwhile, however, and showed a far greater correlation between certain
disease states and HLA class II antigens, and a number of new associations were
also uncovered. A typical example of this evolution were the data obtained in
patients with insulin-dependent diabetes (IDDM). At first, there seemed to be
a weak association between HLA-A1 and then HLA-B8 and IDDM; a similar
association was then uncovered for antigen HLA-DR3. It then became apparent that these antigens constitute one of the most frequent HLA haplotypes in
the Caucasian population. A far stronger association was found, however,
between IDDM and HLA antigens DR3 and DR4 (51). Today, more than 50
human diseases are associated more or less strongly with various products of
the HLA complex; many of these are autoimmune diseases, where a theoretical
explanation for the relationship seems relatively easy. Another number of ill-
nesses do not enter into this category, and the background for their association
with HLA remains obscure.

The third major milestone of HLA has been a consequence of recent
advances in fundamental genetics and of the introduction of molecular biology
techniques to the study of HLA. The HLA complex was localized by Lamm to
the sixth human chromosome as early as 1971 (52). Rapidly thereafter, the
position of its loci on this chromosome, extending from the centromere (DP) to
the telomere (A) was established. The successful application of molecular
biology techniques to tissue typing began in 1984, using recombinant fragment
length polymorphism (RFLP) techniques (53). More direct methods, and particularly the extraordinary sensitivity of the polymerase chain reaction (PCR)
then identified, within a relatively short time, the sequence of a number of
alleles. This process, which continues at present, as the number of alleles of
known sequence continues to grow, along with identification of new mutations
in these sequences. Once again, the HLA community has had to start its studies
from the beginning. It seems clear, however, that this new era will make it possible to define with ever-greater precision the HLA compatibility requirements
for organ, and particularly bone marrow transplantation. Although transplantation has been facilitated greatly by the advent of ever-more powerful
immunosuppressive agents, the long-term outcome continues to depend upon
levels of donor–recipient histocompatibility. Bone marrow transplantation,
which requires an even stricter level of compatibility, will also benefit as our
knowledge of the actual structure of the various determinant antigens continues
to progress. In similar fashion, it will become necessary to review once
again the association between HLA and disease, with ever-better correlations
resulting from the more precise definition of the actual HLA genotypes of the
patients under study.

We have left for last the most astounding of all of the breakthroughs eman-
ating from the 40-year saga of HLA. This has been the fundamental discovery
of the role of molecules of the major histocompatibility complex (MHC) in

immune responsiveness (54). This role was highlighted by the phenomenon of MHC restriction, whereby a response to viral antigens is only possible if there is MHC identity between the infected cells and the killer T lymphocytes involved in the response (55). These findings are directly applicable to the human MHC, and have received corroboration from the crystallographic imaging of the HLA-A2 molecule, sheltering an antigenic peptide in its 'arms' (56). From now on, study of associations between HLA and disease will have to take on a new structural dimension, as we recognize the role of HLA molecules as antigen (peptide) presenters (regardless of whether these peptides are of auto or hetero origin), and the dichotomy between HLA class I and class II antigens becomes fully clarified.

Thus, from the humble pipettes and serology of the 1950s and 1960s, HLA studies have acquired a molecular, that is an atomic dimension, based upon a study of affinities between the various aminoacids which constitute the 'pocket' of the HLA molecule, and those of the peptides which they shelter and present. HLA is now placed at the very heart of the immune response, and the consequences of this new situation remain unexploited, and hold immense potential for the future.

We have tried to present the HLA saga in the most objective manner possible. We have no doubt, however, that this effort has only been successful in part. We beg the forgiveness of those many workers whose contributions may have been omitted or cited incompletely.

Notes and References

1. P. S. Russell and H. J. Winn, *Publication No. 1229*, National Academy of Sciences, USA National Research Council, Washington, DC (1965).
2. H. Balner, F. J. Cleton and J. G. Eernisse (eds), *Histocompatibility Testing 1965*, Munksgaard, Copenhagen (1965).
3. W. Bodmer, F. J. Cleton and J. G. Eernisse (eds), *Histocompatibility Testing 1966*, Munsgaard, Copenhagen (1966).
4. E. S. Curtoni, P. L. Mattiuz and R. M. Tosi (eds), *Histocompatibility Testing 1967*, Williams & Wilkins, Baltimore (1967).
5. P. I. Terasaki (ed.), *Histocompatibility Testing 1970*, Munksgaard, Copenhagen (1970).
6. J. Dausset and J. Columbani (eds), *Histocompatibility Testing 1972*, Munksgaard, Copenhagen (1973).
7. F. Kissmeyer-Nielsen (ed.), *Histocompatibility Testing 1975*, Munksgaard, Copenhagen (1975).
8. W. F. Bodmer, J. R. Batchelor, J. G. Bodmer, H. Festenstein and P. J. Morris (eds), *Histocompatibility Testing 1977*, Munksgaard, Copenhagen (1978).
9. P. I. Terasaki (ed.), *Histocompatibility Testing 1980*, UCLA Tissue Typing Laboratory, Los Angeles (1980).
10. E. Albert, M. P. Baum and W. R. Mayr *et al.* (eds), *Histocompatibility Testing 1984*, Springer-Verlag, Heidelberg (1984).
11. B. Dupont (ed.), *Histocompatibility Testing 1987*, Vols I and II, Springer-Verlag, Heidelberg (1989).

12. K. Tsuji, M. Aizawa and T. Sasazuki (eds), *HLA 1991*, Oxford University Press, Oxford (1992).
13. J. Dausset and A. Nenna, *Compt. Rendus Soc. Biol.* **186**, 1539 (1952).
14. R. Payne, *Meth. Med. Res.* **10**, 27 (1964).
15. R. Payne and M. R. Rolfs, *J. Clin. Investig.* **37**, 1756 (1958).
16. J. J. Van Rood, J. G. Bernisse and A. van Leeuween, *Nature*, **181**, 735 (1958).
17. J. Dausset, *Acta Haematol.* **20**, 156 (1958).
18. J. J. Van Rood, *Thesis*, Leiden State University, Leiden (1962).
19. R. Payne, M. Tripp, J. Weigue, W. Bodmer and J. Bodmer, *Cold Spring Harbor Symp.* **29**, 285 (1964).
20. F. T. Rapaport, H. S. Lawrence, L. Thomas, J. M. Converse, W. S. Tillett and J. H. Mulholland, *J. Clin. Investig.* **41**, 2166 (1962).
21. D. B. Amos, *Brit. J. Exp. Pathol.* **34**, 464 (1953).
22. P. I. Terasaki, M. Mandell, J. van de Water and T. S. Edgington, *Ann. NY Acad. Sci.* **120**, 332 (1964).
23. K. Hirschhorn, F. Bach, F. T. Rapaport, J. M. Converse and H. S. Lawrence, *Ann. NY Acad. Sci.* **120**, 303 (1964).
24. B. Bain, M. R. Vas and L. Lowenstein, *Blood* **23**, 108 (1964).
25. F. H. Bach and K. Hirschhorn, *Science* **143**, 813 (1964).
26. N. R. Schulman, V. J. Marcher, L. Aledort, M. C. Hiller and J. J. Bunter, *Trans. Assoc. Amer. Phys.* **75**, 89 (1962).
27. F. Milgram, K. Kane and E. Witebsky, *J. Am. Med. Assoc.* **192**, 845 (1965).
28. J. Colombani, M. Colombani, A. Bengsam and J. Dausset, in *Histocompatibility Testing 1967* (E. S. Curtoni, P. L. Mattiuz and R. M. Tosi, eds), Williams & Wilkins, Baltimore, (1967), p. 413.
29. F. T. Rapaport, H. S. Lawrence, L. Thomas and J. M. Converse *et al.*, *Ann. NY Acad. Sci.* **99**, 564 (1962).
30. J. G. Gray and P. S. Russell, in *Histocompatibility Testing Publ. 1229*, National Academy of Sciences, National Research Council, Washington, DC (1965), p. 105.
31. J. M. Converse and F. T. Rapaport, *Ann. Surg.* **147**, 273 (1956).
32. F. T. Rapaport and J. M. Converse, *Ann. NY Acad. Sci.* **64**, 386 (1957).
33. F. T. Rapaport and J. M. Converse, *Ann. Surg.* **147**, 273 (1958).
34. F. T. Rapaport and J. Dausset (eds.), *Human Transplantation*, Grune & Stratton, New York (1968).
35. F. T. Rapaport, J. Dausset, L. Legrand, A. Barge, H. S. Lawrence and J. M. Converse, *J. Clin. Investig.* **47**, 2206 (1966).
36. J. J. Van Rood, A. Van Leeuwen and A. Schippers *et al.*, *Histocompatibility Testing Series Haematol.* **11**, 37 (1965).
37. J. Dausset, P. Ivanyi and D. Ivanyi, *Histocompatibility Testing Series Haematol.* **11**, 51 (1965).
38. J. Bodmer, W. F. Bodmer, R. Payne, P. Terasaki and D. Vredroe, *Nature* **210**, 28 (1966).
39. J. J. Van Rood, A. Van Leeuwen and A. Schippers *et al.*, *Histocompatibility Testing Series Haematol.* **11**, 37 (1965).
40. F. T. Rapaport J. Dausset, L. Legrand, A. Barge, H. S. Lawrence, J. M. Converse, *J. Clin. Investig.* **47**, 2206 (1968).
41. F. Kissmeyer-Nielsen (ed.) *Histocompatibility Testing 1975*, Munksgaard, Copenhagen, 1975.
42. J. F. Amiel, in *Histocompatibility Testing 1967* (E. S. Curtoni, P. L. Mattiuz and R. M. Tosi, eds), Williams & Wilkins, Baltimore, (1967), p. 79.
43. J. Dausset, in *Histocompatibility Testing 1967* (E. S. Curtoni, P. L. Mattiuz and R. M. Tosi, eds), Williams & Wilkins, Baltimore, (1967), p. 81.
44. P. I. Terasaki and M. R. Mioxey, *Transplant Reviews* **22**, 105 (1975).
45. D. A. Brewerton, M. Caffey, F. D. Hart, D. C. O. James, A. Nicholls, R. D. Sturrock, *Lancet* **1**, 904 (1973).
46. F. Bach and D. B. Amos, *Science* **156**, 1506 (1967).

47. E. J. Yunis and D. B. Amos, *Proc. Natl Acad. Sci. (USA)* **68**, 3031 (1971).
48. J. Klein and D. C. Schreffler, *Transpl. Rev* **6**, 3 (1971).
49. M. S. Park, P. I. Terasaki, I. D. Bernoco and Y. Iwaki, *Transpl. Proc.* **10**, 823 (1978).
50. R. Rosi *et al.*, *J. Exp. Med.* **148**, 4592 (1978).
51. A. Svejgaard, P. Plato, L. P. Ryder, L. Nielsen and M. Staub, *Transpl. Rev.* **22**, 3 (1975).
52. L. O. Lamm, U. Friedrich, G. B. Petersen, J. Jørgenssen, J. Nielsen, A. J. Therkellen, F. Kissmeyer-Nielsen, *Human Hered.* **24**, 243 (1974).
53. D. Cohen, P. Pall, I. Legall *et al.*, *Immunol. Rev.* **87**, 105 (1955).
54. B. Benacerraf and H. D. McDevitt, *Science* **175**, 273 (1972).
55. R. M. Zinkernagel and P. C. Doherty, *J. Exp. Med.* **144**, 1427 (1975).
56. P. J. Bjorkman, M. A. Saper, B. Samraoui, W. S. Bennett, J. L. Strominger and D. C. Wiley, *Nature* **329**, 512 (1987).

Early Investigations on Antibody Structure and Idiotypy

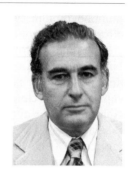

ALFRED NISONOFF

Department of Biology, Rosenstiel Research Center, Brandeis University, Waltham, MA 02254, USA

This memoir will review some of the early research of my laboratory on two subjects – the structure of antibodies and idiotypy – both considered in the context of other contemporary work. This is not intended to be a comprehensive review, and many significant contributions made at the time are necessarily not discussed. My principle collaborators in the early work on structure were William Mandy, Jerry Palmer, Frank Wissler and Richard Hong. The research on idiotypy was initiated in collaboration with Bruce MacDonald, John Hopper, Laura Pawlak, David Hart and Susan Spring.

Structure of Antibodies

Before 1958 the information available on the structure of antibodies was very limited. The molecular weights of IgG and IgM were known and some data were available on amino acid composition. In addition, hydrodynamic measurements, electron microscopy and hapten-binding studies had indicated that IgG is an elongated, flexible molecule with two antigen-binding sites. There was a limited amount of data on N-terminal sequences, but the interpretation was ambiguous because of molecular heterogeneity, the (as yet undiscovered) multichain nature of the molecule, and the fact that many immunoglobulin polypeptide chains do not possess a free N-terminal amino group. A dramatic improvement in our knowledge of the structure occurred during the next five years.

Major contributors to the research were Rodney Porter, Gerald Edelman and their collaborators. (Porter and Edelman shared the Nobel Prize in Physiology or Medicine in 1972.) Porter had worked in Frederick Sanger's laboratory in

IMMUNOLOGY: THE MAKING OF A MODERN SCIENCE
ISBN 0-12-274020-3

Cambridge in the late 1940s and wanted to apply Sanger's methods of protein sequencing to antibodies. Although immunoglobulins could be obtained reasonably free of other proteins, a major obstacle to sequencing was the large size of the molecules (150 kDa for IgG) in addition to the heterogeneity of Ig preparations. (That myeloma proteins are accurate representations of normal immunoglobulins was not yet widely appreciated.) Porter focused his early efforts on the problem of molecular size. His approach was to use proteolytic enzymes in an effort to produce fragments of antibody that retained antigen-binding activity. Using the enzyme papain, he had shown as early as 1950 that antibodies could be degraded into c.40 kDa fragments that had lost their capacity to precipitate the specific antigen but could specifically block precipitation of the antigen by intact antibody (1). He drew the correct inference that univalent fragments of antibody had been separated from the bivalent molecules. (Univalent molecules are of course unable to form a lattice or network but can nevertheless compete for the antigen.) The bivalence of IgG antibodies had been established by Herman Eisen and Fred Karush, using equilibrium dialysis, in 1949 (2). Porter found it difficult to purify active antibody fragments, in part because of the presence of extraneous proteins in the crude papain preparations available at the time. The situation changed when papain was crystallized by Kimmel and Smith in 1954 (3). In 1958 and 1959, using the highly purified enzyme and recently developed methods for protein fractionation, Porter reported the preparation and isolation of Fab (antigen-binding) and Fc (crystallizable) fragments of rabbit IgG (4,5).

Gerald Edelman, at the Rockefeller Institute, was using a complementary approach to antibody structure. Edelman had an M.D. degree and was working toward a Ph.D. in the laboratory of Henry Kunkel. His initial experiments were straightforward, and the results were published as a one-page paper in 1959 (6). He found that reduction of disulphide bonds in human γ-globulin by β-mercaptoethylamine, in the presence of 6 M urea as a denaturing agent, caused a decrease in the apparent average molecular weight from 158 kDa (measured in 6 M urea) to 48 kDa. Similarly treated IgM had an apparent average molecular weight of 41 kDa. This was the first clear evidence that immunoglobulins have a multichain structure. (N-Terminal sequencing had suggested a single-chain structure partly because, as we now know, most of the heavy chains are blocked at the N-terminus.) Edelman extended this work in collaboration with Miroslav Poulik, who had expertise in starch gel electrophoresis acquired in the laboratory of Oliver Smithies. Together they showed that human IgG contains polypeptide chains of two different molecular weights (now designated light (L) and heavy (H)) (7). They reported a molecular weight of 17 kDa for the L chain (accepted value c.22 kDa); that of the H chain was not well characterized. Another major advance was made by Poulik and Edelman (8) and Edelman and Gally (9). They showed that a Bence-Jones (urinary) protein migrated in starch gel at the same rate as the L chain of a myeloma protein of the same patient and that the two proteins had other physical chemical characteristics in common as

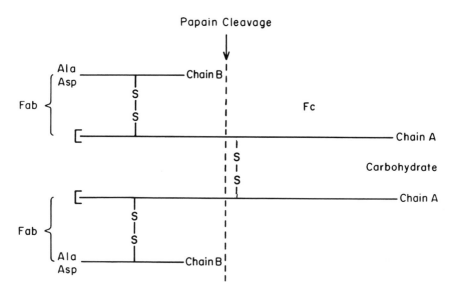

Figure 1 Schematic diagram of the structure of rabbit IgG proposed by Fleischman, Porter and Press (*14*), modified to show the presence of one rather than three disulphide bonds joining the two heavy (A) chains.

well. Thus they discovered that a Bence-Jones protein is a light chain, produced in excess by the same cell line that synthesizes the myeloma protein. In addition to solidifying the concept of the multichain structure of immunoglobulin, this work gave added respectability to the proteins of multiple myeloma and set the stage for a major sequencing effort on immunoglobulin, carried out initially with Bence-Jones proteins and published in 1965 by Hilschmann and Craig (*10*) and by Putnam and his collaborators (*11*).

The now well-known four-chain structure of IgG was established by Porter and coworkers in 1962 and 1963 (*12–14*). Their deceptively simple model, described by Fleischman, Porter and Press in an elegant paper (*14*), delineates the relationships between the Fab/Fc fragments and the H and L chains of the molecule. It also shows spatial relationships among the Fab and Fc fragments as well as the interchain disulphide bonds (see Fig. 1). They demonstrated that an Fab fragment comprises a complete L chain and about half a heavy chain, whereas the Fc fragment is made up of the remaining (C-terminal) sequences of the two H chains and also contains most of the carbohydrate. Contributing to the success of this work was a careful immunological analysis of the relationship among the chains and fragments (*13,14*), and the first reliable determination, by Roger Pain (*15*), of the molecular weight of a H chain (which has a strong tendency to aggregate in neutral solution). Pain's success was probably due in part to the use of relatively mild conditions, developed by Porter, for the separation of H and L chains.

When Porter's paper on papain digestion appeared in 1958, my laboratory was using equilibrium dialysis to investigate the affinity and degree of heterogeneity of rabbit antihapten antibodies. We applied the method to Porter's Fab fragments (then designated fragments I and II) and were able to show virtually complete retention of hapten-binding activity upon fragmentation of an affinity-purified antibody (16) and to demonstrate a valence of 0.9 to 1.0 (17), confirming the conclusion based on inhibition of precipitation. The data also showed that there is little or no co-operativity between the two binding sites, since the hapten-binding curves of Fab and intact antibody were virtually superimposable.

Our work with other proteolytic enzymes was undertaken to test the hypothesis that L-cysteine, present in preparations of papain to protect its activity, might play a direct role in the fragmentation by reducing interchain disulphide bonds. We therefore looked for cleavage in two stages and found that this occurs when pepsin and a reducing agent are used. The work was first reported in 1959 (18). Interestingly, our initial premise, i.e. that cleavage by papain occurs in two stages, later proved incorrect. Because papain cleaves on the N-terminal side of the single interheavy chain disulphide bond in rabbit IgG it liberates Fab fragments without a requirement for reduction of the bond. Direct evidence that the interheavy chain disulphide bond is localized in the Fc fragment was obtained later in collaboration with Frank Inman (19).

We used pepsin at its highest effective pH range (4–5) followed by L-cysteine, 2-mercaptoethylamine, thioglycolate or cyanide at neutral pH, where pepsin is inactive (18,20,21). Pepsin alone caused a reduction in sedimentation coefficient ($s_{20,w}$) from about 7 to 5 (molecular weight 106 kDa (22)), but the antibody remained bivalent. Subsequent reduction caused a further decrease in $s_{20,w}$ to c.3.5, a loss of capacity to precipitate antigen, and acquisition of the ability to block specific precipitation of antigen by the intact rabbit antibody; all these properties corresponded to those of the Fab fragments released by papain. The precipitation-blocking activities of the two types of fragment were shown to be nearly identical on a quantitative basis, and the 3.5S fragments of an antihapten antibody retained hapten-binding activity equivalent to that of the parent γ-globulin molecules (20). Subsequent work showed that the portion of the molecule removed by pepsin corresponds to Porter's fragment III (the Fc fragment), which is partially degraded in the process and will, of course, no longer crystallize. It was determined that only a single disulphide bond links the two 3.5S fragments and that this bond is more readily reduced than any of the other disulphide bonds in the 5S molecule (21).

We found that the 3.5S fragments (later called Fab') liberated by pepsin and a reducing agent can be recombined in high yield, to again produce the 5S molecule, by reoxidation of an intersubunit disulphide bond after removal of reducing agent (22,23). Using affinity-purified antibodies, we observed that the reconstituted 5S molecules (c.100 kDa) were again able to form specific precipitates. This approach led to the first preparations of antibodies of dual specificity (hybrid antibodies), obtained by recombining a mixture of Fab' fragments derived from two affinity-purified rabbit antibodies, specific for ovalbumin and bovine IgG, respectively (24). The recombined 5S molecules failed to precipitate with either antigen alone, but gave a good precipitate when a mixture of the two antigens was used. The failure to precipitate an individual antigen, despite the statistical likelihood that part of the recombined product was bivalent, was attributed to the fact that hybrid antibodies are univalent with respect to either antigen and can therefore block precipitation. For random recombination the expected ratios are 1:2:1, with hybrid antibodies constituting 50% of the product. (Hybrid antibodies were later purified by successive absorption to, and elution from, two matrices, each containing one of the two antigens covalently bound.)

A visual demonstration of the existence of hybrid antibodies was carried out in collaboration with G. Drews and H. H. Fudenberg (25). We took advantage of the elongated appearance under the microscope of chicken erythrocytes (CRBC) as compared to human erythrocytes (HRBC). Bovine γ-globulin and hen ovalbumin were conjugated to CRBC and HRBC, respectively. A mixture of 5S molecules, prepared from affinity-purified antibodies and specific for each of the two protein antigens, agglutinated both types of RBC when added to a mixture; however, individual clusters observed under the microscope contained only CRBC or HRBC. In contrast, a hybridized 5S preparation yielded agglutinates in which each cluster contained both types of red cell.

In collaboration with Jerry Palmer and Richard Hong, we subsequently found that the disulphide bond joining the Fab' fragments in fact links two heavy chains and that it is the most labile S–S bond in the rabbit IgG molecule (26,27). When this bond is selectively reduced, the intact IgG molecule (not treated with enzyme) dissociates into two half-molecules, each containing one complete H and L chain, in saline at pH 2.5; no other dissociating reagent is required. Upon increasing the pH to neutrality, the two half-molecules reassociate to give a 7S product in high yield, with or without reoxidation of the disulphide bond (28). The reassociation occurs, through non-covalent interactions, even if the –SH groups formed upon reduction are blocked. This provides an alternative method for producing antibodies of dual specificity, that does not require enzymatic digestion (27,29). A by-product of the work was that it established the presence of a single interheavy chain disulphide bond in rabbit IgG, rather than three postulated by Porter on the basis that five S–S bonds can be reduced in the absence of a denaturing agent such as urea. The presence of a single interheavy chain disulphide bond was subsequently confirmed by amino acid sequence analysis (30).

The model proposed by Fleischman, Porter and Press, discussed above, shows the Fab fragments in contact with one another, linked only by disulphide bonds. The principal experimental evidence for such an arrangement was the separation of two Fab' fragments from F(ab')$_2$ upon mild reduction after peptic digestion.

Besides providing a source of hybrid antibodies, peptic digestion of anti-bodies of the IgG class has been used by many laboratories (31) because it pro-vides a means of removing the Fc fragment without altering the bivalence of the molecule. It therefore permits identification and study of effector functions that are localized to the Fc region. It was found, for example, that F(ab')$_2$ cannot fix complement, pass through the placenta or bind to Fc receptors. Hybrid anti-bodies have been tested experimentally as a means of targeting drugs to par-ticular tissues.

Idiotypes of Immunoglobulins

Investigations in my laboratory on the topic of idiotypy began in 1968, long after the concept had been established. As pointed out by Silverstein (32), the notion of idiotypy dates back to the work of Paul Ehrlich and others near the turn of the century. Systematic immunochemical studies on idiotype began in 1955 with the work on myeloma proteins of Slater, Ward and Kunkel at the Rockefeller Institute (33). Idiotypy in antibodies induced by immunization was first demonstrated in 1963 by Oudin and Michel (Pasteur Institute) in rabbit antisalmonella antibodies (34) and by Kunkel, Mannik and Williams in anti-bodies specific for human blood group A substance (35). The term 'idiotype' was coined by Jacques Oudin, who applied the designation exclusively to anti-bodies of a particular specificity induced on an individual animal and identified with an antiserum produced in another animal of the same species. The term was soon extended by general usage to include myeloma proteins, antibodies produced in different animals of the same inbred strain, T cell receptors, etc., without restriction on the source of the anti-idiotypic antibodies. This degeneration of his definition was not welcomed by Oudin, whose scientific opinions were not characterized by great flexibility. (This did not prevent him from making three major discoveries: on single-dimensional diffusion methods in agar gel, allotypes and idiotypes, respectively.) A convenient updated defini-tion of idiotype is the collection of idiotopes on an individual antibody molecule.

The structural basis of idiotypy became clear after the discovery of hyper-variable regions in immunoglobulins by Wu and Kabat in 1970 (36); it was immediately apparent that the enormous diversity of antibody specificities should be paralleled by a corresponding diversity of idiotypes.

Our interest in the subject arose from previous investigations on rabbit allo-types carried out in collaboration with the laboratory of Sheldon Dray (37,38). We had helped to establish certain principles of allotypy by applying quantita-tive immunochemical methods to allotype–antiallotype interactions and thought it might prove useful to apply similar methodology to the study of idio-types.

From the standpoint of the timeliness of our research, it is relevant that in

1968 many of the applications of idiotypy remained to be identified, despite the fact that the phenomenon itself had been clearly defined in 1955. As a subject for research, idiotypy was slow to capture the attention of immunologists. A major increase in the amount of research began around 1970, 15 years after the appearance of Kunkel's paper on myeloma proteins. The probable reason for the revived interest was the identification or better understanding of potential applications of research on idiotypy. I will briefly outline some of these applications and our own related research. Discussion of the important contributions of many investigators is necessarily omitted from this brief memoir.

Idiotype as a phenotypic marker for B cell clones

In collaboration with Bruce MacDonald we used idiotype as a marker to investigate the persistence in rabbits of clones of cells producing anti-*p*-azobenzoate antibodies. During prolonged immunization, the same idiotypes, and presumably therefore the same B cell clones, were shown to persist for more than 8 months (*39*). Similar findings were reported by Oudin and Michel (*40*), who used *Salmonella* as the immunogen. In some rabbits we found that the idiotypes initially present were replaced after a few months by new idiotypes, associated with higher affinity for benzoate, that persisted for longer than one year with continued immunization (*41*). Such investigations illustrate the usefulness of idiotype as a clonal marker for examining the fate of B cell and, eventually, T cell clones. We later used idiotype as a marker to demonstrate the dominance of secondary B cell clones in an immunized animal; that is, the inhibition of expression of new, primary clones upon antigenic stimulation, caused by the presence of established secondary B cells of the same specificity (*42*). (A possible explanation is that the secondary cells, being more numerous and of higher affinity, compete successfully for the antigen.)

Recurrent (cross-reactive) idiotypes

The repeated occurrence of the same idiotype in immunoglobulins of the same specificity from different individuals was first reported in 1968 by Williams, Kunkel and Capra (*43*), who showed that cold agglutinins from different patients frequently shared some (generally not all) idiotopes. The presence of recurrent idiotypes in antibodies of inbred mice was first reported by Cohn, Notani and Rice (*44*). Soon afterwards, Eichmann and Kindt found that some members of a partially inbred family of rabbits produced antibodies to a streptococcal carbohydrate that shared some idiotopes (*45*). Our own work on recurrent or cross-reactive idiotypes began with the observation that all adult mice of the A strain produce antibodies to the *p*-azobenzene arsonate (Ars) hapten that share idiotype; in general, 20–70% of the antibody population expresses the cross-reactive idiotype, now designated CRI_A (*46,47*). The postulate (*46,48*) that recurrent idiotypes are associated with germline genes has been confirmed for numerous idiotypes. In the case of CRI_A single V_H and V_L germline genes were shown by Siekevitz et al. (49) and Sanz and Capra (50), respectively, to encode molecules expressing the idiotype. However, nearly all Id-positive monoclonal antibodies, obtained after immunization with the Ars hapten, exhibit somatic mutations (51,52) and higher affinities (53,54) than the germline product. Thus, some mutations can be tolerated without disruption of the idiotype. This question was later investigated systematically for CRI_A by Jacqueline Sharon and collaborators, using site-directed mutagenesis (55,56). Extensive studies on such questions have been carried out with other idiotypes as well. Those of Cesar Milstein, Claudia Berek and their collaborators on murine antibodies to phenyloxazolone have been particularly informative (57–59). Antibodies expressing cross-reactive idiotypes have thus provided a useful frame of reference for studying V gene families, somatic mutation and affinity maturation.

Immunological suppression of idiotypes

This topic is related to Niels Jerne's idiotype network theory (60), which has attracted a great deal of attention. The existence of recurrent idiotypes facilitated studies on idiotype suppression induced by administration of anti-Id antibodies to an inbred mouse before immunization with the relevant antigen. The possibility of immunological suppression of an idiotype was suggested by the earlier work of Rose Mage and Sheldon Dray on allotype suppression (61). We demonstrated long-term in vivo suppression of CRI_A by anti-Id in collaboration with David Hart, Ai-Lan Wang and Laura Pawlak (62). At about the same time, Cosenza and Kohler reported on suppression in vitro of an idiotype associated with antibodies to phosphorylcholine in BALB/c mice (63). In vivo suppression of the latter idiotype was later reported by Strayer et al. (64).

The suppression of idiotype expression by anti-Id is of course a central facet of Jerne's idiotype network hypothesis of regulation of antibody synthesis (60). This hypothesis has been the basis of endless discussion and many experiments. It was inevitable that it should receive serious attention because of the ingenuity of the hypothesis, the persuasiveness and accomplishments of Niels Jerne, and his personal contacts with investigators from around the world in his capacity as Director of the Basel Institute of Immunology. Nevertheless, the importance of idiotype regulation in the normal immune response to an antigen remains controversial, probably owing to a paucity of quantitative supporting data. There is better support for the possibility that regulation mediated by idiotypes in the neonate may play a role in the development of the adult repertoire of B cells (65,66).

An idiotope as an 'internal image' of the epitope of an antigen

A more fruitful part of Jerne's hypothesis was his suggestion that a segment of an anti-Id antibody might sometimes mimic structurally the epitope of an antigen, that is, express an 'internal image' of the antigen. There is now good evidence (summarized in reviews (67–69)) that this can occur, and the concept has led, for example, to the identification of anti-Id antibodies (anti-anti-X) which can react with cellular receptors for X, a finding consistent with a resemblance of the anti-Id to X. Our contribution to this area of research includes the proposal, made in 1981 in collaboration with Edmundo Lamoyi (70), that anti-Id antibodies might be used as vaccines. A similar suggestion was put forward at about the same time by Ivan Roitt and his collaborators (71). In collaboration with Michael Gurish, we used anti-Id antibodies to generate antibodies to pseudorabies virus in mice (72). Many such studies have been carried out with experimental animals (see the reviews in (67–69)). Clinical investigations are in progress, by the IDEC Corporation and by S. Ferrone and his colleagues (73), in which anti-Id antibodies are being used in an effort to cause tumour regression in human melanoma. The original antigen, X, is a proteoglycan of high molecular weight present on the surface of most human melanoma cells. Despite a great deal of research and promising results in experimental animals, it is still an open question whether anti-idiotypes will ultimately prove useful as human vaccines.

I should emphasize the obvious: that the brief bibliography which follows does not begin to cover all the relevant papers. In the case of idiotypy, some of its numerous applications have not been discussed.

Notes and References

1. R. R. Porter, *Biochem. J.* **46**, 479 (1950).
2. H. N. Eisen and F. Karush, *J. Am. Chem. Soc.* **71**, 363 (1949).
3. J. R. Kimmel and E. L. Smith, *J. Biol. Chem.* **207**, 515 (1954).
4. R. R. Porter, *Nature* **182**, 670 (1958).
5. R. R. Porter, *Biochem J.* **73**, 119 (1959).
6. G. M. Edelman, *J. Am. Chem. Soc.* **81**, 3155 (1959).
7. G. M. Edelman and M. D. Poulik, *J. Exp. Med.* **113**, 861 (1961).
8. M. D. Poulik and G. M. Edelman, *Nature* **191**, 1274 (1961).
9. G. M. Edelman and J. A. Gally, *J. Exp. Med.* **116**, 207 (1962).
10. N. Hilschmann and L. C. Craig, *Proc. Natl. Acad. Sci. USA* **53**, 1403 (1965).
11. K. Titani, E. Whitley, L. Avogardo and F. W. Putnam, *Science* **149**, 1090 (1965).
12. J. B. Fleischman, R. H. Pain and R. R. Porter, *Arch. Biochem. Biophys.* (Suppl. 1), 174 (1962).
13. R. R. Porter, in *Symposium on Basic Problems in Neoplastic Disease*, Columbia University Press, New York, (1962), p. 20.
14. J. B. Fleischman, R. R. Porter and E. M. Press, *Biochem. J.* **88**, 220 (1963).
15. R. H. Pain, *Biochem. J.* **88**, 234 (1963).
16. A. Nisonoff and D. L. Woernley, *Nature* **183**, 1325 (1959).
17. A. Nisonoff, F. C. Wissler and D. L. Woernley, *Arch. Biochem. Biophys.* **88**, 241 (1960).
18. A. Nisonoff, F. C. Wissler and D. L. Woernley, *Biochem. Biophys. Res. Commun.*, **1**, 318 (1959).
19. F. P. Inman and A. Nisonoff, *J. Biol. Chem.* **241**, 322 (1966).
20. A. Nisonoff, F. C. Wissler, L. N. Lipman and D. L. Woernley, *Arch. Biochem. Biophys.* **89**, 230 (1960).

21. A. Nisonoff, G. Markus and F. C. Wissler, *Nature*, **189**, 293 (1961).
22. A. Nisonoff, *Biochem. Biophys. Res. Commun.* **3**, 466 (1960).
23. W. J. Mandy, M. M. Rivers and A. Nisonoff, *J. Biol. Chem.* **236**, 3221 (1961).
24. A. Nisonoff and M. M. Rivers, *Arch. Biochem. Biophys.* **93**, 460 (1961).
25. H. H. Fudenberg, G. Drews and A. Nisonoff, *J. Exp. Med.* **119**, 151 (1964).
26. J. L. Palmer and A. Nisonoff, *Biochemistry* **3**, 863 (1964).
27. R. Hong, J. L. Palmer and A. Nisonoff, *J. Immunol.* **94**, 603 (1965).
28. S. R. Stein, J. L. Palmer and A. Nisonoff, *J. Biol. Chem.* **239**, 2872 (1964).
29. A. Nisonoff and J. L. Palmer, *Science* **143**, 376 (1964).
30. I. J. O'Donnell, B. Frangione and R. R. Porter, *Biochem. J.* **116**, 261 (1970).
31. A. Nisonoff, *Current Contents* **24**, 25 (1970).
32. A. M. Silverstein, in *A History of Immunology*, Academic Press, New York (1988), chap. 10.
33. R. J. Slater, S. M. Ward and H. G. Kunkel, *J. Exp. Med.* **101**, 85 (1955).
34. J. Oudin and M. Michel, *C.R. Acad. Sci. Paris* **257**, 805 (1963).
35. H. G. Kunkel, M. Mannik and R. C. Williams, *Science* **140**, 1218 (1963).
36. T. T. Wu and E. A. Kabat, *J. Exp. Med.* **132**, 211 (1970).
37. S. Dray, G. O. Young and A. Nisonoff, *Nature* **199**, 52 (1963).
38. S. Dray and A. Nisonoff, *Proc. Soc. Exp. Biol. Med.* **113**, 20 (1963).
39. A. B. MacDonald, L. Alescio and A. Nisonoff, *Biochemistry* **8**, 3109 (1969).
40. J. Oudin and M. Michel, *J. Exp. Med.* **130**, 619 (1969).
41. A. B. MacDonald and A. Nisonoff, *J. Exp. Med.* **131**, 583 (1970).
42. B. M. Eig, S.-T. Ju and A. Nisonoff, *J. Exp. Med.* **146**, 1574 (1977).
43. R. C. Williams, H. G. Kunkel and J. D. Capra, *Science* **161**, 379 (1968).
44. M. Cohn, G. Notani and S. A. Rice, *Immunochemistry* **6**, 111 (1969).
45. K. Eichmann and T. J. Kindt, *J. Exp. Med.* **134**, 532 (1971).
46. M. G. Kuettner, A. L. Wang and A. Nisonoff, *J. Exp. Med.* **135**, 579 (1972).
47. M. I. Greene, M. J. Nelles, M.-S. Sy and A. Nisonoff, *Adv. Immunol.* **32**, 253 (1982).
48. B. Blomberg, W. Geckeler and M. G. Weigert, *Science* **177**, 178 (1972).
49. M. Siekevitz, S. Y. Huang and M. L. Gefter, *Eur. J. Immunol.* **13**, 123 (1983).
50. I. Sanz and J. D. Capra, *Proc. Natl Acad. Sci. USA* **84**, 1085 (1987).
51. G. Rathbun, I. Sanz, K. Meek, P. Tucker and J. D. Capra, *Adv. Immunol.* **42**, 95 (1988).
52. T. Manser, L. J. Wysocki, M. N. Margolies and M. L. Gefter, *Immunol. Rev.* **96**, 141 (1987).
53. T. F. Kresina, S. M. Rosen and A. Nisonoff, *Mol. Immunol.* **19**, 1433 (1982).
54. T. Rothstein and M. L. Gefter, *Mol. Immunol.* **20**, 161 (1983).
55. J. Sharon, *J. Immunol.* **144**, 4863 (1990).
56. A. Nisonoff, T. M. Oliveira and J. Sharon, *Int. Immunol.* **5**, 1 (1993).
57. C. Berek, G. M. Griffiths and C. Milstein, *Nature* **316**, 412 (1985).
58. C. Berek and C. Milstein, *Immunol. Rev.* **96**, 23 (1987).
59. C. Rada, S. K. Gupta, E. Gherardi and C. Milstein, *Proc. Natl Acad. Sci. USA*, **88**, 5508 (1991).
60. N. K. Jerne, *Ann. Inst. Pasteur (Paris)* **125C**, 373 (1974).
61. R. Mage and S. Dray, *J. Immunol.* **95**, 525 (1965).
62. D. A. Hart, A. L. Wang, L. L. Pawlak and A. Nisonoff, *J. Exp. Med.* **135**, 1293 (1972).
63. H. Cosenza and H. Kohler, *Proc. Natl Acad. Sci. USA* **69**, 2701 (1972).
64. D. S. Strayer, W. M. F. Lee, D. A. Rowley and H. Kohler, *J. Immunol.* **114**, 728 (1975).
65. J. F. Kearney, M. Vakil and N. Solvason, *Cold Spring Harbor Symp. Quant. Biol.* **52**, 203 (1989).
66. C. Victor, C. Bona and B. Pernis, *Ann. NY Acad. Sci.* **428**, 220 (1983).
67. T. Kieber-Emmons, R. E. Ward, S. Raychaudhuri, R. Rein and H. Kohler, *Int. Rev. Immunol.* **1**, 1 (1986).
68. R. L. Mernaugh, R. K. Bright and R. C. Kennedy, *Biotechnology* **20**, 391 (1992).
69. A. Nisonoff, *J. Immunol.* **147**, 2429 (1991).
70. A. Nisonoff and E. Lamoyi, *Clin. Immunol. Immunopathol.* **21**, 397 (1981).

71. I. M. Roitt, D. K. Mal, G. Guarnotta, L. D. de Carralho, A. Cooke, F. C. Hay, P. M. Lydyard, Y. M. Thanavala and J. Ivanyi. *Lancet* i, 1041 (1981).
72. M. Gurish, T. Ben-Porat and A. Nisonoff, *Ann. Inst. Pasteur/Immunol.* **139**, 677 (1988).
73. A. Mittelman, Z. J. Chen, H. Yang, G. Y. Wong and S. Ferrone, *Proc. Natl Acad. Sci. USA* **89**, 466 (1992).

The Contribution of the Cytokine Concept to Immunology

BYRON H. WAKSMAN
New York University Medical Center, and Center for Neurological Diseases, Harvard Medical Center, New York, USA

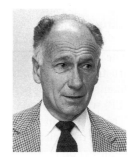

JOOST J. OPPENHEIM
Laboratory of Molecular Immunoregulation, Biological Response Modifiers Program, Division of Cancer Treatment, National Cancer Institute – Frederick Cancer Research and Development Center, Frederick, MD 21702–1201, USA

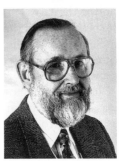

Although the field of cytokines is a popular subdiscipline of immunology today, for a considerable period the study of these non-specific mediators was not accepted by immunologists as worthwhile. The cytokine field is broader in scope than most other subdisciplines of immunology. Its origins are to be found in diverse areas of biology, and many cytokines of current interest to immunologists are also important in developmental biology or have a unique role in specialized organ systems bearing no visible relation to immunology. Cytokines are secreted proteins of 6–30 kDa that function as immunologically non-specific intercellular signals. In contrast with hormones, cytokines usually act over short distances only, in local tissues as bidirectional messengers between leucocytes and somatic cells. Cytokines contribute to the regulation of cell growth and differentiation and to immunologically dependent, as well as independent, inflammatory and repair processes. The diversity in activities of these non-specific mediators delayed their acceptance by immunologists based on the long-term conviction that only reactions between antigenic epitopes and specific combining sites, whether of antibody or of T cells, could be regarded as

IMMUNOLOGY: THE MAKING OF A MODERN SCIENCE
ISBN 0-12-274020-3

properly immunological. However, cellular immunologists who were also interested in the non-specific biological consequences of specific reactions, for example inflammation, killing of 'target' cells, and other aspects of host defence, appreciated the vital role of cytokines.

Early Studies

The attempt to identify a precise starting point of the cytokine field is inevitably frustrating, since individual entities were described and studied at widely different times long before there could be said to be a field. Endogenous pyrogen (EP) was described in 1953 by Bennett and Beeson (1) and the group of interferons (IFN) in 1957 by Isaacs and Lindenmann (2). Yet the correct identification of the cells producing EP by Atkins et al. (3) and the discovery that IFN could act on lymphoid cells by Blomgren et al. (4) and Gisler et al. (5) took place only in the early 1970s. Nerve growth factor (NGF) was also described in 1953 (6). Like EP and the IFNs, NGF became the subject of an immediate growth industry, yet the discovery that NGF could act on B cells and was therefore a cytokine of interest to immunologists had to wait more than a quarter of a century (7).

In most immunologists' minds, the real starting point of the cytokine field was the description of three factors in rapid succession between 1965 and 1967, all produced by lymphocytes responding to an antigenic stimulus: a lymphocyte mitogenic/blastogenic factor (LMF/BF) (8), migration inhibitory factor (MIF) (9,10), and lymphotoxin (LT) (11,12). These discoveries were an inevitable consequence of the new interest in lymphocytes as the principal players in a variety of immune responses (13) and the development of techniques for their in vitro culture (14). These observations led to the convening of pivotal symposia by Lawrence and Landy (15), Stetson (16) and Bloom and Glade (17), and the publication of authoritative reviews by Bloom (18), David and David (19), Atkins and Bodel (20) and Becker and Henson (21).

The MIF and LT discoveries were, however, rooted in a biological discovery made four decades earlier. Rich and Lewis (22) first reported inhibition of cell migration and actual killing of cells (macrophages and fibroblasts) from tuberculin-sensitized guinea-pigs, when these were exposed to tuberculoprotein in explant cultures of spleen or lymph node. Rich (23) made these phenomena the basis of a theory of tuberculin sensitivity/infectious allergy which dominated immunologic thinking in the immediate pre- and post-World War II period.

Rich interpreted his own results as showing that tuberculin sensitivity inevitably resulted in damage or death of sensitive tissues or cells exposed to antigen. However, subsequent studies proved this view to be incorrect because macrophages with intracellular organisms could be shown to survive. Lurie, in

1942 (24), observed that macrophages from tuberculin-sensitized rabbits exhibited an enhanced ability to inhibit the growth of intracellular tubercle bacilli. Suter (25) and Mackaness (26) showed that the activated macrophages from tuberculous animals inhibited the growth of intracellular tubercle bacilli and, coincidentally, other intracellular organisms, such as *Listeria*, as well. Waksman and Matoltsy (27), working for the first time with dispersed cells *in vitro*, added the finding that cultured peritoneal monocytes (containing some contaminating lymphocytes) from sensitized guinea-pigs were 'activated' by the addition of specific antigen. This finding was followed after more than a decade by the definitive demonstration that a macrophage-activating factor (MAF), which, like MIF, was an antigen-induced product of sensitized lymphocytes, was responsible for the macrophage activation (28). This MAF activity, although induced by antigen-stimulated lymphocytes, was shown by Nathan *et al.* (29) to be a non-specific cytokine that acted independently of antigens and antibodies.

Soluble Factors take Centre-stage

The observations that activation of macrophages by soluble cytokines such as MAF or IFN provided the basis for acquired non-specific immunity to infectious organisms shattered the concept that the only major product of antigen-stimulated lymphocytes accounting for host defence consisted of specific antibodies. Macrophage activation by MAF incidentally provided the first demonstration of two concepts which prevail in the cytokine field: first, antigen-specific triggering of an effect which is itself non-specific; and, second, the joint action of two cells communicating and co-operating to fulfil a single biological function.

The studies of cell migration in clotted plasma initiated by Rich also stimulated interest in chemotactic factors influencing the mobilization of leucocytes. Boyden's invention (30) in 1962 of dual-chamber assays of directional migration of cells through porous filters provided the first, sensitive and reproducible method of assessing chemotaxis. This enabled Ward and colleagues (31) to show that antigen-stimulated leucocytes secreted factors that were chemotactic for monocytes.

Furthermore, Rich's observation that explanted cells died when exposed to tuberculoproteins anticipated the discovery of lymphocyte-derived cytotoxic factors. In 1967, Ruddle and Waksman (11), in a study of delayed hypersensitivity, found that sensitized lymphocytes triggered by specific antigen released a factor that killed syngeneic fibroblasts. Granger and Williams (12), almost simultaneously, showed that mitogen-activated spleen cells produced a similar soluble factor which they called 'LT' (lymphotoxin).

The reports of *in vitro* lymphocyte blastogenesis in response to polyclonal stimulants initiated by Nowell (14) motivated Kasakura and Lowenstein (8) to search for mitogenic factors. They were the first to detect lymphocyte-derived blastogenic factors (BF) in the supernatants of mixed allogeneic leucocyte culture. They considered these BF to consist predominantly of major histocompatibility complex (MHC)-unrestricted non-specific lymphocyte mitogenic factors (LMF). They also reported detecting minor 'specific' mitogenic activities and a number of prominent immunologists, who disdained the non-specific cytokines, took up this theme and reported finding antigen-specific helper and suppressor factors in the 1970s and early 1980s. However, these specific factors could never be purified and their molecular structure was never defined. Studies of non-specific LMF led Dumonde and his colleagues in 1969 (32) unilaterally to coin the term 'lymphokines' for the recently described family of lymphocyte-derived mediators. This attention-getting term galvanized the interest of additional immunologists in these intercellular lymphocyte signals.

Many immunologists were surprised to see fever become legitimized as a participant in immunological processes. Yet the first real cytokine activity to be detected was EP (endogenous pyrogen) (33,34). Atkins has traced the concept of a pyrogenic molecule, produced by leucocytes in response to microbes or their products and acting on subcortical centres in the brain, to William Welch at Johns Hopkins, as early as 1888. This idea was first taken up experimentally during World War II by Menkin (35), who carried out a series of studies on various factors derived from inflammatory exudates and was able to purify and crystallize a fever-inducing principle which he called 'pyrexin'. This substance was later shown to be contaminated with bacterial pyrogen. Bennett and Beeson (1), using care to eliminate contaminating bacterial components, reported the presence of a heat-labile pyrogen in acute inflammatory exudates, as well as in saline extracts of disrupted blood leucocytes and from dermal sites of inflammation. An identical pyrogen was shown to be released by macrophages under the influence of sensitized T lymphocytes exposed to antigen (3) and it ultimately became clear that monocytes were a major source of EP in the leucocyte population studied by earlier workers (34).

In an entirely independent but convergent line of research, Gery (36,37) during a sabbatical year in the laboratories of Waksman and Gershon, demonstrated that activated macrophages released a substance stimulatory for thymocytes. Gery called his factor LAF (lymphocyte activating factor); soon after, it was rechristened TAF (T cell activating factor) to distinguish it from the various factors found to act on B cells (as reviewed by Oppenheim and Gery (38). LAF's ability to augment T cell responses to antigen led to the inference that, even though it was macrophage derived, LAF might play an important role in augmenting specific immune responses. Based on similarities in the biological and biochemical properties of LAF and EP, Rosenwasser and Dinarello, the latter a former student of Atkins, proposed the co-identity of these two cytokines (39).

The discovery of tumour necrosis factor (TNF) also illustrates the convergence of unrelated lines of research resulting in the identification of related or identical molecules exhibiting entirely different functional roles (40,41). Almost a decade after the description of lymphotoxin, Lloyd Old and his colleages (42) described a toxic molecule produced by macrophages of BCG-primed mice stimulated with endotoxin. This factor was cytotoxic for certain types of tumour cells and, accordingly, was named TNF. Old traced the discovery of TNF to Coley's use of killed bacteria, notably *Streptococcus pyogenes* and *Serratia marcescens*, as a cancer therapy in some patients as early as 1893. The effective principle in Gram-negative bacterial filtrates ('Coley's toxins') proved ultimately to be lipopolysaccharide endotoxin. Independently, Kawakami and Cerami (43) succeeded in identifying a molecule responsible for wasting in parasitized cattle, which they named 'cachectin'. Cachectin was produced by stimulated macrophages, acted by suppressing lipoprotein lipase in adipocytes, and had the effect of preventing triglyceride clearance. It was not until 1984 that the identity of Ruddle's and Granger's forms of LT was established by Gray *et al.* (44) and of TNF and cachectin by Pennica and her collaborators (45). Concomitantly, Aggarwal (from the same group) reported that TNF and LT use the same binding site, thus justifying the renaming of LT as TNF-β (40).

The Era of Cytokines

Cohen was the first to observe that MIF-like activities could be produced by a variety of non-lymphocytic cell lines. That observation and the detection of macrophage-derived 'monokines' such as LAF led him to propose the more inclusive term 'cytokines' for the family of secreted proteins involved in immunologically mediated inflammatory reactions (46). The term 'cytokine' as used in contemporary immunological research refers to soluble extracellular proteins or glycoproteins that participate in non-specific as well as immunologically dependent inflammatory reactions, cell growth, differentiation, development and repair processes contributing to host defence.

In 1976, the first of a series of International Lymphokine Workshops was convened at a Bethesda Country Club by Cohen, Landy and Oppenheim. By the time of the second meeting, the descriptive phase of cytokine research peaked with the publication of a review by Waksman listing almost 100 apparently distinct biological cytokine activities (47). At this second meeting, held in Ermatingen, Switzerland, in 1979, the initial results obtained with newer techniques for characterizing the biological and biochemical properties of partially purified cytokine molecules fostered the mistaken belief that most cytokine activities could be attributed to only a few molecules and culminated in their renaming as either interleukin 1 or 2 (38). This idea thus led to the substitution of a more neutral interleukin terminology for the numerous assay-oriented and confusing acronyms. Accordingly, a number of immunologists proposed that LAF, BAF and TAF be renamed interleukin 1 (IL-1) and that BF/LMF otherwise also known as T cell growth factor (TCGF) be renamed IL-2. Following considerable controversy this nomenclature was grudgingly accepted, and we are now into the mid-teens! A number of the other cytokines, among them TNF-α, LT (now also known as TNF-β), the IFNs and colony stimulating factors (CSF) escaped being renamed. The initial intent to restrict the interleukin terminology to immunologically targeted lymphokines was very short-lived with the naming of IL-3 by Ihle (48), a lymphokine that acts predominantly as a growth factor for haematopoietic progenitor cells.

Nomenclature continues to present a problem. A subcommittee of the IUIS–WHO nomenclature committee, in 1986, stated two straightforward principles: 'The historical or common usage name of a particular activity can, and should, be retained so as to ensure historical credit where appropriate and to avoid confusion as to which entity is which'; and 'The primary amino acid sequence [is] essential, since this [is] the only information that distinguishes between distinct but highly homogenous molecules' (49). Less than two years later Paul (50), representing the same official body, while inviting suggestions for nomenclature of 'lymphohaematopoietic regulatory proteins', recommended the interim use of the name proposed by those studying a given entity (until exact characterization of the molecule) and recommended that the interleukin nomenclature *not* be continued, but that scientists instead devise other meaningful terms that would be easier to remember than a countless number of interleukins.

The molecular era may be said to have begun soon after the Ermatingen meeting, with the development of newer technologies such as high performance liquid chromatography, microsequencing and the production of monoclonal antibodies to cytokines. This permitted the purification and amino acid sequencing of the minuscule quantities of the more common cytokine activities that could be isolated from culture supernatants. Application of molecular biology further revolutionized studies of cytokines by making available larger quantities of cloned and expressed pure recombinant cytokines. In retrospect, those immunologists on peer review committees who, in the 1970s, refused to fund studies of cytokines as being too phenomenological, failed to anticipate that such studies would provide the necessary bioassays for detecting and identifying the functional activities of purified and recombinant cytokines. The application of molecular technologies has led to the discovery of numerous new cytokines and has modified our concepts concerning the spectrum of activities ascribed to previously described cytokines. The molecular era was initiated in 1980 with the cloning of IFN-α$_1$ by Nagata and coworkers in the laboratory of Weissman (51) and of IFN-β$_1$ which was first cloned by Taniguchi and his colleagues (52). (By now, about 16–20 variants of IFN-α have been identified which interact with the same cell surface receptor and promote antiviral resistance.) This was followed by the cloning of IFN-γ by Gray and colleagues (53). IFN-γ is a potent activator of macrophages and acts in part by inducing the expression of adhesion proteins; therefore, IFN-γ exhibits MIF as well as MAF activity. It is appropriate to note here that David and his colleagues, in an admirable display of scientific persistence, pursued the identification of a less pleiotropic MIF activity and have succeeded in cloning and expressing another molecule which has MIF (as well as MAF) activity, if used as a co-stimulant with phytohaemagglutinin (54).

The following year, 1983, saw the cloning of IL-2 by Taniguchi and collaborators (55). Availability of the recombinant form of IL-2 enabled many investigators to confirm that this cytokine is a major lymphoproliferative cytokine for T, B and NK cells. IL-2 also enhances the activities of lymphoid cells indirectly by inducing the production of a variety of other immunostimulating cytokines such as IFN-γ, TNF and IL-1. Additional lymphoproliferative factors, such as IL-4, IL-6, IL-7, IL-9, IL-10 and IL-12, have since been identified. In 1984 the first of three chains in the IL-2 receptor, IL-2Rα was cloned by Leonard and colleagues (56). These observations were presented at the 4th International Lymphokine Workshop held in 1984 at Schloss Elmau, Germany. One also learned there of the cloning of the first haematopoietic growth factor, IL-3 (multi-CSF), by the laboratory of Young in Australia (57). This was followed by the cloning of GM-CSF by another Australian team led by Gough (58), of M-CSF by Kawasaki et al. (59) and of G-CSF by Souza et al. (60), and, independently, Nakata et al. (61). The 1984 meeting also was the scene of an unanticipated and instructive controversy concerning IL-1. The nucleotide sequence for a 31 kDa molecule, said to be a precursor of IL-1 with IL-1 activity, was reported by Auron and Dinarello (62). Henney and colleagues had cloned the same molecule previously and discarded it because it appeared to be inactive. It later became clear that this molecule is an inactive precursor that is cleaved by an IL-1-converting enzyme to yield the active 17 kDa form of IL-1β. Another team led by Lomedico (63) had cloned another 31 kDa precursor with IL-1 activity which was named IL-1α. When this molecule is cleaved, it yields an active 17 kDa IL-1α that exhibited only 28% homology in amino acid sequence to IL-1β. IL-1α and IL-1β each use the same two receptors and exhibit an enormous range of identical biological activities. Both are produced by most nucleated cell types and act on almost every tissue in the body. They are, however, not unique in having a multiplicity of biological effects, since TNF-α is similarly pleiotrophic. Although TNF uses receptors distinct from those of IL-1, it has many activities that overlap those of IL-1 and acts synergistically with IL-1. For example, it is now clear that since both IL-1 and TNF induce fever, EP activity is attributable not only to IL-1, but can also be ascribed to TNF, as well as IFN and IL-6, all of which are pyrogenic (as reviewed by Dinarello (64)).

During 1984 the two cytotoxic factors, LT (TNF-β) by Pennica (45) and TNF (designated TNF-α) by Gray (44), were also cloned and expressed. TNF-α and TNF-β are encoded at adjacent sites on the same chromosome within the MHC. These cytotoxins showed only 28% homology in their amino acid sequences, but nevertheless use the same receptor binding sites. The first of the cytokines which proved subsequently to have potent non-specific immunosuppressive and anti-inflammatory effects, namely transforming growth factor β (TGF-β), was identified and cloned the following year by Derynck et al. (65). This was followed by the recognition that other cytokines, such as IL-4 and IL-10, have negative regulatory effects.

In the mid-1980s, Leonard and Oppenheim became aware that the neutrophil and monocyte chemotactic activities previously detected in partially purified preparations of IL-1 were absent from purified recombinant preparations of IL-1 and, therefore, might be due to novel cytokines contaminating the partially purified preparations of natural IL-1. Yoshimura and colleagues (66) then proceeded to isolate and purify these 'contaminant' chemoattractant cytokines, and this culminated in the cloning of a monocyte-derived neutrophil chemotactic factor (MDNCF), otherwise known as neutrophil attracting protein 1 (NAP 1), by Matsushima et al. (67). Retrospectively, it was realized that the gene and sequence for MDNCF had been previously identified by gene cloning techniques by Schmidt and Weissman (68). This represents one of the first examples of molecular phenomonology; the identification of proteins without a function. Although cytokine-like molecules and receptors are being first identified with ever-increasing frequency by gene cloning approaches, the pathophysiological relevance of these peptides remains in abeyance until cellular immunologists identify some of their functions. MDNCF subsequently was observed to chemoattract T lymphocytes as well as neutrophils and accordingly was renamed IL-8 (69). This molecule has proven to be a member of a superfamily containing over 14 distinct structurally related chemoattractants acting on every inflammatory cell type. These chemoattractant cytokines are now called 'chemokines'. They regulate the adhesion of leucocytes to endothelial cells, diapedesis and migration of infiltrating leucocytes into inflammatory sites.

It is beyond the scope of this historical review to discuss the cloning of the IL-6 family (70,71), or of the many other cytokines acting on T and B cells. The cloning of cytokine receptors initiated by Leonard with the IL-2Rα (56) initiated studies of the nature of other cytokine–receptor interactions and of the mechanisms of cytokine-induced signal transduction pathways. The development of homologous recombination technology has enabled molecular biologists to develop knock-out mice deficient in selected cytokine or other receptors. This development, ironically, has led molecular biologists back into the animal room and has yielded new and unexpected findings concerning the actual pathophysiological roles of a number of the cytokines. Particularly striking has been the resultant demonstration of a high degree of redundancy of some of the cytokines. Nature seems to have provided compensatory alternative mediators for many of the cytokine functions engaged in host defence processes. These results will occupy us in the 1990s and provide wonderful material for future histories.

A Burgeoning Discipline

At the cytokine and lymphokine workshops, convened annually since 1984, an ever-increasing number of cytokines and receptor molecules have appeared on the immunological stage. These meetings have galvanized the rapid progress in cytokine research and culminated in the founding of the International Cytokine Society in 1993. An ever-increasing number of scientists, more than it was possible to credit in this review, have contributed to the extraordinary progress in cytokine studies from the phenomenological to the molecular stage over the past three decades. The workshops have conveyed many new principles, including recognition of the intimate and overlapping interactions among intercellular signals that marshall non-specific inflammatory and specific immunological responses in host defence and repair processes. It has become clear that cytokines generated in the course of immunological reactions exert a profound influence on such non-immunological processes as haematopoiesis, tissue repair, and the neuroendocrine systems. Indeed, cytokine-like growth factors such as TGF-β and PDGF play major roles in development and, in addition, contribute to the regulation of immune functions. Cytokines provide the intercellular communication links between the immune system and other tissues and organs. The field of cytokines has been enthusiastically adopted by biotechnology companies and is in the forefront of clinical applications of immunology. Thus, the study of cytokines has helped to propel immunology from the limited arena of immunological specificity to larger concerns of the cell biology, biochemical, molecular and clinical aspects of host defence.

Notes and References

1. I. L. Bennett, Jr and P. B. Beeson, *J. Exp. Med.* **98**, 493 (1953).
2. A. Isaacs and J. Lindenmann, *Proc. R. Soc. London, Ser. B* **147**, 258 (1957).
3. E. Atkins, J. D. Feldman, L. Francis and E. Hursh, *J. Exp. Med.* **135**, 1113 (1972).
4. H. Blomgren, H. Strander and K. Cantell, *Scand. J. Immunol.* **3**, 697 (1974).
5. R. H. Gisler, P. Lindahl and I. Gresser, *J. Immunol*, **113**, 438 (1974).
6. R. Levi-Montalcini and V. Hamburger, *J. Exp. Zool.* **123**, 233 (1953).
7. U. Otten, P. Ehrhard and R. Peck, *Proc. Natl Acad. Sci. USA* **86**, 10 (1989).
8. S. Kasakura and L. Lowenstein, *Nature* **208**, 794 (1965).
9. B. R. Bloom and B. Bennett, *Science* **153**, 80 (1966).
10. J. R. David, *Proc. Natl Acad. Sci. USA* **56**, 73 (1966).
11. N. H. Ruddle and B. H. Waksman, *Science* **157**, 1060 (1967).
12. G. A. Granger and T. W. Williams, *Nature* **218**, 1253 (1968).
13. J. L. Gowans, *J. Physiol.* **146**, 54 (1959).
14. P. C. Nowell, *Cancer Res.* **20**, 462 (1960).
15. H. S. Lawrence and M. Landy, *Mediators of Cellular Immunity*, Academic Press, New York, (1969).
16. C. A. Stetson, *Am. J. Pathol.* **60**, 435 (1970).
17. B. R. Bloom and P. R. Glade, *In vitro Methods in Cell-Mediated Immunity*, Academic Press, New York (1971).

18. B. R. Bloom, *Adv. Immunol.* **13**, 102 (1971).
19. J. R. David and R. A. David, *Prog. Allergy* **16**, 300 (1972).
20. E. Atkins and P. Bodel, *New Engl. J. Med.* **286**, 27 (1972).
21. E. L. Becker and P. M. Henson, *Adv. Immunol.* **17**, 93 (1973).
22. A. R. Rich and M. R. Lewis, *Proc. Soc. Exp. Biol. Med.* **25**, 596 (1927–1928).
23. A. R. Rich, *The Pathogenesis of Tuberculosis*, 2nd edn, Charles C. Thomas, Springfield, IL (1941).
24. M. B. Lurie, *J. Exp. Med.* **75**, 247 (1942).
25. E. Suter, *J. Exp. Med.* **97**, 235 (1953).
26. G. B. Mackaness, *J. Exp. Med.* **120**, 105 (1964).
27. B. H. Waksman, and M. Matoltsy, *J. Immunol.* **81**, 220 (1958).
28. J. J. Mooney and B. H. Waksman, *J. Immunol.* **105**, 1138 (1970).
29. C. F. Nathan, M. L. Karnovsky and J. R. David, *J. Exp. Med.* **133**, 1356 (1971).
30. S. V. Boyden, *J. Exp. Med.* **115**, 453 (1962).
31. P. A. Ward, H. G. Remold and J. R. David, *Science* **163**, 1079 (1969).
32. D. C. Dumonde, R. A. Wolstencroft, G. S. Panayi, M. Matthew, J. Morley and W. T. Howson, *Nature* **224**, 38 (1969).
33. E. Atkins, *Physiol. Rev.* **40**, 580 (1960).
34. E. Atkins, in *Interleukin-1, Inflammation and Disease* (R. Bomford and B. Henderson, eds), Elsevier, Amsterdam (1989), pp. 3–15.
35. V. Menkin, *Science* **100**, 337 (1944).
36. I. Gery, R. K. Gershon and B. H. Waksman, *J. Immunol.* **107**, 1778 (1971).
37. I. Gery and B. H. Waksman, *J. Exp. Med.* **136**, 143 (1972).
38. J. J. Oppenheim and I. Gery, *Immunol. Today* **14**, 232 (1993).
39. L. J. Rosenwasser, C. A. Dinarello and A. S. Rosenthal, *J. Exp. Med.* **150**, 709 (1979).
40. J. Vilcek and B. B. Aggarwal (eds), *Tumor Necrosis Factors: Structure, Function and Mechanism of Action*, Marcel Dekker, New York (1992).
41. W. Fiers and W. A. Buurman (eds): *Tumor Necrosis Factor: Molecular and Cellular Biology and Clinical Relevance*, Karger, Basel (1993).
42. E. A. Carswell, L. J. Old, R. L. Kassel, S. Green, N. Fiore and G. Williamson, *Proc. Natl Acad. Sci. USA* **72**, 3666 (1975).
43. M. Kawakami and A. Cerami, *J. Exp. Med.* **154**, 631 (1981).
44. P. Gray, B. B. Aggarwal, C. V. Benton, T. S. Bringman, W. J. Hensel, J. A. Jarrett, D. W. Leung, B. Moffet, P. Ng, L. P. Svedersky, M. A. Palladino and G. R. Nedwin, *Nature* **321**, 721 (1984).
45. D. Pennica, G. E. Nedwin, J. S. Hayflic, P. H. Seeburg, R. Derynck, M. A. Palladino, W. J. Kohr, B. B. Aggarwal and D. V. Coeddel, *Nature* **312**, 724 (1984).
46. S. Cohen, P. E. Bigazzi and T. Yoshida, *Cell. Immunol.* **12**, 150 (1974).
47. B. H. Waksman, *Pharmacol. Ther. A* **2**, 623 (1978).
48. J. N. Ihle, L. Pepersack and L. Rebar, *J. Immunol.* **126**, 2184 (1981).
49. K. A. Smith, *Immunol. Today* **7**, 321 (1986).
50. W. E. Paul, *Immunol. Today* **9**, 366 (1988).
51. S. Nagata, H. Taira, A. Hall, H. Johnsrud, M. Streuli, J. Escodi, W. Boll, K. Cantell and C. Weissmann, *Nature* **284**, 316 (1980).
52. T. Taniguchi, M. Sakai, Y. Fujii-Kariyama, M. Muramatsu, S. Kobayashi and T. Sudo, *Proc. Jap. Acad.* **B55**, 464 (1979).
53. P. W. Gray, D. W. Leung, D. Pennica, E. Yelverton, R. Najarian, C. C. Simonsen, R. Derynck, P. J. Sherwood, D. M. Wallace, S. L. Berger, A. D. Levinson and D. V. Goeddel, *Nature* **285**, 503 (1982).
54. W. Y. Weiser, T. A. Temple, J. S. Witek-Ciannotti, H. G. Remond, C. C. Clark and J. R. David, *Proc. Natl Acad. Sci. USA* **86**, 7522 (1989).
55. T. Taniguchi, H. Matsui, T. Fujita, C. Takaoka, N. Kashima, R. Yoshimoto and J. Hamuro, *Nature* **302**, 305 (1983).
56. W. J. Leonard, J. M. Depper, G. R. Crabtree, S. Rudikoff, J. Pumphrey, R. J. Robb, M. Kronke, P. B. Svetlik, N. J. Peffer, T. A. Waldmann and W. C. Green, *Nature* **311**, 626 (1984).

57. M. Fung, A. J. Hapel, S. Ymer, D. R. Cohen, R. M. Johnson, J. D. Campbell and I. C. Young, *Nature* **307**, 233 (1984).
58. N. M. Gough, H. Gough, D. Metcalf, A. Kelson, V. Grail, N. A. Nicola, A. W. Burgess and A. R. Dunn, *Nature* **309**, 763 (1984).
59. E. S. Kawasaki, M. B. Ladner, A. M. Wang Jr, Van Arsdell, M. K. Warren, M. Y. Coyne, V. L. Schweickart, M.-T. Lee, K. J. Wilson, A. Boosmam, E. R. Stanley, P. Ralph and D. F. Mark, *Science* **230**, 291 (1985).
60. L. M. Souza, T. C. Boone, J. Gabrilove, P. H. Lai, J. M. Zsebo, D. G. Murdock and V. R. Chazin *et al.*, *Science* **232**, 61 (1986).
61. S. Nakata, M. Tsuchiya, S. Asano, Y. Kaziro, T. Yamazaki, O. Yamamoto, Y. Hirata, N. Kubota, M. Oheda, H. Homura and M. Ono, *Nature* **319**, 415 (1986).
62. P. E. Auron, A. C. Webb, L. J. Rosenwasser, S. F. Mucci, A. Rich, S. M. Wolff and C. A. Dinarello, *Proc. Natl Acad. Sci. USA* **81**, 7907 (1984).
63. P. T. Lomedico, V. Gubler, C. P. Hellman, M. Dukovich, J. G. Giri, Y. Pan, K. Collins, R. Semionow, A. O. Chua and S. B. Mizel, *Nature* **312**, 458 (1984).
64. C. A. Dinarello, Fever, in *Interleukin-1, Inflammation and Disease* (R. Bomford and B. Henderson, eds), Elsevier, Amsterdam (1969), pp. 175–190.
65. R. Derynck, J. A. Jarrett, E. Y. Chen, D. H. Eaton, J. R. Bell, R. K. Assoian, A. B. Roberts, M. B. Sporn and D. V. Goeddel, *Nature* **316**, 701 (1985).
66. T. Yoshimura, K. Matsushima, S. Tanaka, E. A. Robinson, E. Apella, J. J. Oppenheim and E. J. Leonard, *Proc. Natl Acad. Sci. USA* **84**, 9233 (1987).
67. K. Matsushima, K. Morishita, T. Yoshimura, S. Lavu, Y. Kobayashi, W. Lew, E. Apella, H. F. Kung, E. Leonard and J. J. Oppenheim, *J. Exp. Med.* **167**, 1883 (1988).
68. J. Schmidt and C. Weissmann, *J. Immunol.* **139**, 250 (1987).
69. C. G. Larsen, A. O. Anderson, E. Appella, J. J. Oppenheim and K. Matsushima, *Science* **243**, 1464 (1989).
70. T. Hirano, K. Yasukawa, H. Harada, T. Taga, Y. Watanabe, T. Matsuda, S. Kashiwamura, K. Nakajima, K. Koyama, A. Iwamatsu, S. Tsunasawa, F. Sakayama, H. Matsui, Y. Takahara, T. Taniguchi and T. Kisimoto, *Nature* **324**, 73 (1986).
71. A. Zilberstein, R. Ruggieri, J. H. Korn and M. Revel, *EMBO J.* **5**, 2529 (1986).

Somatic Generation of Antibody Diversity

SUSUMU TONEGAWA
Center for Cancer Research, Massachusetts Institute of
Technology, 77 Massachusetts Avenue, Cambridge,
MA 02139–4307, USA

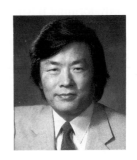

By the beginning of the 1970s, immunologists agreed that an individual vertebrate synthesizes many millions of structurally different forms of antibody molecules even before it encounters an antigen. Moreover, Gerald Edelman and Rodney Porter had shown that a typical antibody molecule is composed of two identical light chains and two identical heavy chains (*1,2*). It had also been found that each of these two types of chain exhibits great sequence variability in the amino terminal region between one antibody molecule and the next and no sequence variability in the carboxyl terminal regions (*3*). These two regions were then referred to as the variable, or *V*, and the constant, or *C*, regions. However immunologists and geneticists were divided for many years into two schools of thought with respect to the issue of whether the genetic diversity required for the synthesis of these proteins is generated during evolution, and is carried in the germline, or during development, in which case it would be present in somatic but not germline cells. One school of thought held that the germline must include a separate gene for every polypeptide that ultimately appears in an antibody molecule (*4*). In this germline theory, antibody or immunoglobulin genes are expressed in exactly the same way as those for any other protein, and no special gene-processing mechanisms are needed. On the other hand, the model requires an enormous number of immunoglobulin genes inherited from the parents. While the four-chain structure of an immunoglobulin molecule allows diversity to be generated by chain paring, the number of genes required for both light and heavy chains is still very large. One major difficulty for germline theories of antibody diversity was the observation that all antibody polypeptide chains of a given type share a common genetic marker (allotype) that segregates as a single Mendelian gene. If there were many thousands of light and heavy

This article is based on a Nobel Lecture delivered at Kalorinsha Institute on 8 December 1987.

IMMUNOLOGY: THE MAKING OF A MODERN SCIENCE
ISBN 0-12-274020-3

chain genes, how could the same genetic marker in all of these genes have been maintained?

The second theory supposed that there are only a limited number of antibody genes in the germline, and that these genes somehow diversify as the antibody-forming B lymphocytes emerge from their stem cells. In other words, the diversification of antibody gene sequences takes place in specialized somatic, or body, cells rather than being carried from generation to generation by the germ cells (5–7). One attraction of this latter theory is that it relieves the host of the need to commit a disproportionately large fraction of the inherited genes to code for antibodies, but the theory demands an unprecedented mechanism for diversifying the inherited genes somatically.

Arguments for and against these contrasting ideas were made both verbally and in written form for many years. However, all of these arguments were based on the interpretation of amino acid sequences of immunoglobulin polypeptide chains or on the generally accepted principles of evolution and genetics. No direct evidence for either view had been obtained. This was because no technique was available that would allow an analysis of the fine structure of specific genes from higher organisms.

Gene Counting

In the early 1970s, the technology for purifying a specific eukaryotic mRNA was just becoming available. Furthermore, a method to determine the number of copies of a specific gene by kinetic analysis of nucleic acid hybridization had already been established (8,9). These technical developments led some scientists, including myself, to think that one can experimentally determine the number of immunoglobulin genes contained in a germline genome and thereby decide which of the two major theories of antibody diversity is correct. The validity of this approach is based in part on the fact that the V region of a given chain type, while being different, exhibits a high degree of amino acid sequence homology. It was therefore thought that an mRNA coding for a specific immunoglobulin polypeptide chain would hybridize not only with its own gene but also with many other immunoglobulin genes, if they existed in a germline genome.

I thus obtained mouse myeloma cells and put my effort to purifying immunoglobulin mRNA and carrying out the hybridization studies. However, the initial studies focusing on the mouse κ light chain and heavy chain genes gave ambiguous results. The difficulties were threefold: uncertainty about the purity of the mRNA used as the hybridization probe; a lack of knowledge of the extent to which a probe will hybridize with the related but not identical genes; and the precise effect of sequence differences on hybridization kinetics. Thus, it turned out to be nearly impossible to make a convincing interpretation of the data obtained in these early studies in relation to the issue of the evolutionary versus somatic generation of antibody diversity.

One subsequent series of experiments which I carried out on genes coding for the mouse λ light chains, however, was very encouraging (10). Using an mRNA preparation that was more than 95% pure, I could show that the mouse λ light chain gene is reiterated no more than the β globin gene. The latter gene had been shown to be essentially unique. Fortunately, Weigert, Cohn and their coworkers had identified at least eight different V_λ region sequences among BALB/c-derived myelomas (11). Since the V regions were highly homologous, differing by only one, two or three amino acid residues, it was very likely that the corresponding genes would cross-hybridize extensively if they existed separately in the germline genome. Furthermore, statistical analysis of λ light-chain-secreting myelomas strongly suggested that a BALB/c mouse has the capacity to synthesize many more than the eight different V_λ regions identified. Thus, the number of the mouse λ genes determined experimentally (no more than a few) was far smaller than the number of different V_λ regions (at least eight, most probably many more) detected in proteins. On the basis of these results I was convinced that a somatic diversification occurs in this gene system.

Rearrangement

In the meantime, I became aware that some immunologists had been speculating that immunoglobulin polypeptide chains may be encoded by two separate DNA segments, one each for the V and C regions. Drawing an analogy from the elegant Campbell model (12) on the integration and excision of a phage λ genome, Dryer and Bennett had further suggested that one of many 'V genes' may be excised out from the original chromosomal position and joined with the single 'C gene' in an immunoglobulin-producing B cell (13). This model successfully explained the maintenance of the common genetic marker in all immunoglobulin polypeptide chains of a given type by postulating a single C gene for that cell type. Although a somatic recombination between the 'V and C genes' is an inherent aspect of the model, it is clearly a version of the germline theory of antibody diversity because the model assumed that the germline genome carries many 'V genes', one for every V region that an organism can synthesize.

When the Dryer and Bennett model was published in 1965, it was not accepted widely by biologists. This is understandable because the model was built on two hypotheses, both of which violated the then current dogmas of biology. These are the principles of one gene encoding one polypeptide chain, and of the constancy of the genome during ontogeny and cell differentiation. My personal reaction to the model when I learned of it in the early 1970s was also that of scepticism. However, at the same time I thought that the model might be testable if one were to use restriction enzymes. While in Dulbecco's laboratory, I had heard of Daniel Nathans' breakthrough in the analysis of the

SV40 genome by an application of the then newly discovered restriction enzymes (14). As one who used to struggle to define the transcriptional units of this DNA virus I was keenly aware of the power of these enzymes for the analysis of DNA structure. However, an extension of the restriction enzyme analysis from a viral genome of 5×10^3 base pairs to the 2×10^9 base pair genome of an eukaryote as complex as a mouse, required the use of an additional trick for the detection of a specific DNA fragment in a vast array of irrelevant fragments. An obvious solution seemed to lie in the combination of an electrophoretic separation of enzyme-digested DNA and the sensitive technique of nucleic acid hybridization. I discussed with Charlie Steinberg the need for developing a method that allows an *in situ* detection of a specific DNA sequence among the electrophoretically fractionated DNA fragments, but we really could not come up with a good idea worthy of exploring. As we all know, a very simple and elegant method ideal for this purpose was later developed by Edward Southern (15).

A few weeks passed by before I accidentally saw in one of the Institute's cold rooms a huge plexiglass tray in which someone was fractionating serum proteins by starch gel electrophoresis. I thought one may be able to fractionate a sufficient amount of digested DNA in a gel of such dimensions, so that DNA eluted from gel slices could be used for liquid phase hybridization. A quick calculation seemed to indicate that the experiment was feasible. Nobumichi Hozumi, a postdoctoral fellow in my laboratory, and I therefore decided to give it a try although we were keenly aware of the intense labour required by this type of experiment. As hybridization probes we used purified κ or λ light chain mRNA (V + C probe) and its 3'-half fragment (C probe) that had been iodinated to a high specific activity. The rationale of the experiment was as follows. First, if an immunoglobulin polypeptide chain is encoded by two 'genes', V and C, in the germline genome, it is highly probable that treatment with a restriction enzyme will separate these DNA sequences into fragments of distinct size, thus allowing their electrophoretic separation. Second, if a somatic rearrangement joins the V and C 'genes' it is also highly probable that the myeloma DNA digested with the same restriction enzyme will contain a DNA fragment carrying both V and C 'genes'.

The results obtained were clear-cut. To our pleasant surprise the patterns of hybridization of the embryo (a substitute of germline) DNA and a κ-myeloma DNA were not only drastically different but also perfectly consistent with the occurrence of separate V and C 'genes' and a joined V plus C gene, respectively (16). We were of course aware of the alternative interpretations of the results, such as fortuitous modification of the enzyme cleavage sites in one of the two types of DNA. However, we considered these alternative explanations of the results unlikely because they all required multiple fortuitous events. Our confidence was fortified soon afterwards as the development of Southern blot techniques allowed us to carry out more extensive analysis using a variety of restriction enzymes and myeloma cells.

Joining of Gene Segments

While the experiments with restriction enzymes were informative, details of the rearrangement were difficult to come by with this approach. Fortunately, recombinant DNA technology was just becoming available and was the ideal means for this purpose. Debates on the possible hazards of this type of research were flaring, initially in the USA and shortly afterwards in European countries. In order to make sure that our research would not become a target of controversy, Charlie and I got in touch with Werner Arber at the University of Basel who was co-ordinating recombinant DNA research activities in Switzerland. A small informal work group was set up by the local researchers interested in this technique. The consensus of the group which was supported by most of the other Swiss researchers was that we should all follow the practices and guidelines being adopted in the USA. We met about once a month and exchanged information regarding both ethical and practical aspects of the technology.

On the basis of the previous experiments attempting to count immunoglobulin genes, I thought that it would be wise to start with the mouse λ light chain system, the simplest of all chain types that had been studied. Our goal was to clone the V_λ and C_λ 'genes' in the germline state from embryonic cells as well as the rearranged V plus C 'genes' from a λ myeloma, and to determine the relationship between these genomic DNA clones by electron microscopy and DNA sequencing. No precedent existed at that time for cloning 'unique' eukaryotic genes. We therefore had to devise a few tricks as we attempted to clone the first immunoglobulin gene. For instance, our available probe at that time was again 95% pure mRNA rather than a cDNA clone. This situation made the screening of a large number of DNA clones difficult because of the high background. To avoid this problem we pre-enriched the λ gene-containing genomic DNA fragments as much as possible using preparative R-loop formation (17,18), so that the DNA library constructed would have the clone of interest at a high frequency.

Starting with the embryonic DNA we could isolate a clone that clearly hybridized specifically with the λ mRNA (18). When an electronmicroscopist, Christine Brack, who had just joined us from the Biozentrum of the University of Basel, examined the mixture of this clone and λ mRNA that had been annealed under an appropriate condition, she found a beautiful R loop from which about a half of the mRNA strand protruded. This and additional analysis convinced us that we had cloned a V_λ 'gene' to which no C 'gene' was contiguously attached, thus confirming at the DNA clone level that the V and C 'genes' are indeed separate in the germline genome. A subsequent DNA sequencing study carried out in collaboration with Allan Maxam and Walter Gilbert of Harvard University revealed that this DNA clone corresponded to the V 'gene' for the λ_2 subtype (19).

In the meantime Minoru Hirama, another postdoctoral fellow, succeeded in preparing λ and κ cDNA clones. Once these probes became available isolation

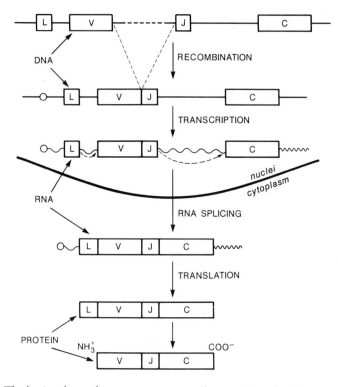

Figure 1   The basic scheme for rearrangement and expression of an immunoglobulin light chain gene. At top is an arrangement of the gene segments on a germline genome. Somatic rearrangement links the *V* and *J* gene segment and generates a complete light chain gene shown just below the germline genome. The entire gene containing the leader exon (*L*), the *V* region (*V* and *J*), the *C* region exon (*C*), and the introns present between these exons are transcribed into a pre-mRNA in the nuclei of the B cell. The pre-mRNA is processed by RNA splicing as it is transported from the nuclei to the cytoplasm. The resulting mRNA, devoid of introns, is translated in the endoplasmic reticulum into a nascent polypeptide chain, from which a mature λ light chain is generated after cleavage of the signal peptide.

of the genomic clones became much easier. My assistant Rita Schuller and I isolated a number of genomic DNA clones from λ and κ chain-synthesizing myelomas as well as from embryos (*20,21*). Analysis of these DNA clones by electron microscopy, by restriction enzyme mapping, and by DNA sequencing not only confirmed the somatic rearrangement of immunoglobulin genes but also revealed some striking features of their arrangement and rearrangement (Fig. 1). These can be summarized as follows:

(1) Although the *V* and *C* 'genes' are rearranged and are much closer to each other in myeloma cells than in embryo cells, they are not contiguous and

are separated by a few kilobases of DNA sequence that does not participate in coding of the polypeptide chain. This untranslated DNA sequence
present within the rearranged, complete immunoglobulin gene was unanticipated and was also among the first demonstrations of an intron in
eukaryotic genes (22).

(2) The V 'gene' found in the germline genome is about 13 codons short when
it is compared to the length of the conventionally defined V region. The
missing codons were found in a short stretch of DNA referred to as a J or
joining) gene segment that is located many kilobases away from the incomplete V 'gene' (referred to as a V gene segment) and a few kilobases
upstream of the C 'gene' (also referred to as a C gene segment). In myeloma
cells the rearrangement event attaches the J gene segment to the V gene
segment and thereby creates a complete V region 'gene' (20,23).

(3) The signal peptide is encoded in yet another DNA segment referred to as
the L (or leader) exon that is separated from the V gene segment by a short
intron (19,23).

Finding that the V_λ 'gene' was split into two gene segments, V_λ and J_λ, in the
germline genome was completely unexpected. But as soon as this discovery was
made its implication for the somatic generation of antibody diversity was
obvious. If the germline genome carries multiple copies of different V and J gene
segments, the number of complete V 'genes' that can be generated by random
joinings between these two types of gene segments would be much greater than
the total number of the inherited gene segments. Thus, contrary to the Dryer
and Bennett original concept, DNA rearrangement can provide a major means
for the somatic diversification of antibody molecules. The amino acid sequence
data of the κ light and heavy chains were consistent with this concept (24,25).
Indeed, the nucleotide sequence analysis of the mouse κ chain gene complex
carried out both in my laboratory and in Phillip Leder's laboratory at the United
States National Institutes of Health confirmed that a germline genome contains
multiple V and J gene segments and that these gene segments are joined in different combinations in each myeloma cell (20,26). Four different J_κ gene segments were found several kilobases upstream of the C_κ gene segment. The exact
number of V_κ gene segments is unknown even today, but it is estimated to be
200 to 300 (27).

Heavy Chain Genes

Inasmuch as an immunoglobulin heavy chain is also composed of V and C
regions, it was reasonable to expect that its gene also would undergo the type
of DNA rearrangement described for the light chain genes. This supposition
was confirmed by Leroy Hood and his coworkers at California Institute of
Technology and by ourselves (Fig. 2) (28,29). As in κ genes, four J gene segments were found several kilobases upstream of the C gene segments coding for

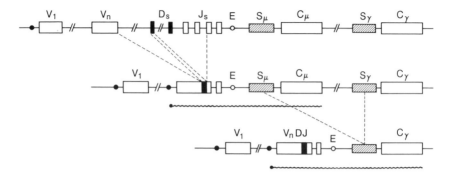

Figure 2   Organization of the immunoglobulin heavy chain family. At the top, middle and bottom are organization in a germline genome, in a genome of B cells synthesizing a μ class heavy chain and in a genome of a plasma cell synthesizing a γ class heavy chain, respectively. A mouse haploid genome carries several hundred different V gene segments, about a dozen D gene segments, four J gene segments, and one copy of C gene segment for each of the eight different classes or subclasses of immunoglobulin heavy chains. In a virgin B cell one copy each of the V, D and J gene segment pools have been linked up and the joined VDJ DNA sequence is transcribed into a pre-mRNA together with the C_μ gene segment. In different B cells of the same organism, a different set of V, D and J gene segments are usually hooked up and expressed. As the virgin B cell differentiates either to a plasma cell or to a memory B cell (see Fig. 5) the second type of somatic recombination called 'switch recombination' often occurs between a region (S_μ) located upstream of the C_μ gene segment and another region (S_γ) located upstream of the C_γ gene segment.

the C region of the μ class heavy chain. Multiple V gene segments were also identified.

While these features of the organization of heavy chain genes are essentially the same as those of the light chain genes, one observation made during these studies suggested that the somatic assembly of gene segments plays an even more prominent role in the diversification of heavy chains than of light chains. It was found that from one or two to a dozen amino acid codons, present in the V–J junction region of the assembled gene, are not found in either of the corresponding germline V or J gene segments (30,31). This suggested that a third type of short gene segment referred to as D (or diversity) might participate in the somatic assembly of a heavy chain gene. Indeed, Hitoshi Sakano and Yoshi Kurosawa, two postdoctoral fellows in my laboratory, soon discovered about a dozen D gene segments (32,33) which were subsequently mapped in a region upstream of the J cluster in the germline genome (34,35). Thus, the construction of a complete heavy chain V 'gene' requires two DNA recombinational events, one joining a V with a D gene segment and the other the same D with a J gene segment.

Recombination Rules

The joining of *V–J* or *V–D–J* involves a site-specific recombination. It might therefore be expected that these gene segments would carry sequences in the vicinity of the joining ends that are recognized by a putative site-specific recombinase. Furthermore, such recognition sequences are likely to be common for all gene segments of a given type (for example V_κ segments), because they all seem to be capable of joining with the common set of gene segments of the appropriate type (for example, J_κ segments). Indeed, a heptamer and a nonamer sequence are conserved in the region immediately downstream of each V_κ gene segment (Fig. 3) (*36,37*). Sequences complementary to the V_κ heptamer and nonamer were also found in the region immediately upstream of each of the

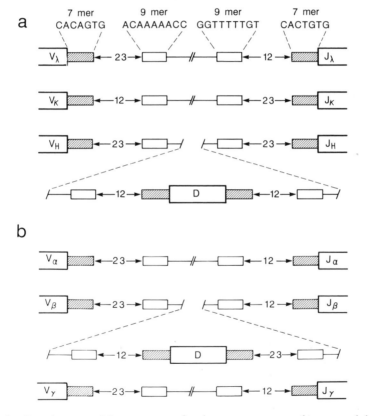

Figure 3   Putative recognition sequences for the rearrangement of immunoglobulin and T cell receptor genes. The conserved heptamer and nonamer sequences and the length of the spacer between these sequences are schematically illustrated for immunoglubulin (a) and for T cell receptor (b) gene families. The sequences shown at the top of (a) and (b) are consensus sequences. Individual sequences may deviate from these consensus sequences by a few nucleotides.

four J_κ gene segments. The same sets of sequences were also found in the corresponding regions of the V_λ and J_λ gene segments (36). When the heavy chain V and J gene segments were analysed subsequently, they too had the common conserved sequences (30,31). Furthermore, D gene segments carry the heptamer and nonamer sequences both upstream and downstream (32,33). Another interesting feature of these putative recognition sequences is the fact that the length of the spacer between the heptamer and nonamer is either 12 or 23 base pairs (30,31). In addition, a gene segment carrying a recognition sequence with one type of spacer is able to join only with a gene segment with the spacer of the other type. This 12/23 base pair spacer rule seems to be adhered to strictly. Little is currently known about the recombinase, but proteins with an affinity to the heptamer or nonamer have been identified in the extract of Abelson virus transformed pre-B-cell lines in which the rearrangement occurs in vitro at a relatively high frequency (38,39). Since then, a pair of genes, RAG-1 and RAG-2, whose protein products are essential for V–(D)–J joining has been identified and cloned in David Baltimore's laboratory (40,41).

Diversity Generated at the Joins

The deduced amino acid sequence of a germline J_κ gene segment was compared with the determined amino acid sequences of those κ chains that are encoded in part by that J_κ gene segment. The joining site is not prefixed but rather shifts toward upstream or downstream by several base pairs in different joining events (36,37). This flexibility in the precise site of the joining was subsequently found to be characteristic of the joining ends of other gene segments rather than of just J_κ gene segments (31). It applies even when the same pair of gene segments were joined in different B cell percursors, such that the completed V 'genes' are likely to have slightly different codons in the junction regions.

The V–D and D–J junctions exhibit diversity of yet another type. We found that up to a dozen base pairs of essentially random sequence are inserted in these junctions, apparently without a template, during the breakage and reunion of the recombining gene segments (32,33). While the precise mechanism is not yet known, the terminal deoxynucleotide transferase which is found in early B lymphatic nuclei, or an enzyme with similar characteristics, is thought to play a role in this phenomenon (42).

The part of the V region affected by the above two diversification mechanisms is limited. But this does not mean that they do not play a significant role in the determination of antibody specificity. On the contrary, the junctions encode the most variable two of the six loops of polypeptides that make up the antigen binding region of the antibody molecule (Fig. 4). Furthermore, specific cases are known where the affinity of an antibody to a defined antigen is drastically altered by a slight change in one junction sequence (43). Thus, the junctional variation also is a potent somatic generator of antibody diversity.

Somatic Mutation

When F. Macfarlane Burnet proposed the clonal selection theory, he recognized the need for some kind of random genetic process in order to generate antibodies able to bind specifically to the vast variety of antigens (44). He considered somatic mutations as the most plausible mechanism. Subsequently, this idea was adopted and forcefully presented by many including Joshua Lederberg, Niels Kaj Jerne and Melvin Cohn (5–7).

The amino acid sequence data accumulated by Martin Weigert in Melvin Cohn's laboratory at the Salk Institute provided an excellent opportunity to examine directly the role of somatic mutations in antibody diversity (7,11). They had analysed the λ_1 light chains derived from 18 myelomas. All the mice were of an inbred strain, BALB/c, and so should have been genetically identical. They found that twelve of the $V_{\lambda 1}$ regions were identical but that the other six differed both from the majority sequence and from one another by only one, two, or three amino acid residues. They proposed that BALB/c mice may carry only one germline $V_{\lambda 1}$ 'gene' which codes for the majority sequence, and that all the other $V_{\lambda 1}$ regions observed are encoded by somatic mutants of this single $V_{\lambda 1}$ 'gene' that arose in B cell development. As I have already mentioned in an earlier section, our gene-counting experiment by hybridization kinetics suggested that the germline BALB/c genome carries no more than a few $V_{\lambda 1}$ 'genes'. This number was reduced to one when we re-evaluated the copy number by the more reliable Southern blotting method (20). The final proof of somatic mutation in $V_{\lambda 1}$ came when we cloned and sequenced the sole germline $V_{\lambda 1}$ segment and the rearranged λ_1 genes expressed in a myeloma (23). As Weigert and Cohn guessed, the nucleotide sequence of the germline $V_{\lambda 1}$ gene segment corresponded to the major amino acid sequence, while the λ_1 gene expressed in the myeloma had been altered by single base changes.

Since this work, several subsets of κ light and heavy chains and their germline, V gene segments have been analysed by cloning and sequencing (45–48), and have all confirmed that somatic mutations further amplify the diversity encoded in the germline genome. Particularly revealing was the analysis carried out by Patricia J. Gearhart, Leroy Hood and their coworkers for the V_H regions associated with the binding of phosphorylcholine (PC). They demonstrated that single base changes can be extensive and yet are restricted to the joined VDJ sequences and the immediately adjacent regions (49,50).

Developmental Control of Rearrangement and Hypermutation

Why have two extraordinary somatic genetic mechanisms, recombination and hypermutation, evolved in the immune system in order to carry out what appears to be one task – namely, to diversify antibodies? The answer may be the differential roles of these two genetic mechanisms. Thanks to the efforts of

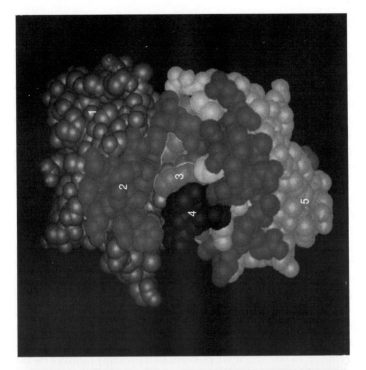

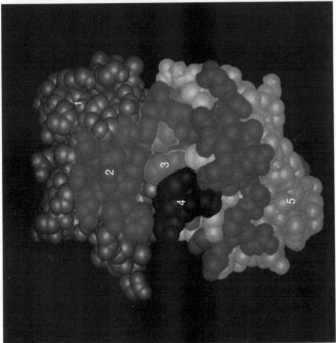

Figure 4 (caption opposite)

several independent groups of cellular and molecular immunologists, a general picture is emerging that describes the relationship between the states of B cell development and the occurrence of somatic recombination or mutation (Fig. 5) (51–57). Somatic recombinations contributing to diversity are initiated first for the heavy chain and then for the light chain during the differentiation of progenitor cells, and the completion of somatic recombination is accompanied by the appearance of virgin B cells (58–60). These B cells form clones each of which is composed of cells bearing homogenous IgM molecules as surface receptors. Thus, somatic recombination is completed *prior to* any possible interaction of a B cell with antigens.

When an antigen enters lymphatic tissue for the first time, it will be screened by these virgin B cells. The small fraction of these B cells that happen to have sufficient affinity for the antigenic determinants in question will respond and follow either of two pathways: they will produce the primary antibody response, or they will contribute to the generation of memory B cells. In the former pathway, the selected B cells will proliferate and differentiate into antibody-secreting plasma cells. During this process, the C region of the heavy chain can switch from μ to another class, but mutation is rare in either the heavy or the light chain V region. Consequently, the antibodies secreted by plasma cells in the primary response would largely have the same V regions as the immunoglobulin receptors on the virgin B cells from which they derive.

By contrast, immunoglobulin remains in the cell surface receptor form during the other pathway taken by the antigen-activated virgin B cells, namely the generation of memory cells. During this process, the hypermutation

---

Figure 4 Space-filling, stereo image of antibody combining site. Atomic coordinates of mouse immunoglobulin MOPC 603 (62) were used to produce the picture. The heavy chain variable domain is colour-coded dark grey, and the light chain variable domain light grey. The hypervariable regions (except the V_H third hypervariable region) are blue, the heavy chain segment coded for by the *D* gene is red, and the heavy and light chain segments coded for the *J* genes are yellow. The *D* segment corresponds virtually exactly to the third heavy chain hypervariable region; hypervariable regions were defined as in Novotney *et al.* (63) except for the heavy chain second hypervariable region, which is marked as defined by Kabat *et al.* (25). The antigen of this particular immunoglobulin, phosphoryl choline, binds into the cavity in the middle of the picture between the V_H and V_L domains, making contacts to amino acid residues belonging to the V_H and *J* segments of the heavy chain and the V_L structures of antibodies which bind the protein antigen lysozyme (64, 65). There, the contact areas contributed by the *D* segment amount to 50% and 24%, respectively, of the total heavy chain contact area. This image was computer generated by Jiri Novotny using the program SPHERE of Robert Bruccoleri. Because of reproduction difficulties, a black-and-white version of the original colour photograph is shown: 1, heavy chain variable domain; 2, hypervariable regions; 3, heavy and light chain *J* regions; 4, heavy chain *D* region; 5, light chain variable domain.

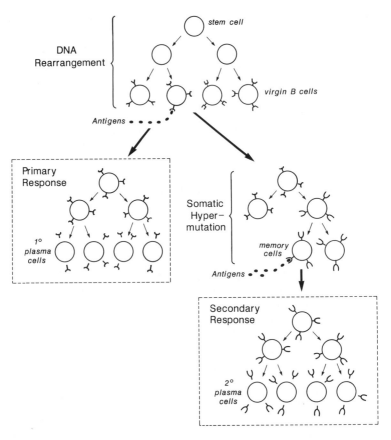

Figure 5   Differentiation of B cells. Note that the receptors present in the memory cells and the antibody molecules secreted by the plasma cells of the secondary response have a tighter fit to the antigen than the receptors on the ancestral virgin B cells or the antibodies secreted by the plasma cells of the primary response. See text for the full explanation.

apparatus appears to be most active and the rate of the mutation approaches 10^{-3} base substitution per cell per generation. Antigen selects, in a stepwise fashion, better and better fitting mutants, so that the immunoglobulins on the surface of memory B cells achieve a substantially higher affinity than the immunoglobulins on the ancestral virgin B cells. Switch recombination also occurs frequently during this process too. When the same antigen as the one that elicited the primary response re-enters the body, the memory B cells are selectively propagated and differentiate into plasma cells. This is the so-called 'secondary antibody response' which, therefore, consists of high affinity antibody of 'mature' isotype; these antibodies show extensive somatic mutation in their V regions. Somatic mutations appear to cease after memory cells are generated, and little or no further mutation takes place during the secondary antibody response.

This scheme of B cell differentiation can be rephrased as follows. An organism is prepared for infection with pathogens bearing virtually any antigens with a large variety of resting B cells. These B cells bear unique immunoglobulin receptors encoded by one copy each of complete light and heavy chain genes that have been constructed by a random or quasirandom assembly of the inherited gene segments. Since the assembly occurs independent of antigens and since the inherited gene segments are not usually selected during evolution for precise fit to particular antigens, the antibody secreted by the plasma cells derived directly from the selected resting virgin B cells during a primary antibody response usually have a relatively low affinity. By contrast, the frequent single base changes that occur during the generation of memory B cells provide the organism with a great variety of finely altered immunoglobulin receptors from which only those with the best fit to the antigen in question will be selected. Since the plasma cells generated during the secondary antibody response are mostly direct descendants of these memory B cells having no further alterations in the antigen-combining sites, these antibodies usually exhibit a much higher affinity for antigen than do primary antibodies. This explains the long-known phenomenon of affinity maturation of antibodies during the course of repeated immunizations (61).

Thus, somatic creation of antibody genes can be viewed as a two-step process. In the first step, blocks of gene segments are employed to build, in an antigen-independent fashion, a set of genes coding for antibodies of great diversity but with low affinity. In the second step, once the antigen is defined, a small selected set of B cells bearing low-affinity antibodies as cell surface receptors undergo somatic mutations with the result that a fraction of them develop a higher affinity to that antigen and can be selected for further expansion. This process improves the ability of the immune system to detect a low concentration of antigens. One wonders what happens to those cells in which mutation did not improve affinity. A recent study suggests that at least some of these cells may be set aside for selection by different antigens (56). Thus somatic mutation may also contribute to the repertoire of receptors specific for antigens not previously introduced into an immune system.

Concluding Remarks

Use of restriction enzymes and recombinant DNA methods allowed resolution of a long-standing and central issue in immunology, the genetic origins of antibody diversity. It turned out that an organism does not inherit even a single complete gene for antibody polypeptide chains. Rather, the genetic information is transmitted in germline as no more than several hundred gene segments. Through a series of specialized somatic recombinations occurring specifically during the differentiation of B lymphocytes, these gene segments are assembled into tens of thousands of complete genes. Somatic hypermutation occurring in these assembled genes further diversifies antibody polypeptide chains, so that B cells displaying immunoglobulin receptors having a better fit to a given antigen can be selected in a later phase of B cell differentiation. Thus, in the immune system, organisms have exploited two major processes for modification of DNA, recombination and mutation, as a means to diversify somatically the limited amount of inherited genetic information in order to cope with the vastly diverse antigen universe.

Why has somatic diversification been necessary in the evolution of the immune system? Micro-organisms and substances produced by them are the primary source of biologically relevant antigens against which vertebrates need to produce antibodies for survival. Since the generation time of micro-organisms is several orders of magnitude shorter than that of vertebrates, the former can produce generic variants much faster than the latter. Thus, if genetic alterations in the germline genome were to be the only source of antibody diversity, vertebrates would be unable to deal effectively with the rapidly changing world of antigens. Somatic diversification allows the individual organism to generate a virtually limitless number of lymphocyte variants. Like organisms in an ecosystem, these lymphocytes are subject to selection by antigens and the fittest will survive. Thus, as Jerne and Burnet were aware, the individual immune system can be conceived of as a kind of Darwinian microcosm.

Acknowledgements

The work summarized in this article is the result of collaboration with many colleagues, students and technical assistants. I wish to extend my sincere thanks to every one of them. I also extend my thanks to the Hoffman LaRoche Company which so generously supported my work in Basle. My special thanks are extended to Charles A. Janeway Jr, Nancy Hopkins and Yohtaroh Takagaki for many useful comments on the manuscript, to Jiri Novotny for preparing Fig. 4, and to my secretary, Eleanor Lahey, Basle, for her tireless devotion.

Notes and References

1. R. R. Porter, *Science* 180, 713 (1973).
2. G. M. Edelman, *Science* 180, 830 (1973).
3. N. Hilschmann and L. C. Craig, *Proc. Natl Acad. Sci. USA* 53, 1403 (1965).
4. L. Hood and D. W. Talmage, *Science* 168, 325 (1970).
5. J. Lederberg, *Science* 129, 1649 (1959).
6. N. K. Jerne, *Eur. J. Immunol.*, 1, 1 (1971).
7. M. Cohn, B. Blomberg, W. Geckeler, W. Raschka, R. Riblet and M. Weigert, in *The Immune System: Genes, Receptors, Signals* (E. E. Sercarz, A. R. Williamson and C. F. Fox, eds), Academic Pres, New York (1974), p. 89.

8. A. H. Gelderman, A. V. Rake and R. J. Britten, *Proc. Natl Acad. Sci. USA* **68**, 172 (1971).
9. J. O. Bishop, *Biochem. J.* **126** 171 (1971).
10. S. Tonegawa, *Proc. Natl Acad. Sci. USA* **73**, 203 (1976).
11. M. Weigert, M. Cesari, S. J. Yonkovich and M. Cohn, *Nature* **228**, 1045 (1970).
12. A. Campbell, *Adv. Genet.* **11**, 101 (1962).
13. W. J. Dryer and J. Bennett, *Proc. Natl Acad. Sci. USA* **73**, 3628 (1965).
14. J. J. Danna, G. H. Sack Jr and D. Nathans, *J. Mol. Biol.* **78**, 363 (1973).
15. E. Southern, *J. Mol. Biol.* **98**, 503 (1975).
16. N. Hozumi and S. Tonegawa, *Proc. Natl Acad. Sci. USA* **73**, 3628 (1976).
17. M. Thomas, R. L. White and R. N. Davis (1976). *Proc. Natl Acad. Sci. USA* **73**, 2294 (1976).
18. S. Tonegawa, C. Brack, N. Hozumi and R. Schuller, *Proc. Natl Acad. Sci. USA* **74**, 3518 (1977).
19. S. Tonegawa, A. M. Maxam, R. Tizard, O. Bernard and W. Gilbert, *Proc. Natl Acad. Sci. USA* **75**, 1485 (1978).
20. C. Brack, M. Hirami, R. Lenhard-Schuller and S. Tonegawa, *Cell*, **15**, 1 (1978).
21. R. Lenhard-Schuller, B. Hohn, C. Brack, M. Hirama and S. Tonegawa, *Proc. Natl Acad. Sci. USA* **75**, 4709 (1978).
22. C. Brack and S. Tonegawa, *Proc. Natl Acad. Sci. USA* **74**, 5652 (1977).
23. O. Bernard, N. Hozumi and S. Tonegawa, *Cell* **15**, 1133 (1978).
24. M. Weigert, L. Gatmaitan, E. Loh, J. Schilling and L. Hood, *Nature* **276**, 785 (1978).
25. E. A. Kabat, T. T. Wu, H. Bilofsky, M. Reid-Miller and H. Perry, *Publication No. 91-3242*, US Department of Health and Human Services Publication, Washington, DC (1983).
26. J. G. Seidman, A. Leder, M. Nau, B. Norman and P. Leder, *Science* **208**, 11 (1978).
27. S. Cory, B. M. Tyler and J. M. Adams, *J. Mol. Appl. Genet.* **1**, 103 (1981).
28. M. Davis, K. Calame, P. Early, D. Livant, R. Joho, I. Weismann and L. Hood, *Nature* **283**, 733 (1980).
29. R. Maki, A. Traunecker, H. Sakano, W. Roeder and S. Tonegawa, *Proc. Natl Acad. Sci. USA* **77**, 2138 (1980).
30. P. Early, H. Huang, M. Davis, K. Calame and L. Hood, *Cell* **19**, 981 (1980).
31. H. Sakano, R. Maki, Y. Kurosawa, W. Roeder and S. Tonegawa, *Nature* **286**, 676 (1980).
32. H. Sakano, Y. Kurosawa, M. Weigert and S. Tonegawa, *Nature* **290**, 562 (1981).
33. Y. Kurosawa, H. von Boehmer, W. Haas, H. Sakano, A. Traunecker and S. Tonegawa, *Nature* **290**, 565 (1981).
34. Y. Kurosawa and S. Tonegawa, *J. Exp. Med.* **155**, 201 (1982).
35. C. Wood and S. Tonegawa, *Proc. Natl Acad. Sci. USA* **80**, 3030 (1983).
36. H. Sakano, K. Huppi, G. Heinrich and S. Tonegawa, *Nature* **280**, 288 (1979).
37. E. E. Max, J. G. Seidman and P. Leder, *Proc. Natl Acad. Sci USA* **76**, 3450 (1979).
38. B. D. Halligan and S. V. Desiderio, *Proc. Natl Acad. Sci. USA* **84**, 7019 (1987).
39. R. J. Agutera, S. Akira, K. Okagaki and H. Sakano, *Cell* **51**, 909–917 (1987).
40. D. G. Schatz, M. A. Oettinger and D. Baltimore, *Cell* **59**, 1035 (1989).
41. M. A. Oettinger, D. G. Schatz, C. Gorka and D. Baltimore, *Science* **248**, 1517 (1990).
42. F. Alt and D. Baltimore, *Proc. Natl Acad. Sci. USA* **79**, 4118 (1982).
43. T. Azuma, V. Igras, E. Reilly and H. N. Eisen, *Proc. Natl Acad. Sci. USA* **81**, 6139 (1984).
44. F. M. Burnet, *The Clonal Selection Theory of Acquired Immunity*, Cambridge University Press, London (1959).
45. A. L. M. Bothwell, M. Paskind, M. Reth, T. Imanishi-Kari, K. Rawesky and D. Baltimore, *Cell* **24**, 624 (1981).
46. S. Crews, J. Griffin, H. Huang, K. Calame and L. Hood, *Cell* **25**, 59 (1981).
47. D. Givol, R. Zakut, K. Effron, G. Rechavi, D. Ram and J. B. Cohen, *Nature* **292**, 426 (1981).
48. E. Selsing and U. Storb, *Nucl. Acids Res.* **9**, 5725 (1981).
49. P. J. Gearhart, N. D. Johnson, R. Douglas and L. Hood, *Nature* **291**, 29 (1981).
50. S. Kim, M. Davis, E. Sinn, P. Patten and L. Hood, *Cell* **27**, 573 (1981).
51. B. A. Askonas and A. R. Williamson, *Eur. J. Immunol*, **2**, 487 (1972).

52. C. Berek, G. M. Griffiths and C. Milstein, *Nature* **316**, 412 (1985).
53. D. McKean, K. Huppi, M. Bell, L. Standt, W. Gerhard and M. Weigert, *Proc. Natl Acad. Sci. USA* **81**, 3180 (1984).
54. K. Okumura, M. H. Julius, T. Tsu, L. A. Herzenberg and L. A. Herzenberg, *Eur. J. Immunol.* **6**, 467 (1976).
55. M. Sablitzberg, C. Kocks and K. Rajewsky, *EMBO J.* **4**, 345 (1985).
56. M. Sickevitz, C. Kocks, K. Rajewsky and R. Dildrop, *Cell* **48**, 757 (1987).
57. L. J. Wysocki, T. Manser and M. L. Gefter, *Proc. Natl Acad. Sci. USA* **83**, 1847 (1986).
58. R. Maki, J. Kearney, C. Paige and S. Tonegawa, *Science* **209**, 1366 (1980).
59. P. P. Perry, D. E. Kelley, C. Coleclough and J. F. Kearney, *Proc. Natl Acad. Sci. USA* **78**, 247 (1981).
60. M. G. Reth, P. A. Ammirati, S. J. Jackson and F. W. Alt, *Nature* **317**, 353 (1985).
61. H. N. Eisen and G. W. Siskind, *Biochemistry* **3**, 3996 (1964).
62. Y. Satow, G. H. Cohen, E. A. Padlan and D. R. Davis, *Mol. Biol.* **190**, 593 (1986).
63. J. Novotny, R. E. Bruccolei, J. Newell, D. Murphy, E. Harber and M. J. Karplus, *J. Biol. Chem.* **258**, 14433 (1983).
64. A. G. Amit, R. A. Mariuzza, S. E. V. Phillips and R. Poljak, *Science* **233**, 747 (1986).
65. S. Sheriff, E. W. Silverton, E. A. Padlan, G. H. Cohen, S. J. Smith-Gill, B. C. Finzel and D. R. Davies, *Proc. Natl Acad. Sci USA* **84**, 8075 (1987).

Tracking an Imaginary Monster: Isolating T Cell Receptor Genes

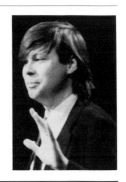

MARK M. DAVIS
Howard Hughes Medical Institute and the Department of
Microbiology and Immunology, Stanford University School of
Medicine, Beckman Center, Room B221, Stanford, CA
94305–5428, USA

By the early 1970s, it was clear that lymphocytes could be subdivided into two categories: B cells, which bear cell surface immunoglobulins (Ig) and can be turned into antibody secreting factories; and T cells, a much more mysterious category which were primarily responsible for phenomena such as delayed type hypersensitivity, B cell 'help' and graft rejection. Both B and T lymphocytes seemed capable of antigen recognition and a particularly sensational aspect of the T cell version, discovered in 1974 by Zinkernagel and Doherty and others (see this volume), was that at least some T cells required both a specific antigen and a particular MHC type simultaneously (1). This dual recognition requirement was clearly different than antibody mediated recognition and stirred considerable interest as to how this was accomplished. Through the mid- to late 1970s and through the early 1980s, arguments raged back and forth in the noisy and confused fashion that seems to characterize many of these early immunological debates. Sentiment crystallized along two major lines concerning the nature of what came to be known as 'the T cell receptor'. The first group thought that both antigen and MHC could be recognized by a single receptor binding site, whereas the second argued that having two receptors, one for antigen and one for the MHC, made more sense. This two-receptor model seemed the most popular, as one could easily imagine an antibody-like molecule being used for antigen recognition and some generic non-rearranging receptor family governing the MHC part. Also, the available data seemed to stack up quickly in favour of the 'two-receptor' camp. The first of these were the papers of Binz et al. (2) as well as Rajewsky and Eichmann (3), who used anti-idiotype antisera made from antigen-specific antibodies to block T cell responses that were specific for that antigen. This suggested that not only was the antigen receptor component of T cell recognition like an antibody, but that

IMMUNOLOGY: THE MAKING OF A MODERN SCIENCE
ISBN 0-12-274020-3

it was actually an antibody or at least the *V* regions thereof. Parallel data also appeared from the work of Marchalonis, who reported the isolation of an 'IgT' molecule using similar antisera (*4*). Later work by Frances Owen gave strong impetus to this paradigm by showing the apparent existence of T-cell-specific 'constant' regions distal to the IgH locus on mouse chromosome 12, also using antisera (*5,6*). Thus the 'two-receptor' camp seemed to have established that one component of the T cell receptor used antibody *V* regions together with T-cell-specific constant regions.

In parallel with progress on this front was work on antigen specific suppressor factors, which could be chronicled in a separate book by itself, but for the sake of brevity it can be said that many groups reported the isolation of antigen-specific suppressor factors. These generally consisted of two chains, one of which had antigen-binding properties and the other having a serological epitope mapping to the *I–J* locus in the mouse H-2 region (in between genes for class II MHC molecules) as reviewed by Dorf and Benacerraf (*7*).

Despite this apparent progress, the credibility of both the IgT story and the antigen-specific suppressor work had largely collapsed by 1982. Exhaustive attempts by the groups of Hood and Tonegawa, among others, had utterly failed to find any evidence of Ig *V* or *J* region usage by any T cell clones (*8*). Especially shocking was the very rapid 'walk' through the *I* region by Michael Steinmetz in Lee Hood's group which found, in essence, that there was no *I–J* region (*9*). Thus by 1982–1983, a sense of desperation began sinking into the immunology community regarding the nature of the T cell receptor. It seemed that the slate had to be wiped clean and some completely new approaches taken. Many molecular biologists were also bitter at their cellular immunology collaborators for leading them down a garden path. A very funny chronicle of this period of recrimination was captured by Antonio Continho and Tommy Meo (*10*) who, in classic murder-mystery style, invited short retrospectives from many of the people who had contributed to this early T cell receptor work and then attacked them (and the field in general) in an overview. The one molecular biologist who had remained calm enough to contribute a piece was Tasuku Honjo, who, in obvious frustration, compared the T cell receptor to an 'imaginary monster' from Japanese mythology (*10*). A somewhat more measured piece on the same theme was contributed by Jensenius and Williams entitled 'Paradigm Lost' (*11*).

A Portrait of the Artist

Blissfully unaware of this intellectual ferment, I had been simultaneously wrapping up my undergraduate studies and fencing career at Johns Hopkins University in Baltimore in 1974. There I had had the good fortune to work in synthetic organic chemistry with Dr Peter Y. Johnson. This type of chemistry is good for the part-timer in research, as things happen quickly and you often know where you stand experimentally within days or at most weeks. 'P.Y.', as he was known, had an infectious enthusiasm and drama about him that also helped pull me into the research business. It was in his laboratory that I first realized that I had some talent for bench work. After a year or so, though, I found myself unable to relate to the organic chemistry theory behind the experiments I was doing and moved to Michael Beer's laboratory in the Biophysics Department in the adjacent building, where I felt much more in the swing of things intellectually – as I was no longer in the somewhat arcane and dry chemical world, but in an increasingly exciting one of DNA and proteins and developing cells. The clinching argument to moving was also the fact that, whereas chemists almost always have to wash their own glassware, biologists never do! In any event, from these first experiences in chemistry and molecular biology, I found myself arriving in Pasadena, California, in the autumn of 1974 to begin graduate school. In my six years there, I had the unusual good fortune (although it seemed otherwise at the time) of having two successive Ph.D. supervisors in two different areas (I often frighten present or prospective graduate students now with this scenario). My first victim was Eric Davidson, a wild but very smart character who rode a motorcycle to the laboratory everyday and wore a leather jacket with a large green frog (*Xenopus laevis*) on the back, which was the logo for the 'tiger toads', his personal football team. He had learned to play the five-string banjo in the backwoods of Appalachia and was a fabulous player with, at last count, three albums of folk music to his credit. Although born and raised in New York, he was happy to affect a hillbilly accent whenever he felt the occasion called for it, such as when he was serving straight whiskey to laboratory members in his office or playing the banjo at parties.

Coming directly from the relatively staid East Coast, it was quite a shock to meet such people (although I had been warned about California in general terms). But of more importance was the fact that Eric was working in the very interesting area of developmental biology, specifically sea urchin embryogenesis, and trying to apply molecular techniques to understand how gene expression is controlled. As with all the very best people, he had a fine sense of rigour and intellectual breadth. Moreover, he held all his students to this same high standard, and we were forced to become educated and well-read. Of particular importance to this narrative is the fact that it was there that I learned the arcane science of nucleic acid hybridization and participated in some of the earlier experiments to count the number of genes being expressed in different stages of sea urchin development. This also turned out to be an excellent background for recombinant DNA projects, which is what I soon found myself working on because, after several years with Eric, the combination of my project going poorly and Eric's impatience with my slapdash experimental style persuaded me to move down the hall to Leroy Hood's laboratory.

This was plunging into the immunological thicket, but I had known Phil Early, a graduate student there for some years, who was working in the then 'jumping' area of Ig gene cloning. Phil was the only one working on a cloning project in Lee's laboratory at the time and it was obviously going to need more hands to be competitive. Lee was also just the right kind of supervisor for me at the time as, while he kept us inspired and braced up during the rougher parts, he generally left us alone to work through the various problems. This was 1977, and Tonegawa had just published his initial description of Ig gene rearrangement and Leder and Seidman at the NIH were weighing in as well. As it turned out, Phil and I worked very well together and, with a lot of help from Tom Maniatis and Norman Davidson and members of their groups at Caltech, we managed to get in some interesting work of our own in the area of $V(D)J$ rearrangements in IgH genes and class switching. In any event, this was my first exposure to immunology, and was relatively painless, as antibodies are easily the best understood molecules in the immune system. The various issues surrounding cellular immunology were relatively dark and mysterious and those of us on the molecular side of the fence had the greatest difficulty understanding what the various experiments were about.

Still, this view from afar must have interested me, as when it came time to finish up in Lee's laboratory I felt it was important to move away from immunoglobulin genes and into this more cellular area of immunology. Mitch Kronenberg, a fellow graduate student in Lee's laboratory and the only person there who seemed to be following this part of the field, suggested William Paul at NIH as a postdoctoral mentor. This also made sense as my girlfriend (and soon afterwards wife), Yueh-hsiu Chien, had just taken a position at NIH. I immediately liked Bill when I visited and found the Laboratory of Immunology a lively and congenial place. Furthermore, it was a hotbed of cellular immunology, with all the arguments of the day being discussed constantly and usually with an unusual clarity that even I could get the gist of. This issue of communication is very important, as much of the data of the time were discussed in terms too obscure for people outside the area. However, I think that, as in all branches of science, the smarter and better-trained people tend to be clearer about what they are doing and thus are much easier to understand than the other kind. So it was that the 'LI', as it is known, really had a high concentration of excellent people. I also think a lot of it was due to Bill's leadership of the unit, which was, and remains today, rigorous and fair. Although at first I had the vague notion that I would do a purely cellular immunology project, when I actually reached the LI and began talking to people there, such as Ron Schwartz and John Kung, the universal message I got was that all the easy cellular experiments had been done and that what was needed most were molecular reagents to sort out the next steps. In particular, Ron emphasized the mysteries of T cell recognition where, as chronicled above, the repeated efforts (and claims of success) to isolate the receptor for antigen (known, familiarly, as the T cell receptor) had failed miserably. This advice convinced me to work on a general cloning strategy for genes which mediated important immune functions, and to at least toy with the idea of solving the T cell receptor problem.

The Strategy

In my days with Eric Davidson, many groups, including his, had measured the differences in gene expression between different tissues by synthesizing cDNA, or the equivalent, from one messenger RNA population and 'subtracting' it with mRNA from another. This makes use of the ability of reverse transcriptase to make a DNA copy of an RNA, usually starting from the poly A 'tail' at the 3' end. The ability to count genes comes from the work of Wetmur and Davidson, and Britton, Bishop and others, who realized that the rate of annealing between two complementary bits of DNA (or an RNA:DNA hybrid) could be a direct measure of the number of different species (12). Thus an mRNA population which hybridizes ten times more slowly than another at some standard concentration has ten times as many different species. In any event, there were hundreds of reports of gene counting in the literature, all showing relatively large differences, even between resting and growing cells. Once gene cloning became possible, this type of activity quickly died, as molecular biologists could attack specific questions directly, gene by gene. But, in thinking about that work, I realized that no one had looked at closely related cells, such as B and T lymphocytes, where the differences in gene expression might be very small. The smaller the difference, the easier it would be to isolate the genes representing this difference, for two reasons. The first reason is the obvious one, that there would be fewer genes to analyse. The second reason is not so obvious: a probe representing 2% of the gene expression would, when purified, be 50 times enriched for the different sequences – and easily enough to get over a technical barrier to screening clone libraries with labelled cDNAs. This was because people had found empirically that cDNAs which vary by less than 0.1 or 0.05% in a population could not be reliably detected in screening clone libraries, yet most genes are expressed as rare mRNAs with 5–20 copies per cell (c.0.01–0.001% of all mRNAs) (12).

Thus to have a 'net' broad enough to find all the genes that differ between two cell types, it would be important to have a strong enrichment for the cDNAs of interest. In the example of a 2% difference, the 50-fold enrichment that you would obtain in purifying such a probe would elevate even the least abundant cDNA species into the detectable range ($50 \times 0.001 = 0.05\%$). B and T cells are the perfect pair of cells to work with in this respect as they derive from common precursors and have many similar cellular properties. Another very convenient aspect is that there are many cloned tumour cell lines and hybridomas available to start with.

Thus, as I 'weighed my options' in those early days at the LI, I became more and more convinced that B and T cells would have fairly minor differences in their gene expression and that labelled cDNA probes representing these differences might quickly yield interesting genes. Which genes exactly to go for first was less clear, as regulatory genes, recombinases and T cell receptors were all worthy objectives at the time. The main thing to me at the time was that this would be a way to short-circuit the standard cloning strategy of the day, which was to identify and isolate a protein, sequence it and then design degenerate oligonucleotides to screen libraries – a very long and drawn out process and likely to be impossible for many rare abundance class genes. Once a gene was in hand, it seemed that one could reasonably and quickly work 'backwards' to the protein and a variety of other studies. Now, with more experience, I can say that it takes quite a long time to do all that, but at the time I had no experience of working with proteins of any kind, except restriction endonucleases and some of the other handy enzymes which you could conveniently buy. I also think that all immunologists were amazed at the rapid resolution of most of the questions surrounding antibody diversity in the late 1970s, which was largely made possible by recombinant DNA technology. This even led, I think, to the optimistic extreme where it was thought that just by cloning the gene for something, you could answer all the questions about its function.

When I discussed this idea with Bill Paul, he immediately saw the potential and encouraged me to go ahead with it, even though I think he had hoped I would do something more directly related to his interests in B cell related cytokines and the mouse *xid* defect. His response was relatively typical of most immunologists in that they saw that this might be a good way of bringing molecular biology to bear on some very difficult problems. In contrast, the typical response of molecular biologists was one of dismissal, in that I was adopting an obscure and even 'old-fashioned' technology with no well-defined objective (that is, a specific gene) in sight. I think also that many molecular biologists had concluded in the 1970s that hybridization analysis had not got them anywhere and there was also a rapidly expanding new generation of 'clone age' molecular biologists who had missed the relatively brief era of hybridization kinetics and were keen to dismiss what they barely understood in favour of the 'strategies du jour'. In any event, my own sense that this was the right thing to do and Bill's encouragement were all I needed to plunge ahead, first working with RNA from spleen and thymus tissue. One or two experiences with the difficulty of getting RNA from these tissues, as well as purifying B and T cells from them, convinced me that lymphoma lines were the way to go. Bill put me in touch with Dick Asofsky and Jin Kim, who had characterized a number of spontaneous and chemically induced B and T cell lymphoma lines.

My first real results came in December 1980, when I made some labelled cDNA from EL-4, a well-known T cell line, and hybridized it with mRNA from BAL 17, a B cell line from Kim and Asofsky. As I completed the last points in the hybridization curve, I realized that virtually all of the T cell cDNA could react with the B cell mRNA and that only about 2% of the gene expression was different. By isolating that 2% and analysing its hybridization pattern, I estimated that only about 100–200 genes with average size messages were expressed by the EL-4 cell and absent in the B cell. At this point, I knew that it was going to be a useful approach, although for what I did not know, partly just because the number of things worth cloning in lymphocytes kept growing daily. I set about solidifying and extending the observation. Jin Kim would thaw out her lines and get them growing, then give them to me to expand and make mRNA. I soon amassed a repertoire of four or five B and T cell RNAs and did various subtractions. I found that essentially any B cell differed from any T cell by 2% of its gene expression, as well as the reverse (T*-B), as I had done initially. I also found that cells within the B or T lineage differed by very little (less than 0.5%) and that the B*-T and T*-B differences were representative of normal B and T cell mRNA populations and thus were not tumour artefacts.

I noted these findings briefly in a meeting report (13) and have always intended to publish the full-blown version, but events moved so quickly afterwards that this may be in eternal limbo. Later on at Stanford, Alan Krensky, Jan Jongstra, Carol Clayberger and I found that B and T tumour cells seem to lose a significant fraction of their specific gene expression versus factor dependent cell lines (14). Thus transformation and adaptation to cell culture may require the loss of large numbers of genes.

Reduction to Practice

In the spring of 1981 my efforts in this subtraction approach were in full swing. Bill was extremely supportive, so much so that he assigned a very able technician, Ellen Nielsen, to work with me, as well as a postdoctoral fellow, David Cohen, and gave me complete autonomy to take things wherever I wanted them to go. I realized that the crucial step was to use these specific cDNAs to isolate genes and I was helped in thinking about this by talking to Tom Sargent, who had been a fellow graduate student and friend at Caltech and had come to Igor Dawid's laboratory at NIH. He mentioned an observation of his that cDNAs tended to have enough of a 'hairpin' sequence at the 3' end to allow a second strand to be synthesized by DNA polymerase. We both realized that this made it very easy to make a clone 'library' from subtracted cDNA, as one could take subtracted cDNA, double-strand it and clone it directly into plasmids by the standard methods. Being able to screen cDNA libraries already enriched for the species of interest had a great attraction, so we both started working on this methodology, Tom on the *Xenopus* system (14) and David Cohen in my group, who took cDNA from a helper T cell hybridoma obtained from Ellen Heber-Katz in Ron Schwartz's laboratory and subtracted it with a B cell mRNA.

When David finished making this T-cell-specific library, he asked what the next step was. I remember saying he should probe the library with T*-B probe and try to isolate a T cell receptor gene. By this time (summer 1981), it was already becoming clear that the first attempts to isolate genes from T cells which had antibody 'pieces' such as Js or Vs had failed (8), leading me to think that whatever T cells expressed for the purposes of antigen-MHC co-recognition must be T-cell specific. Yet in order to generate many specificities, it seemed likely that such a gene would rearrange its pieces in some way analogous to antibodies, thus a good assay for a T cell receptor gene would be rearrangement in T cells versus some non-lymphoid DNA. Despite my best sales efforts, David was not convinced that this was what he wanted to do, and started to work on B cell-specific genes, which ultimately led to the isolation and characterization of XLR (15), an interesting family of nuclear proteins encoded on the X and Y chromosomes (whose function is not yet known). Meanwhile, I took up the T cell receptor challenge, making a series of probes and screening David's library. I had great trouble, however, in getting clones which were truly T-cell specific, partly because I was trying to use 'dot blots' of candidate clones to survey expression patterns. This turned out to be completely irreproducible and I have had a strong dislike for dot blotting ever since.

Luckily, I was rescued from my ineptitude by the arrival of Stephen Hedrick in the beginning of 1982. Steve had been working very successfully in Ron Schwartz's laboratory across the hall, but became convinced that molecular biology was the way forward and was anxious to learn how it was done. He also was unshakeable in his desire to take a shot at cloning the T cell receptor. Although he had only had experience in cellular immunology, he had no trouble mastering even the most complicated molecular techniques quickly. Unfortunately, I chose this time to make one of my more serious strategic blunders. That is, I decided to take up the suggestion of Ron Schwartz that the quickest way to the T cell receptor genes would be to subtract helper T cell hybrids (T_h) with suppressor T cells (T_s) hybrids. We obtained a T_s cell line from Masaru Taniguichi, and Steve quickly turned out beautiful hybridization curves showing that there was only a 0.3% difference in gene expression between our T_h and T_s cells. We immediately started screening David's T cell specific library and isolated a number of clones. Unfortunately, these clones and the subtracted probes had an almost random pattern of expression with respect to B and T cells. After about six months of work with results of this sort, we concluded that the T_s had reverted to its fusion partner origins and did not really represent a distinct subset of T cells, if indeed it ever had.

The Home Stretch

In any event, we returned to our T-B strategy with the added wrinkle that I had come across in the literature a very elegant method, described by Bernard Mechler and Terry Rabbitts (16), for making membrane-bound polysomal RNA. Unlike the standard (and fairly useless) method of pelleting membrane fractions (and thus bound polysomes) this procedure floated them upwards in a sucrose density gradient. This was not only aesthetically more pleasing, but results in a much better fractionation. Since T cell receptors must be in the membrane polysomes, which includes all secreted or cell membrane proteins, we immediately incorporated this into our screening procedure and thus made T^*_{mb}-B probes to screen the T-B library. Plunging ahead with this, by the beginning of 1983 we had screened and rescreened some 40 cDNAs. We were then presented with the problem of how to distinguish between those that were the same and those that were different. Luckily, Leona Fitzmaurice, who worked with Rose Mage down the hall and who was the only other certified molecular biologist in the LI at the time, had thoroughly mastered the art of running RNA on methyl-mercury gels and making Northern blots. Nowadays, people (including myself) are very wary of methyl-mercury, so those are still the best looking Northerns that my laboratory has ever obtained. Bands were sharp and clear, and the derivatized ABT paper could be used over and over again with many different probes. As our candidate cDNA clones were quite small, averaging just 300 nucleotides, we could not hope to see overlapping sequences reliably, so we just used Northern blots to see which gave the same patterns for mRNA.

After some months of this, by the end of the winter 1983 we had whittled down the initial group of 40 clones to 10 distinct ones. Using a rat Thy 1 cDNA obtained from Jack Silver (a former Hood-ite) we were able to establish that one of our 10 clones was the mouse Thy 1. This encouraged us enormously, as Thy 1 is a very rare sequence (0.001% of the clones in cDNA library from thymocytes generously provided by Christophe Benoist, then in Len Herzenberg's laboratory at Stanford, one of the few molecular biologists to take my approach seriously). Southern blotting also began in earnest, although here again there was quite a guessing game, as it is impossible to know which restriction digests might reveal a particular rearrangement and which ones will not. We settled on a number of different ones, including Pvu II, not a particularly robust (or cheap) restriction enzyme but one that had been lucky for us in a completely unrelated Southern analysis project of David Cohen's. As always with this technique, there were various technical problems (false alarms due to partial digests, and so forth), but ultimately we were able to get good Southern blots with multiple digests for all but one of the clones. Unfortunately, none of those nine clones showed any rearrangement.

At that time things were definitely heating up in the 'receptor wars', as we called them. This was because a number of groups including Kappler and Marrack, Reinherz and Schlossman, Jim Allison and also Larry Samelson in Ron Schwartz's group had all made monoclonal antibodies against 'clonotypic' T cell surface molecules. These molecules looked suspiciously like T cell receptors in that they varied from T cell to T cell and occurred as disulphide linked heterodimers (dubbed α and β) (17–21). Also, we were running out of time, as I was preparing to leave for a job at Stanford and Steve was giving job seminars all around the country, ultimately landing one at the University of California, San Diego. For some reason, I had also agreed to help teach the cloning course at Cold Spring Harbor in May, and was thus out of action for three weeks.

Finally, we were in town long enough to try again with our last clone, TM 86. The timing is distinct, as Chien and I were just getting ready to drive up to my father's house in Connecticut for the 4th July weekend when I got a call Sunday morning from Steve: 'You should come and look at this,' I think he said, 'this looks like the real thing'. I rushed over (we lived less than one mile away from NIH) and agreed that TM 86 looked like a classic rearranging gene. Steve had stopped by the laboratory on his way to the zoo, and I do not know how long his kids had to wait in the car. As for me, we went ahead with our visit to my father's house but I told him that we would have to leave the next day, instead of later as planned. The next few weeks were frantic – we went through tons of Southern blots with all sorts of T cell and non-T cell DNAs. We had already prepped-up full-length clones corresponding to TM 86 from Benoist's thymocyte libraries, and sequencing was well underway. My time there was up, however, as we were due to fly to Palo Alto on 20 July. We flew in and immediately got to work, borrowing equipment from Hugh McDevitt's laboratory next door. Luckily, Chien had decided to work with me at Stanford, so we were able to move reasonably quickly. Meanwhile, the laboratory at NIH with Steve, Ellen and David was still going strong and over the next few months completed several sequences and computer searches. It was clear that this gene was very immunoglublin-like with V, C and J region elements and more homologous to immunoglobulins than to anything else. The C region, in particular, was as much like C_K as C_κ was to C_λ. Also looking at the different cDNA sequences, we found distinct J regions assorting independently. The evidence was overwhelming that this must be one of the chains of a T cell recognition molecule.

A Grand Tour

In the second week of August, however, there was yet another interruption. As a very nice going away present, Bill had put my name forward to join a small group of immunologists who were going to visit immunology centres in mainland China and give a series of symposia. Always interested in travel opportunities, I accepted and, as an afterthought, the agency arranging the travel suggested I also attend the International Congress of Immunology in Kyoto right after the meeting. I had never been to Japan either, so that seemed like a good idea as well. In any event, off I went with Stuart Schlossman, Tony Fauci, Mike Frank and Eng Tan among others on a 10-day trip to Beijing and Shanghai. It was a very interesting trip for both touristic and cultural reasons. One was how poor it was compared to Taiwan, which Chien had taken me to two years before. Another was how, despite all the propaganda about the 'people's' this and that, the society had this very heirarchial, if not outright feudal character. The science was pretty limited for me as it was all very applied, being directed towards markers for specific diseases and so forth. The feeling was largely mutual, as I gave a talk in Beijing that apparently none of our hosts understood. They were sufficiently concerned about this that they assigned me a special translator in Shanghai who went over my talk with me the night before. Even then there was apparently a lot of confusion, as the head of the institute there interrupted the translator to give her own rendition, but even then there were no questions after my talk.

But this was no longer my primary concern. When the NIH first arranged flights for my trip, they had not obtained a confirmed reservation leaving Shanghai for Kyoto, but I had been assured that one would come through by the time I got there. Thus it came as a shock to be told at the airline office in Shanghai that no there were no flights open until September! It looked as if I might miss the Kyoto Congress. I was becoming increasingly agitated and tried to pressure my hosts to get me something, anything that would get me to Japan. But they seemed unable to help. Early Saturday morning, I knew, there was a direct CAAC flight to Osaka (near Kyoto), as several of my colleagues were on it. I insisted that I was going to the airport with them and would try to get on that flight or any flight that was leaving China that day. The young secret policeman in charge of our stay in Shanghai tried to dissuade me from getting into the taxi by telling me that the plane was overbooked and that they would have to throw off ten passengers with confirmed reservations. I thanked him for the information but went anyway. At the airport there was a mob scene, but whatever was on the sign waved by our guide helped to get us through. He came back with the same story that I had heard on leaving the hotel – no chance of getting on. 'I'll just wait', I said, 'and see what comes up', or words to that effect. I still wonder what he thought of my stupidity. The plane was delayed for many hours. After the better part of a morning sitting around on the luggage in the hot and crowded airport, they called me up to the desk and asked me if I wanted 'smoking or non-smoking'. I was ecstatic, and after waiting a few more hours for the plane to actually get going, I could not help noticing that there were half a dozen empty seats on the plane. Later, I was told that a whole tour group of immunologists who were on their way to the Kyoto meeting from Shanghai had had all their reservations mysteriously vanish from the CAAC's computer (in Tokyo) and that it took some people until the middle of the next week to make it to Kyoto.

But the fun was not yet over. On arriving in Osaka airport, I was asked for my visa. 'What visa?' I must have replied, brightly. This made me many new friends in airport security and they took me to a back room (no bare light bulbs though, just a big office area), where they tried to impress upon me the seriousness of my crime. One thing that must surely have baffled them is why I was so cheerful during our several hours together. The simple reason was that I was so happy to have gotten out of Shanghai at all that this little visa difficulty did not look like a problem. They did not see it that way of course and my principal interrogator asked me over and over again why I thought I could just come waltzing into Japan without a visa. I replied truthfully that nobody had told me and, incredibly lamely, that I had gone all over Europe without one some years before. I knew that they could not be too seriously concerned about me when

I saw that they had my name in a large book of all the foreigners who were coming to the congress. Also, when they asked if I knew any upstanding Japanese citizens who could vouch for my good character, I could immediately name Tasuku Honjo, who I knew from my antibody gene cloning days. The conclusion is interesting for those seeking to understand how the bureaucratic mind works. It was explained to me that in order to stay in Japan, I must apply for a temporary visa. This, however, would automatically be denied because you could not land at a Japanese airport without having one already. I could, however, appeal against this decision to the Minister of Justice. I signed various forms (which could have said anything) and my friend went off to some other part of the building. Five minutes later he was back. The Minister had given the 'thumbs up' sign (or its Japanese equivalent) and I was free to terrorize the populace! Prior to the meeting I had talked to the chair of the most relevant section, Harvey Cantor, and he had tentatively agreed to let me speak in the middle of the week. Leon Rosenberg from Stanford brought me some new slides from Steve and Ellen in Bethesda, summarizing their sequence comparisons and a computer search they had done. I had freely discussed what we had done all through the meeting, so many people were 'primed' for the actual talk. It was certainly the biggest audience by far that I had ever spoken to, 4000 or so, but I tried to keep calm and present the facts as I knew them. After I got through it, Masaru Taniguichi and Susumu Tonegawa told the Japanese media that this was big news and they immediately clustered around me to get the story. I have no idea what they wrote, but it was in all the papers the next day, along with the obligatory picture of my head. Many people have told me afterwards that it was from my talk in Kyoto that they really thought the T cell receptor saga at last had started to yield to molecular biology.

Taking a slightly different approach, Tak Mak at the Ontario Cancer Institute in Toronto, isolated a human equivalent of our mouse β gene and we published simultaneously in March of 1984 in *Nature* (22–24). The γ gene discovery by Tonegawa followed a few months later using our protocol (at the time thought to be α) (25) and Tonegawa's paper and ours on the α chain were published in October 1984, again in the same issue of *Nature* (26,27). Some years later (1987), the partner to the γ chain, δ was discovered by Yueh-hsiu Chien at Stanford (28) and this completed the set of four TCR genes that we know today. While the αβ form of the T cell receptor heterodimer seems solely devoted to recognizing peptide–MHC complexes, the γδ form, which is expressed on an entirely different set of T cells, has more antibody-like recognition properties (29), and its function is still very mysterious.

Epilogue

To conclude, I have tried to select elements that I think are important in understanding how it all happened. I am sure that I have left out important bits, but maybe I will remember these later. I think the importance of our discovery of that first T cell receptor gene was that it gave the first glimpse of what Honjo had earlier called an 'imaginary monster'. The complete DNA sequence gave a clear snapshot of what the polypeptide would look like and how it could confer specificity. That this was so antibody-like was not so important at the time, but that we had breached a major bottleneck to understanding the mechanisms of T cell recognition was. It also helped to re-form a consensus in favour of a one-receptor model, where a single site could recognize both antigen and MHC simultaneously. Also, the virtue of having a gene gives you many lines of attack not available to those working the antibody–protein angle. What was also gratifying to many people on a sociological and aesthetic level, was that we were this tiny little group that nobody had ever heard of working in a department with no reputation in molecular biology. We had been competing with large and well-oiled laboratories, and had won the first round in the T cell receptor sweepstakes.

Notes and References

1. R. M. Zingernagel and P. C. Doherty, *Nature* **248**, 701 (1974).
2. H. Binz, H. Wigzell and H. Bazin, *Nature* **264**, 639 (1976).
3. K. Rajewsky and K. Eichmann, *Contemp. Topics Immunobiol.* 7, 69 (1977).
4. J. J. Marchalonis, *Contemp. Top. Mol. Immunol.* 5, 125 (1976).
5. F. L. Owen, R. Riblet and B. A. Taylor, *J. Exp. Med.* 153, 801 (1981).
6. M. Spurll and F. L. Owen, *Nature* **293**, 742 (1981).
7. M. E. Dorf and B. Benacerraf, *Ann. Rev. Immunol.* 2, 127 (1984).
8. M. Kronenberg, M. M. Davis, G. Siu, J. A. Kapp, J. Kappler, P. Marrack, C. W. Pierce and L. Hood, *J. Exp. Med.* 158, 210 (1983).
9. M. Steinmetz, K. Minard, S. Horvath *et al.*, *Nature* **300**, 35 (1982).
10. A. Coutinho and T. Meo, *Scand. J. Immunol.* 18, 79 (1983).
11. J. C. Jensenius and A. F. Williams, *Nature* **300**, 583 (1982).
12. B. Lewin, *Gene Expression*, vol. 2, 2nd edn, Wiley, New York (1980).
13. M. M. Davis, D. I. Cohen, E. A. Nielsen, A. D. DeFranco and W. E. Paul, in *B and T cell tumors (UCLA Symposium)* (E. Vitetta and C. F. Fox, eds), vol. 24, Academic Press, London (1982), p. 215.
14. J. Jongstra, T. J. Schall, B. J. Dyer, C. Clayberger, J. Jorgensen, M. M. Davis and A. M. Krensky, *J. Exp. Med.* 165, 601 (1987).
15. D. I. Cohen, A. D. Steinberg, W. E. Paul and M. M. Davis, *Nature* **314**, 372 (1985).
16. B. Mechler and T. H. Rabbitts, *J. Cell Biol.* 88, 29 (1981).
17. J. P. Allison, B. MacIntyre and D. Block, *J. Immunol.* 129, 2293 (1982).
18. S. C. Meuer, K. A. Fitzgerald, R. E. Hussey, J. C. Hogdon, S. F. Schlossman and E. L. Reinherz, *J. Exp. Med.* 157, 705 (1983).
19. K. Haskins, R. Kubo, J. White, M. Pigeon, J. Kappler and P. Marrack, *J. Exp. Med.* 157, 1149 (1983).
20. L. E. Samelson, R. N. Germain and R. H. Schwartz, *Proc. Natl Acad. Sci. USA* 80, 6972 (1983).
21. J. Kaye, S. Porcelli, J. Tite, B. Jones and C. A. Janeway, *J. Exp. Med.* 158, 836 (1983).
22. Y. Yanagi, Y. Yoshikai, K. Leggett, S. P. Clark, I. Aleksander and T. W. Mak, *Nature* **308**, 145 (1984).

23. S. M. Hedrick, D. I. Cohen, E. A. Nielsen and M. M. Davis, *Nature* **308**, 149 (1984).
24. S. M. Hedrick, E. A. Nielsen, J. Kavaler, D. I. Cohen and M. M. Davis, *Nature* **308**, 153 (1984).
25. H. Saito, D. M. Kranz, Y. Takagaki, A. D. Hayday, H. N. Eisen and S. Tonegawa, *Nature* **309**, 757 (1984).
26. Y. Chien, D. M. Becker, T. Lindsten, M. Okamura, D. I. Cohen and M. M. Davis, *Nature* **312**, 31 (1984).
27. H. Saito, D. M. Kranz, Y. Takagaki, A. C. Hayday, H. N. Eisen and S. Tonegawa, *Nature* **312**, 36 (1984).
28. Y. Chien, M. Iwashima, K. Kaplan, J. Elliott and M. M. Davis, *Nature* **327**, 677 (1987).
29. H. Schild, N. Mavaddat, C. Litzenberger, E. W. Ehrich, M. M. Davis, J. A. Bluestone, L. Matis, R. K. Draper and Y-h. Chien, *Cell* **76**, 1 (1994).

Immunology and Medicine

Organ Transplantation and the Revitalization of Immunology

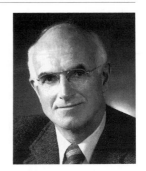

JOSEPH E. MURRAY

Harvard Medical School, Brigham and Women's Hospital,
108 Abbot Road, Wellesley Road, MA 021812, USA

Over 150 years ago Pasteur wrote: 'No category of science exists to which one could give the name of applied science. Science and application of science are linked together as a fruit is to the tree that has borne it.' Salvatore has expanded Pasteur's concept: 'There are no divisions in science, only one humanity.' As a surgeon–scientist who has spent a professional lifetime seeking new knowledge in both laboratory and hospital, I support their holistic viewpoints.

Barriers between scientific disciplines can impede progress. Some bioscientists consider that bench science is more difficult, more intellectual, more 'pure and scientific' than clinical science. In my opinion, such an attitude is intellectual provincialism. A good example of the oneness of science is the development of organ and tissue transplantation. After World War II, surgeons and physicians on both sides of the Atlantic refused to accept the dogma that human organ transplantation would never be possible. Bench scientists had difficulty understanding the determined optimism of clinicians who were willing to study and test any type of treatment that might help desperately ill patients, for example extensive thermal burns requiring skin transplants, and terminally uraemic patients needing new kidneys.

The conference at which this volume was conceived, an informal meeting of scientists, historians, and philosophers, reinforced my previous conviction that clinical scientists are essential for progress in medicine. An opening speaker opined that the current rebirth of immunology occurred at the Cold Spring Harbour Symposium of 1967. Apparently he was unaware of the several Transplantation Conferences sponsored biennially by the New York Academy of Science in the 1950s and 1960s. Another speaker asked rhetorically: 'When did the transplanters begin to include immunology into their meetings?' This astonished me, considering that from the early 1950s transplant conferences

IMMUNOLOGY: THE MAKING OF A MODERN SCIENCE
ISBN 0-12-274020-3

included topics of immunology, genetics, zoology, pathology, biochemistry, surgery and internal medicine, as well as haematology and plastic surgery. A later speaker, reluctantly admitting that surgeons have contributed to immunology, commented on the 'luck' of the transplant surgeons. I quickly responded that no conscientious surgeon depends on luck. Success in surgery demands laborious preparation, scholarly homework and, for transplanters, a zeal to challenge the impossible. Medawar, the acknowledged doyen of transplantation, always credited surgeons for their powerful roles in the extraordinary progress of transplantation.

Early in my career I was advised not to waste my time on research on organ transplantation; instead, I should wait for the basic scientists to solve the problem. Fortunately, I paid no attention. Joining the renal transplantation team at the Peter Bent Brigham Hospital under George W. Thorn, Physician-in-Chief, and Francis D. Moore, Surgeon-in-Chief, I made a firm commitment to laboratory and clinical research. Professors Albert Coons and Bernard Davis, our colleagues at Harvard Medical School, Department of Microbiology, were originally sceptical about the project, but over the years they became more interested, and ultimately admired our success in making clinical transplantation a reality.

Background of Human Organ Transplantation

There were three routes to transplantation: studies of kidney disease and hypertension, studies of skin grafts and twins and surgery. Although renal transplantation had been performed sporadically during the first half of this century (1,2), planned programmes for human organ transplantation started only in the late 1940s. At that time, clinicians in Paris, London, Edinburgh and Boston began renal transplantation in non-immunosuppressed human recipients, in spite of the warnings and pessimistic predictions of many scientists and experienced clinicians. Both Loeb (3) and Medawar (4) claimed that human allotransplantation would never be possible because the roots of individuality were so deep and impenetrable. But, encouraging experiences with short-term functioning human renal allotransplants occurred from time to time. We in Boston and two superb groups in Paris had obtained temporary function of human renal allografts (5,6); Lawlor and coworkers in Chicago actually reported 'success' in a patient (7), a report which was later rescinded.

Thorn had long been interested in the well-known association of renal disease to hypertension, a condition for which there was no effective treatment. After World War II, he invited Willem W. Kolff from the Netherlands to Boston to demonstrate a dialysis machine that he (Kolff) had developed during his forced confinement by the Germans (8). Carl W. Walter, a Brigham surgeon and engineer, helped to improve the design (9), and thus the Kolff–Brigham 'artificial kidney' was devised. It was first used in patients in 1948 and set the stage for extensive, innovative approaches to both acute reversible renal disease and end-stage kidney failure. Because renal dialysis was only a temporary substitute for renal function, it was logical to seek a more permanent therapy. (Chronic dialysis was not developed until ten years later, in 1958, in Seattle (10)). During a Grand Rounds at the Brigham, Thorn stated that the best way to treat hypertension would be to remove both kidneys. The audience gasped. The seed for the Brigham renal transplant programme had been planted.

In 1932, E. C. Padgett of Kansas City reported the use of skin allografts from familial and unrelated donors to treat severely burned patients. Although none of these skin allografts survived permanently, they remained long enough to be life-saving. The survival time of the allografts was difficult to determine; some melted away slowly and were replaced by adjacent normal skin, whilst others were rejected rapidly. Skin grafts from family members seemed to survive best. None survived permanently. The only certainty was established when, in 1937, J. B. Brown of St Louis achieved permanent survival of skin grafts exchanged between monozygotic twins (11). This observation, although restricted in application, was the only ray of light in the problem of tissue and organ replacement until Gibson and Medawar demonstrated that a second allograft from the same donor was rejected more rapidly than the first (12). This report of the 'second set' phenomenon established that the rejection process was not immutable; instead, it implied an allergic or immunological process which potentially might be manipulated.

Dizygotic twins also play a significant role in the history of organ transplantation. In 1779, John Hunter, always curious about experiments of nature, presented before the Royal College of Surgeons his observations of the physical characteristics of the freemartin, the female member of differently sexed dizygotic twin cattle (13). In 1917, F. R. Lillie of Woods Hole dissected placentas of several pairs of freemartin cattle and noted intermingling of blood between them. Because of the sterility of the female, it was natural that most subsequent studies related to endocrine aspects of the freemartin (14). In 1945, R. D. Owen, then at Wisconsin, now at Caltech, noted the coexistence of different red cell blood types in these cattle and published on the tolerogenic consequences of placental intermingling of circulation (15). He cited Lillie as the key reference.

Owen's report brought the freemartin to the attention of the immunologists. In 1951, D. Anderson and coworkers reported successful experimental skin allografts between the freemartin and the normal twin male (16). The freemartin story culminated in the report of R. E. Billingham, L. Brent and P. Medawar in 1953 that described acquired immunological tolerance in mice (17). In their paper they acknowledged that their experimental protocol had a counterpart in the twin cattle model of Owen. Although not applicable clinically, the experimental production of acquired immunological tolerance in mice was still another source for optimism in the quest for successful human renal transplantation. Sir Michael Woodruff, pioneer transplant surgeon in

Edinburgh, confirmed the freemartin concept in humans when he found a pair of twins – one male, the other female – who shared each other's differing red cell types. Postulating a shared placental circulation between the two, he cross-skin-grafted them successfully (*18*).

In the early 1900s, A. Carrel, a French surgeon working at the Rockefeller Institute, developed techniques for suturing blood vessels in dogs. Carrel and his coworker C. C. Guthrie then transplanted kidneys and even entire heads in these animals. Although they recognized that autografts survived longer than allografts or xenografts (*19*), they did not conceptualize the rejection process. They did comment that loss of function of the allotransplants seemed to be a result of neither infection nor infarction, but was something different.

After World War II, W. J. Dempster (*20*) and M. Simonsen (*21*) published extensively on canine renal transplantation, concentrating on the biology and biochemistry of allograft rejection. They showed that skin and kidney allografts possess a common antigen that could sensitize a recipient to a subsequent allo-graft of either tissue from the same donor. At this time there was a tacit assumption that renal autografts would ultimately deteriorate, possibly from lack of nerve supply, lymphatics, or both. From a physiological point of view, if human renal transplantation were to be successful, researchers needed to establish that renal transplants in the absence of an immunological barrier could function *permanently*. Therefore, among my first laboratory projects, I developed a reproducible canine *autograft* model that resulted in normally functioning renal autografts for years (*22*).

The Identical Twin Transplant

Our team was well prepared when, in the autumn of 1954, D. Miller of the US Public Health Service referred to John P. Merrill, the nephrologist in the Brigham transplant programme, a patient with severe renal disease. Miller suggested there might be the opportunity for renal transplantation because the patient had a healthy identical twin brother. We possessed the necessary surgical and medical skills. Here was a chance to transplant an immunologically compatible kidney. The only remaining problem was the ethical decision to remove a healthy organ from a normal person for the benefit of someone else. This was a first in medical history and a review of the literature would not help!

After consultations with other physicians and clergy, we decided to offer the opportunity to the recipient and donor. The donor asked whether the hospital would be responsible for his health care for the rest of his life if he decided to donate his kidney. J. Hartwell Harrison, urologist and surgeon for the donor, answered that the hospital could not make such a commitment. But he then hastened to ask the donor if he thought that any physician on our team would ever refuse to take care of him if he needed help? The donor then realized that his future medical care depended on our sense of professional responsibility rather than on legal assurances. We have maintained close contact with the family over the years and they have become true friends. Once the decision to operate was made, an extra professional burden fell on the surgeon for the donor, because his patient is expected to survive. In contrast, the surgeon for the recipient is operating on a patient otherwise doomed to die; nor could the nephrologist be faulted for his inability to cure the nephritis. The transplanted kidney functioned immediately. By the next morning, the patient's eyes were alert and his appetite returned. He was discharged from the hospital within a few weeks. We had achieved success by bypassing, not solving, biological incompatibility (23,24).

In 1982, 28 years later, Medawar, then interested in the problem of cancer and its possible relationship to immunology, stressed the need for scientifically oriented clinicians dealing with cancer. He wrote: '. . . physicians will arise who feel just as much at home in the laboratory as in the cancer ward. Just one brilliant break is needed – akin to that first brilliant kidney transplant at the Peter Bent Brigham Hospital in Boston – and then recruits will come forward by the hundreds' (25).

Our success stimulated world-wide laboratory attempts to breach the immunological barrier. Among the many experimental protocols were total X-ray treatment followed by marrow infusion, immunoparalysis by consecutive graftings, immunological enhancement or adaptation by exposure of the host or graft to antigen before the transplant, matching of donor and recipient by red or white cell typing, and the use of drugs such as toluene and nitrogen mustard as immunosuppressants.

In conjunction with Gustave Dammin, Professor of Pathology, we allografted pieces of skin from various donors onto volunteer uraemic recipients. Survival of the allografts was prolonged by weeks but was never permanent. This suggested that the uraemic state itself was immunosuppressive (26). In mice and rabbits, total body irradiation with X-rays followed by bone marrow infusion from single or multiple donors was able to prolong survival of skin grafts from the marrow donors for months (27).

During these years, we transplanted several more pairs of identical twins. One identical twin recipient, transplanted in 1956, completed a pregnancy two years later (28). She is now a grandmother and the longest surviving renal transplant recipient. Her donor, also a grandmother, is likewise in good health.

In January 1959, a dizygotic twin in terminal uraemia had a kidney transplant from his brother after having received a sublethal dose of total body X-radiation. Skin grafts had previously established their immunological incompatibility. After a complicated postoperative course, he recovered to lead an active, normal life for more than 25 years. This was the world's first successful human allograft. He was, however, the only one of 12 patients on this protocol whose kidney functioned beyond three months. When immunosuppressive drugs became available (29–31), we stopped using the total body–X-ray–marrow protocol.

Later in 1959, J. Hamburger in Paris had similar success with a dizygotic twin recipient after sublethal X-ray treatment. Between 1959 and 1962, he and Rene Kuss, working independently in Paris, produced five long-surviving kidney recipients using non-twin donors – siblings, a cousin, and, in two of Kuss's cases, non-relatives. The recipient of the cousin is still alive, and a member of the French parliament (32).

Immunosuppressive Drugs

The real breakthrough came with the introduction of immunosuppressive drugs by R. Schwartz and W. Dameschek in 1959. They were able to prevent rabbits from producing antibody to bovine γ-globulin by giving the drug 6-mercaptopurine (6-MP) at the time of antigen presentation. The same drug dosage five days before or five days after antigen presentation produced a normal antibody response. This 'drug-induced tolerance' remained after drug treatment was stopped, even though the animals could later produce antibody to another protein, human serum albumen. Thus, the tolerance was specific for the antigen given at the time of drug administration (33).

R. Y. Calne in London (34) and C. Zukoski and coworkers in Virginia (35) tested this drug in the canine renal transplant model and had encouraging results. On the advice of P. B. Medawar, in 1960 Calne came to Boston to work in the Department of Surgery, under F. D. Moore, at Harvard and the Brigham. Calne introduced us to G. H. Hitchings and G. B Elion of the Burroughs Wellcome laboratories, who became enthusiastic collaborators. After Calne's arrival, and with drugs from Burroughs Wellcome, the improvement in canine allograft survival was rapid and dramatic; we soon had bilaterally nephrectomized dogs living on solitary renal allografts that survived for years. One recipient produced a normal litter sired by a drug-treated allografted male. Another was able to recover from a severe infection of the mandible, demonstrating he was not an immunological cripple, a state we feared might result from prolonged use of the drugs (36).

Other drugs were provided by Hitchings and Elion; B-W 322, the imidazole derivative of 6-MP, seemed to have the best therapeutic index. This drug, now known as azathioprine or Imuran, has been used ever since to support organ transplantation. Currently, newer and more effective drugs are available, but azathioprine is still widely used.

Reassured by our laboratory results with these transplants in dogs, we started using the drugs in humans. A patient who received a renal transplant from a cadaver in April 1962 and was treated with azathioprine survived for over one year, the first successful cadaveric transplant (37,38). W. E. Goodwin and coworkers at the University of California in Los Angeles introduced corticosteroids as an adjunct to the treatment (39). Subsequently, several transplantation groups world-wide began their own productive transplantation programmes. By 1965, one-year survival rates of allografted kidneys from living related donors approached 80%, and survival rates of kidneys from cadavers approached 65%. Regional and national donor procurement programmes were established along with a Human Renal Transplant Registry (40).

Optimism and enthusiasm were high, as new drugs and other methods of immune suppression were tested along with refinements in tissue typing and improved organ preservation. Antilymphocyte serum and globulin prepared in horse, sheep and rabbit, along with thoracic duct drainage of lymphocytes, were among the promising regimens tested. To date, more than 300 000 human renal transplants have been performed world-wide.

Other Organs

Success with renal allografts naturally led to attempts to transplant other organs. F. D. Moore and coworkers developed a surgical technique for orthotopic canine liver transplantation (41), as did T. E. Starzl and coworkers. Starzl subsequently performed the first successful human liver allografts (42). Calne, returning to Cambridge, England, also gained extensive human liver transplantation experience. For almost 15 years, both Starzl and Calne and their coworkers performed most of the world's human liver transplants (43). Today, transplantation of the liver is done around the world and is the second most frequently performed transplant operation.

The heart was the next organ to be transplanted. R. Lower and N. Shumway had developed the surgical technique in dogs in 1960 (44) and were planning a careful programme for cardiac transplantation in humans. After C. N. Barnard's first human cardiac transplant in South Africa in 1967, other cardiac surgeons with little or no immunological background rapidly accumulated large numbers of heart-transplanted patients, only to see them all die of rejection within a few months. This period, from 1968 to 1970, was transplantation's darkest hour because of the careless application of technical procedures with insufficient laboratory background. The sole redeeming feature in heart transplantation was the continuation of Shumway's programme at Stanford, which achieved permanent success in 1970 (45). Today, with the development of newer drugs, cardiac transplantation is a recognized and accepted form of treatment. Single and double lung transplants have followed, as well as combined heart–lung transplants.

Transplantation of the pancreas, with or without an accompanying renal graft, is now possible for some patients. Multiple organ transplants in combination with liver and parts of the intestinal tract have also been successful. In 1992, there were 9659 kidney, 2997 liver, 2161 heart, 551 pancreas and 48 heart-lung transplants performed in the USA alone (46).

Ironically, allografts of skin, the tissue used classically in most of the early studies of transplantation, have proven to be the most difficult to transplant.

Skin is the ultimate protection of the individual against the environment and, therefore, over time, has evolved into our strongest barrier against foreign proteins. The earlier conventional wisdom was that the fate of skin allografts predicted the results of other transplants. Commenting on the contrasting survival rates of skin and kidney allografts in immunosuppressed dogs, Medawar proclaimed, with his customary flair, that the success of organ transplantation has 'overthrown the doctrinal tyranny of skin grafts' (47).

Consequences Beyond Transplantation

In less than 40 years, organ transplantation has produced exciting insights about complex biological and clinical problems. Bench scientists have become more interested in clinical problems, and clinical investigators have increased their understanding and activity in basic studies. The boundaries between immunology, microbiology, genetics, cellular and molecular biochemistry, and pharmacology have become porous. Co-operation between bench and bedside has led to progress on many fronts – for example, more effective immunosuppressive agents, increased understanding of autoimmune disease and the association of the immunosuppressed state with neoplasia.

National and international collaborations have been established for the preservation and distribution of organs and have spawned vital forums for the exchange of ideas. With clinical success came the need for better organ preservation, and today donor organs can be preserved long enough to be shipped world-wide, if necessary (48).

Another unforeseen result of transplantation was the central role that histocompatibility antigens, originally recognized as markers for animal and human transplantation, play in many unrelated diseases. For example, the histocompatibility antigen DR2 is linked to narcolepsy and B27 to ankylosing spondylitis. Susceptibility to juvenile-onset diabetes is linked to A1, B8, DR3 and DR4, whereas resistance is linked to DR2.

Successful transplantation is most likely when donor organs are in optimal condition. The former criteria for death – cessation of spontaneous breathing and heartbeat – prevented organ use before their function began to deteriorate. The concept of brain death, formulated by a committee at Harvard Medical School in 1968 in response to the needs of transplant teams, now guides these decisions not only for transplant centres but also for intensive care units worldwide (49).

Liver transplants have allowed the treatment and 'cure' of inborn errors of metabolism, such as μ-1-antitrysin defect, Wilson's disease and tyrosinaemia. Liver replacement not only can cure liver failure but can also correct the various extrahepatic symptoms that are the results of metabolic aberrations. Liver transplantation now is being done in patients with liver-based metabolic diseases that produce severe generalized symptoms, even if the liver is otherwise normal in function and appearance (50). The very success of transplantation has created a scarcity of donor organs that, in turn, has led to their unethical allocation. In some areas, the buying and selling of organs has become acceptable (51). The solution to this unexpected and, by most standards, degrading situation does not lie in ethics, politics or even religion, but in the professional standards of surgical and medical care and in the cultural environment of the region.

Animal research has been absolutely indispensable for the development of clinical organ transplantation. The first twin transplant was a complete surgical success only because it was perfected in operations on hundreds of dogs. Without the experience derived from genetically pure strains of mice, human tissue-typing almost certainly could not have been possible or, at best, would have been set back several decades.

Although thousands of lives have already been saved by the use of various immunosuppressive regimens, serious complications still occur as a result of treatment. An increased incidence of *de novo* neoplasia in long-term survivors has been reported, a result presumably of decreased immune surveillance on the part of the recipient (52).

The ultimate aim in transplantation is to achieve an immunological tolerance between donor and recipient, eliminating entirely the need for drugs. There are signs both in the laboratory and in humans that the liver itself may produce tolerogenic factors that may reduce or eliminate the need for immunosuppression (53).

Organ transplantation has progressed rapidly from the impossible to the commonplace. The complementary roles of clinical and laboratory research have produced profound changes in patient care and laboratory disciplines, and transplantation teams with clinical and laboratory expertise now exist worldwide. Although kidney transplantation began this progression, subspecialties have developed for liver, heart, lung, pancreas, intestine and marrow. Paediatric transplantation, for example, requires special skills and facilities.

Our increased understanding of cellular and humoral immunity, autoimmunity and human tissue typing, combined with imaginative and skilful surgical experimentation, have revolutionized patient care. This cascade of progress began with an apparently simple, clear-cut aim: to find a way to replace a destroyed or missing organ. The field of transplantation with its revitalizing effect on immunology could not have occurred without the input of clinical scientists.

Notes and References

1. J. E. Murray, *Les Prix Nobel 1990* (1991), Nobel Foundation, Stockholm, p. 204.
2. F. D. Moore, *Transplant: The Give and Take of Tissue Transplantation*, Simon and Schuster, New York (1972), pp. 66–79.
3. L. Loeb, *Biological Basis of Individuality*, Thomas, Springfield, IL (1945).

4. P. Medawar, *Uniqueness of the Individual*, Methuen, London (1957).
5. L. Michon, J. Hamburger, N. Economos, P. Delinotte, G. Richet, J. Vaysse and B. Antoine, *Presse Med.* **61**, 1419 (1953).
6. R. Kuss, J. Teinturier and P. Milliez, *Mem. Acad. Chir.* **77**, 755 (1951).
7. R. H. Lawlor, J. W. West, P. H. McNulty, E. J. Clancy and P. P. Murphy, *J. Am. Med. Assoc.* **147**, 45 (1951).
8. W. Kolff, *Acta Med. Scand.* **117**, 120 (1944); *Ann. Intern. Med.* **62**, 608 (1965).
9. F. D. Moore, *Transplant: The Give and Take of Tissue Transplantation*, Simon & Schuster, New York (1972), pp. 66–79.
10. W. E. Quinton, D. Dillard and B. Scribner, *Trans. Am. Soc. Artif. Intern. Organs* **6**, 104 (1960).
11. J. B. Brown, *Surgery* **1**, 558 (1937).
12. T. Gibson and P. Medawar, *J. Anat.* **77**, 299 (1942–1943).
13. J. Hunter, *Philos. R. Soc. London, Part I (Communication 20)* **69**, 279 (1779).
14. F. R. Lillie, *Science* **43**, 611 (1916).
15. R. D. Owen, *Science* **102**, 400 (1945).
16. D. Anderson, R. E. Billingham, G. H. Lamkin and P. B. Medawar, *Heredity* **5**, 379 (1951).
17. R. E. Billingham, L. Brent and P. B. Medawar, *Nature*, **172**, 603 (1953).
18. M. F. A. Woodruff and B. Lennox, *Lancet*, **ii**, 476 (1959).
19. A. Carrel and C. C. Guthrie, *Science* **23**, 394 (1906).
20. W. J. Dempster, *Brit. J. Surg.* **40**, 477 (1953).
21. M. Simonsen, J. Buemann, A. Gammeltoft, F. Jensen and K. Jorgensen, *Acta. Pathol. Microbiol. Scand.* **32**, 1 (1953).
22. J. E. Murray, S. Lang, B. J. Miller and G. J. Dammin, *SG&O* **103**, 15 (1956).
23. J. E. Murray, J. P. Merril and J. H. Harrison, *New Engl. J. Med.* **262**, 1251 (1960).
24. J. P. Merrill, J. E. Murray, J. H. Harrison and W. K. Guild, *J. Am. Med. Assoc.* **160**, 277 (1956).
25. P. Medawar, *Pluto's Republic*, Oxford University Press, London (1982), p. 158.
26. G. J. Dammin, N. P. Couch and J. E. Murray, *Ann. NY Acad. Sci.* **64**, 967 (1957).
27. J. E. Murray, R. E. Wilson, J. B. Dealy, N. Sadowski and J. Corsen, in *International Colloquium on the Biological Problems of Grafting*, University of Liège, Belgium, vol. 12 (1959), p. 354.
28. J. E. Murray, J. P. Merrill and J. H. Harrison,. *Ann. Surg.* **148**, 343 (1958).
29. R. Calne, *Lancet* **i**, 417 (1960).
30. C. Zukoski, H. M. Lee and D. M. Hume, *Surg. Forum* **11**, 470 (1960).
31. R. Calne, G. P. J. Alexandre and J. E. Murray, *Ann. NY Acad. Sci.* **99**, 743 (1962).
32. C. Grammes and K. Haglund, *J. NIH Res.* **4**, 71 (1993).
33. R. Schwartz and W. Dameshek, *Nature* **183**, 1682 (1959).
34. R. Calne, *Lancet* **i**, 417 (1960).
35. C. Zukoski, H. M. Lee and D. M. Hume, *Surg. Forum* **11**, 470 (1960).
36. R. Calne, G. P. J. Alexandre and J. E. Murray, *Ann. NY Acad. Sci.* **99**, 743 (1962).
37. J. E. Murray, J. P. Merrill, J. H. Harrison, R. E. Wilson and G. J. Dammin, *New Engl. J. Med.* **268**, 1315 (1963).
38. J. P. Merrill, J. E. Murray, F. Takacs, E. B. Hager, R. E. Wilson and G. J. Dammin, *J. Am. Med. Assoc.* **185**, 347 (1963).
39. W. E. Goodwin, J. J. Kaufman, M. M. Mims, R. D. Turner, R. Glassock, R. Goldman and M. M. Maxwell, *J. Urol.* **89**, 13 (1963).
40. J. E. Murray, B. A. Barnes and J. C. Atkinson, *Transplantation* **5**, 752 (1967).
41. F. D. Moore, L. L. Smith, T. K. Burnap *et al.*, *Transpl. Bull.* **6**, 103 (1959).
42. T. Starzl, C. G. Groth, L. Brettschneider *et al.*, *Ann. Surg.* **168**, 392 (1968).
43. R. Calne and R. Williams, *Br. Med. J.* **4**, 535 (1968).
44. R. Lower and N. Shumway, *Surg. Forum* **11**, 18 (1960).
45. E. Dong, R. B. Griepp, E. B. Stinson and N. E. Shumway, *Ann. Surg.* **176**, 503, (1972).
46. *UNOS Update* **9**, 36 (1993).
47. P. B. Medawar, *Br. Med. J.* **21**, 97 (1965).
48. F. Belzer, *Lancet* **ii**, 536 (1967).

49. Ad Hoc Committee of the Harvard Medical School to Examine the Definition of Death, *J. Am. Med. Assoc.* **205**, 337 (1968).
50. T. Starzl, A. J. Demetris and D. van Theil, *New Engl. J. Med.* **321**, 1014 (1989).
51. W. Land and J. B. Dossitor (eds), *Organ Replacement Therapy: Ethics, Justice, Commerce,* Springer-Verlag, Berlin (1991).
52. I. Penn and M. E. Brunson, *Trans. Proc.* **20**, 885 (1988).
53. R. Y. Calne, R. A. Sells and J. R. Pena, *et al., Nature* **223**, 472 (1969).

Immediate Hypersensitivity: A Brief History

ZOLTAN OVARY

*Department of Pathology, New York University Medical School,
and the Kaplan Comprehensive Cancer Center, 550 First Avenue,
New York, NY 10016, USA*

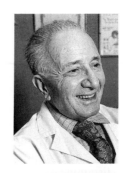

SHUICHI FURUSAWA

*Department of Pathology, New York University Medical School,
and the Kaplan Comprehensive Cancer Center, 550 First Avenue,
New York, NY 10016, USA*

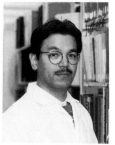

Hypersensitivity has been known since antiquity. One of the most sensational stories is that of Girolamo Gardano, the great renaissance mathematician (the 'father of statistics') and physician, who in 1552 cured the asthma of John Hamilton, the Archbishop of St Andrews, Scotland, by taking away his swan-feathered pillows (1).

By the beginning of this century immunology was very popular because of the Pasteurian vaccinations. The popularity was not the result of the fundamental experiments of Pouilly le Fort on anthrax; it was the consequence of the effective vaccination against rabies developed by Pasteur. The Tsar of Russia had sent to Pasteur several Russian peasants bitten by a rabid wolf. These peasants did not die and it was considered a wonderful success. The Tsar was very grateful and sent to Pasteur a large sum of money, which helped build the Parisian Pasteur Institute. This event was widely publicized and people thought that in a few years vaccination would eliminate infectious diseases. Well, smallpox has been eliminated, but now we have AIDS!

The discovery of Portier and Richet in 1902 (2), made while cruising on the yacht *Princesse Alice II* as guests of Prince Albert I of Monaco, was contrary to the dogma. The dogma stated that: (1) an infectious disease and its symptoms

IMMUNOLOGY: THE MAKING OF A MODERN SCIENCE
ISBN 0-12-274020-3

depend on a specific microbe, and (2) injection of dead or attenuated microbes is followed by specific immunity. Portier and Richet discovered that when a certain substance was reinjected, it could provoke severe illness and death. The symptoms were always the same in the same species and did not depend on the substance used. The important fact was that the substance had to be reinjected. Richet coined the word 'anaphylaxis' to describe this syndrome.

Progress was rapid. In 1906, Maurice Nicolle showed that anaphylaxis can be transmitted passively and the substance which transmits anaphylaxis passively is antibody (3). In 1906, von Pirquet coined the word 'allergy' for human hypersensitivity reactions (4). Later, Coca coined the word 'atopy' to express the fact that some people have allergic reactions to substances which are generally not harmful for others (5). In the early 1910s, Schultz and Dale showed that the symptomatology is caused mainly by liberated histamine (6). Histamine has two main pharmacological actions: it contracts smooth muscles, and it increases the permeability of small veins. Schultz and Dale used the contraction of smooth muscles to study anaphylaxis.

However, it was observed soon after that symptoms of 'classical anaphylaxis' can be provoked by a single injection using the supernatant of a mixture of fresh, even non-immune, sera with some substances. It was thought that 'anaphylatoxins' were liberated (7). In the 1920s it was believed that the disturbance of the colloidal state of the serum (colloidoclasie) liberated anaphylatoxin (8). It was only in the mid-1950s that A. Osler and I, at the Johns Hopkins University, found that the symptoms are caused by breakdown products of activated complement (C3a and C5a) which, it turned out, liberate histamine from mast cells (9).

An important discovery was made by Prausnitz in 1921; that is, transmission of anaphylactic sensitivity to his own skin with the serum of his colleague Kustner (10). It thus became possible to study human hypersensitivity experimentally with the Prausnitz–Kustner (PK) reaction. The importance of histamine liberation in human allergic reactions led Bovet to the discovery of synthetic antihistamines (Bovet and Straub 11), for which Bovet was later awarded the Nobel prize.

Mast cells play a pivotal role in allergic reactions. They have high affinity receptors for immunoglobulin E (IgE) on their membrane (12). They store several very active substances such as histamine, serotonin (in rodents) and other substances in inactive form, for instance the 'slow reactive substance of anaphylaxis' (SRS-A) (13,14) which is even more potent than histamine. Piper (15) and Samuelsson (16) later showed that the SRS-As are degradation products by the lipoxigenase pathway of arachidonic acid, a finding that won the Nobel prize for Samuelsson.

Recently, emphasis has been put on the so-called 'late-phase reaction' (17), that is the clinical manifestations several hours after an acute asthmatic attack, caused by the release of different mediators. These mediators attract different cellular elements to the site from the blood and produce serosal infiltrations. These elements might produce chronic pathological changes.

In 1942, Merrill Chase made the fundamental discovery that delayed (tuberculin type) hypersensitivity reactions could be transferred by living lymphocytes and that immediate (anaphylactic) type reactions are transferred by antibody (18).

Using the action of histamine on the permeability of small veins, we developed passive cutaneous anaphylaxis (PCA) (19). PCA proved to be a useful technique for studying experimentally anaphylactic reactions in animals for the next 20 years. The discovery of monoclonal antibodies by Milstein and Kohler (20), permitted the development of sensitive *in vitro* methods, such as ELISA, for the detection of antibodies (21).

Delineating the Role of Antibody

I started to do immunological research in 1948 in Rome, Italy, with Guido Biozzi. As I am very allergic to cats I started to study histamine release *in vivo* during local anaphylactic reactions. It was still 'the golden age of immunochemistry'!

In 1954, Michael Heidelberger recommended me to Manfred Mayer at the Johns Hopkins University, so I went to Baltimore. The field of immunology was still small enough that I knew most of the researchers personally, beginning with Portier, who was my teacher, and Prausnitz (22). What follows after 1949 in this short historical review will be my own rather personal (perhaps biased) story.

Porter started by using papain to study the structure of γ-globulin in 1959 (23). He showed that two types of fragment were produced – one which still had the combining site for the antigen (Fab) and one which could not combine with the antigen, but was crystallizable (Fc). It is curious that nobody had recognized it at that time, but this was because a portion of the antibody was constant! Porter then developed his now classic 'four-chain model' of the antibody molecule. He showed that two identical A and two identical B chains (later called heavy (H) and light (L) chains) make up the γ-globulin (or antibody) molecule (24).

The next great discovery was that of Hilschmann (25) who showed that the C-terminal half of the light chain is constant. Later it was shown that the heavy chain also had a variable and a constant portion. Intrachain cysteines delimit the so-called 'domains' in these chains. Afterwards, all proteins with similar domains were classified as proteins of the immunoglobulin family. It was first thought that every domain carries a different function or property. However, even for the immunoglobulins this is not always the case, and among other proteins of the immunoglobulin family it is far from universal.

Using the papain digest fragments of rabbit IgG antibody molecules, Karush and I could show that the biological activities are carried by the Fc fragment (26). In our case it was the fixation of the Fc fragment to mast cells. This was the first work showing a role of the Fc fragment.

In 1961, using Porter fragments from anti-hapten antibodies and mono- and bivalent haptens, I showed that to trigger histamine liberation from mast cells two receptors must be cross-linked (27). Our discovery of cross-linking of membrane proteins, as first step of cellular activation, turned out to be of critical importance as the initial step in cellular activation events such as cytokine production and secretion of different messengers.

In 1959, Burnet published his book on the clonal selection theory of acquired immunity, which revolutionized immunological thinking (28). Also in 1959, on the recommendation of my friend Baruch Benacerraf, I was offered a post in the Department of Pathology at the New York University Medical School, which I gladly accepted. With Benacerraf, I showed in 1963 that, in order to boost antibody production against haptenated carriers, the same carrier must be used (29). We discovered this 'carrier effect' well before the complexity of the lymphocyte population was understood. In fact, it was only several years later that T cells were discovered (30–32). In 1970, Mitchison showed that the T cells recognize the carrier moiety of the antigen (33).

In 1962 and 1963, working with Benacerraf and Kurt Bloch, I showed that in the guinea-pig, two types of IgG molecule exist and only one, IgG1, can transmit anaphylactic sensitivity (34–36). This observation was contrary to the dogma of the unitarian theory of antibodies and was an impetus for research into other similar cases.

In 1965, my friends Kimishige and Terry Ishizaka whom I met at the Johns Hopkins University in the late 1950s, then working in Denver, showed that human allergy is caused by a class of immunoglobulin not previously known, named by them IgE (37). This was another turning point in allergy research. The discovery of a human myeloma-producing IgE molecule in Sweden (38) made possible the development of sensitive in vitro bioassays to measure human IgE. The discovery was fortuitous because the threat of hepatitis and AIDS made PK tests no longer possible.

In 1975, Kohler and Milstein made a marvellous discovery, the production of monoclonal antibodies (39), for which they were awarded the Nobel prize. This discovery was one of the important factors contributing to major advances in immunological research. Monoclonal hapten-specific IgE antibodies could be generated (40–42). Meanwhile, the allotype of murine IgE was described (43). Finally, even monoclonal antibody against murine IgH-7[a] (an allotype of IgE) was generated (44).

The Advent of Molecular Immunology

One of the most sensational discoveries of modern immunology was made by Tonegawa (45), who showed that the genes for the immunoglobulin molecule in the germline configuration consisted of separate elements. Those elements that are used to form the protein are called 'exons' and those which separate the exons are known as 'introns'. The immunoglobulin chains are the product of several exons: V and J for the light chain, and V, D and J for the heavy chain variable portions. In the germline, the V segments can be quite numerous; they are divided into many families. The constant portion is composed of several exons, corresponding to each domain. The last exon of each constant gene has alternative forms: one for secreted immunoglobulin and, $3'$ to this, the exon for the membrane immunoglobulin. Although the immunoglobulin molecule is the final product of separated genetic elements, the exons, the introns are not unimportant, as they contain different elements such as promoters and enhancers.

Membrane immunoglobulin is non-covalently associated with two polypeptide chains: α and β. The α chain is the same for all isotypes (46). The exact function of these chains is not yet known, but they probably serve as signal transductors.

Honjo later showed that the first exon of each constant region (except for IgD) is preceded by a portion he called s, which is important for the switch from one class of immunoglobulin to another class (47).

Though antibody was described by Behring and Kitasato in 1890 (48), it was only in 1935, 45 years later, that Heidelberger showed that antibodies can be weighed and therefore they are 'real substances' and not abstract 'properties' (49). If we look at the discoveries from 1935 to the present time, we can appreciate the exponential progress of knowledge in immunology.

In 1983 the mouse (M. Davis (50,51) and human (T. Mak (52)) T cell receptors were isolated and cloned. They are made up of two chains (α and β) and the chains are similar to those of the immunoglobulin L and H chains in that they possess variable and constant portions.

The T cell receptor is non-covalently associated with the CD3 complex composed of one γ, one δ, one ε and two covalently linked ζ chains. It is thought that this complex is important for signal transduction (53).

Cell Interactions

There are two great classes of T cells in adult animals (54), now called CD4 (or helper) and the CD8 (or cytotoxic/suppressor) T cells. For antibody production the CD4 cells play the important role. Mosmann and Coffman later showed that the CD4 cells, depending on the lymphokines they secrete, could be divided in Th1 and Th2 subtypes. The Th1 cells produce interleukin-2 (IL-2) and γ-interferon (IFN-γ), among other lymphokines, but not IL-4 and IL-5. In contrast, the Th2 cells produce IL-4 and IL-5, but not IL-2 and IFN-γ (55). For IgE production IL-4 is essential (56), while Th1 cells are important for delayed-type hypersentivity reactions.

When antigen is injected it is taken up by phagocytic macrophages. The antigen is processed in the peripheral endosomal compartments by macrophages and a certain portion of the carrier moiety (generally a small peptide, of 9–11 amino acids) will go into the groove of a major histocompatibility complex (MHC) class II molecule. This groove is formed by the amino terminal variable portions of the α and β chains of the class II molecule (57,58). This complex of class II molecule plus antigen peptide is recognized by those T cells which bear specific T cell receptors. Macrophages, as 'professional antigen presenting cells', may take up and present any antigen. The end result of the encounter between an antigen-presenting cell and a T cell will be T cell proliferation and/or secretion of lymphokines. B cells can also take up antigen. However, unlike 'professional antigen-presenting cells', B cells take up only those antigens for which they are specific, that is, antigens recognized by the membrane immunoglobulin. The antigen which is taken up by this B cell is then processed similarly to antigen taken up by the macrophage.

Antigen processing became a new field of research, developed by Marrack and Kapler (59), Grey (60), Unanue (61) and others.

Control of IgE Production

If the B cell presenting the antigen encounters a T cell and the receptor of this T cell recognizes the complex of MHC class II plus antigen fragment, the T cell becomes activated to secrete interleukins. A complex phenomenon is initiated, the end result of which is antibody production by the B cells, antibody of the same specificity present on the B cell surface. It is possible that a switch phenomenon will occur and the antibody will not be of the same class but of a class more distant from the amino terminal of the constant chain, 3' from the V region. There are many unresolved questions concerning this 'switch'. Are both of the CD4 T cell subsets (Th1 and Th2) necessary? If so, which encounters the B cell first – the Th1 or Th2 cell? Is reiterated action of T cells, or the lymphokines secreted by these T cells, important for the switching of every isotype? For IgE production, we showed in 1983 that multiple encounters with T cells are necessary (62). However, at this time Th1 and Th2 cells had not yet been described. With the exception of the last question, on which we have some information, the above questions are not yet answered. One thing seems to be unanimously accepted: cognate interaction of T (more precisely CD4 T cells) and B cells is necessary for the initiation of antibody production. The stimulation of B cells by cognate interaction of T cells is an *in vivo* phenomenon. *In vitro*, this B cell stimulation can be achieved by lipopolysaccharides (LPS).

A resting, virgin B cell, with IgM and IgD on its surface, after processing and presenting antigen to a CD4+ T helper cell, begins to multiply and then to secrete epitope-specific IgM, or becomes a memory cell. However, this is an oversimplification, as an activated B cell can secrete antibody and multiply (63). The end-stage cell, the plasma cell, does not multiply, but secretes considerably greater amount of antibody than the dividing cell. We do not know how many times a B cell divides before it becomes a plasma cell or a memory cell. We have only indirect data, such as somatic mutations (64) which show that the cells have divided. We do not know what the impetus is which determines the end of the multiplication and the transformation into a plasma cell or into a memory B cell. The plasma cell has no surface immunoglobulin. This fact, at least, is well established.

We have seen above that the cell also has another choice. Instead of secreting an antibody molecule it can become a memory cell. We are also completely ignorant of what determines this choice. We know that the memory cell is a long-lived B cell (65) and we know that the memory cells go to the germinal centres of lymphoid organs (such as lymph nodes and spleen). A germinal centre is oligoclonal. In other words, although it contains a great number of B cells, these generally derive from one to three ancestor cells (66,67). Finally, the cell may also die. The cause and pathways of this apoptosis are not well understood.

Do IgE memory cells exist? Working with murine cells and separating them into IgE and IgG1 surface immunoglobulin positive cells and culturing these cells with T helper cells, antigen presenting cells and antigen, we could show IgE production from surface IgE$^+$ cells, but also from cells carrying membrane IgG1, but not IgE, molecules. However, we could not find IgE production by cells not having either membrane IgE and IgG1 molecules. In other words, cells lacking surface IgE and surface IgG1 did not produce IgE antibody. Therefore, IgE production can be from two types of cell population: those expressing membrane IgE, but lacking membrane IgG1, and those lacking membrane IgE but expressing IgG1 cells (Takahama, Ovary and Furusawa (unpublished results)). A separate view on memory B cells was proposed in 1989. According to this view the 'primary antibody-forming cells and secondary B cells are generated from separate precursor cell subpopulations' (68).

The first antibody secreted is of the IgM isotype. For production of IgE, a Th2 cell must be involved, as IL-4 is a prerequisite for IgE production (69). The importance of IL-4 for IgG1 and IgE production was first shown by Vitetta (70) and Paul (71). Several laboratories showed that IL-4 is crucial for IgE production (70–74). LPS-stimulated B cells were used to show the importance of IL-4 for IgE production, even *in vivo* (71). There are interleukins that have an opposite action, namely they are inhibitory: IFN-γ is a potent suppressor of IgE production (72,74) and, under certain conditions, IL-2 is also inhibitory (74).

The specificity of the antibody is determined by the variable portions of the light and heavy chains. This portion of the antibody molecule is encoded by the V, D and J for the heavy chain and V and J for the light chain, as mentioned above. The specificity of the antibody remains the same during the entire life of the B cell. However, due to somatic mutations, the affinity of the antibody may increase or decrease.

The isotype is determined by the constant portion of the heavy chain. A cell, which started to produce IgM antibody, can switch to produce another isotype. The DNA encoding this new isotype is situated 3' on the germline DNA. How does the B cell change the isotype which it produces? How does the switch occur? As our subject is hypersensitivity, we are concerned here only with the switch to IgE. IL-4 is a crucial element in IgE production. Studying cells producing IgE, an interesting hypothesis was put forward by Stavnezer (75) and Severinson (76), namely that the IL-4 (or the factors activated by the action of IL-4) might make the DNA at the switch region accessible to the enzyme switch recombinase. Though this enzyme has not yet been cloned, its action is well accepted.

At the beginning of the switch to IgE production, the first change observed is the production of a germline RNA starting upstream to the first constant IgE exon. The germline DNA starts at the Iε motif (70), which is 5' from the first IgE exon. The mature IgE RNA is synthesized only later. The mRNA transcribed from the germline DNA is 2.2 kb long, while the mature IgE RNA is 1.7 kb long. Therefore they can easily be identified. However: 'The precise role of germline transcription with respect to directed class switching remains to be elucidated' (77).

Does the switch from IgM go directly to IgE or is there first a switch from IgM to IgG1 and then a second switch from IgG1 to IgE? Sakano and collaborators found, using *in vitro* cultures, circular DNA containing intermediary exons between IgM and IgG1, as well as others containing intermediary exons between IgG1 and IgE, but no circular DNA with intermediary forms between IgM and IgE (78–80). These experiments strongly suggest that the switch from IgM to IgE goes through IgG1. However, they are not a proof that the direct switch from IgM to IgE never occurs. Another possibility is that the switch is not in *cis* but in *trans*, namely that the IgE exons of the other chromosome are used. Experiments with transgenic mice have shown this possibility (81).

The production of IgE can be suppressed by IL-2 (74) and by IFN-γ (73,74). We have shown that in certain conditions T helper cells, probably Th1 cells (although at that time this distinction had not yet been established), might bring about suppression of IgE production (82,83). It was advocated that suppression of IgE production might be promoted also by suppressor factors (84,85), secreted by T cells (perhaps by CD8 T cells). However, these factors have not yet been cloned satisfactorily.

Acknowledgements

This work was supported by Grant AI–03075 from the National Institute of Health, Japanese Ministry of Education, and Fund ZO–64–1–4409.

Notes and References

1. G. Gardano, *De Vita Propria* (1574). (English trans.: J. Gardan, *The Book of My Life*, E. P. Dutton, New York (1930).)
2. P. Portier and C. Richet, *C.R. Soc. Biol.* **54**, 170 (1902).
3. M. Nicolle, *Ann. Inst. Pasteur, Paris* **21**, 128 (1907).
4. C. v. Pirquet, *Munch. Med. Wochenschr.* **53**, 1457 (1906).
5. A. F. Coca and R. A. Cooke, *J. Immunol.* **8**, 163 (1923).
6. H. H. Dale, *J. Pharmacol.* **4**, 267 (1913).
7. J. Bordet, *C.R. Soc. Biol.* **47**, 1490 (1913).
8. F. Widal, *Progr. Med.* **36**, 48 (1921).
9. A. G. Osler, H. G. Randall, B. M. Hill and Z. Ovary, *J. Exp. Med.* **110**, 311 (1959).
10. C. Prausnitz and H. Kustner, *Zentralbl. Bakt.* **86**, 160 (1921).
11. D. Bovet and A.-M. Straub. *C.R. Soc Biol.* **6**, 119 (1937).
12. H. Metzger, G. Alcaraz, R. Hohman, J. P. Kinet, V. Pribuda and R. Quarto, *Ann. Rev. Immunol.* **4**, 419 (1986).
13. J. Harkavy, *Arch. Intern. Med.* **67**, 709 (1941).
14. W. E. Brocklehurst, *Prog. Allergy* **6**, 539 (1962).
15. P. J. Piper, M. N. Samhoun, J. R. Tippins Jr, H. R. Morris, C. M. Jones and G. W. Taylor, *Int. Arch. Allergy Appl. Immunol.* **66** (Suppl. 1), 107 (1981).
16. B. Samuelsson, *Int. Arch. Allergy Appl. Immunol.* **66** (Suppl. 1), 98 (1981).
17. G. O. Solley, G. Gleich, R. Jordan and A. Schroetzer, *J. Clin. Invest.* **58**, 408 (1976).
18. M. W. Chase, *Proc. Soc. Exp. Biol. Med.* **59**, 134 (1945).
19. Z. Ovary, *Prog. Allergy*, **5**, 460 (1958).
20. G. Kohler and C. Milstein, *Nature* **256**, 495 (1975).
21. E. Engvall and P. Perlman, *Immunochemistry* **8**, 871 (1971).
22. Carl Prausnitz emigrated to the Isle of Wight in the mid-1930s and took up his mother's name: Giles. I met him in 1954 in London at the Founding meeting of the Collegium Internazionale Allergologicum.
23. R. R. Porter, *Biochem. J.* **73**, 119 (1959).
24. R. R. Porter, in *Symposium on Basic Problems in Neoplastic Disease* (A. Gelhorn and E. Hirschberg, eds), Columbia University Press, New York (1962), pp. 177–194.
25. N. Hilschmann and L. C. Craig, *Proc. Natl Acad. Sci. USA* **53**, 1903 (1965).
26. Z. Ovary and F. Karush, *J. Immunol.* **83**, 146 (1961).
27. Z. Ovary, *C.R. Acad. Sci.* **253**, 282 (1961).
28. Macfarlane Burnet, *The Clonal Selection Theory of Acquired Immunity*, Wanderbilt University Press, Nashville, TN (1959).
29. Z. Ovary and B. Benacerraf, *Proc. Soc. Exp. Biol. Med.* **114**, 72 (1963).
30. H. N. Claman, E. A. Chaperon and R. F. Triplett, *J. Immunol.* **97**, 828 (1966).
31. R. Good, A. P. Dalmasso, C. Martinez, O. K. Archer, J. C. Pierce and B. W. Papermaster, *J. Exp. Med.* **116**, 773 (1962).
32. J. F. A. P. Miller, G. F. Mitchell and N. J. Weiss, *Nature* **214**, 292 (1967).
33. N. A. Mitchison, *Eur. J. Immunol.* **1**, 18 (1971).
34. B. Benacerraf and Z. Ovary and K. J. Bloch and E. C. Franklin, *J. Exp. Med.* **117**, 937 (1963).
35. Z. Ovary, B. Benacerraf and K. J. Bloch, *J. Exp. Med.* **117**, 951 (1963).
36. K. J. Bloch, F. M. Kourilsky, Z. Ovary and B. Benacerraf, *J. Exp. Med.* **117**, 965 (1963).
37. K. Ishizaka and T. Ishizaka, *J. Immunol.* **99**, 1187 (1967).
38. S. G. O. Johansson and H. Benich, *Immunology* **12**, 281 (1967).
39. G. Kohler and C. Milstein, *Nature* **256**, 495 (1975).
40. I. Bottcher, M. Ulrich, N. Hirayama and Z. Ovary, *Int. Arch. Allergy Appl. Immunol.* **61**, 248 (1980).
41. F. Liu, J. W. Bohn, E. L. Ferry, H. Yamamoto, C. A. Molinaro, I. A. Sherman, N. R. Klinman and D. H. Katz, *J. Immunol.* **124**, 2728 (1980).

42. Z. Eshhar, M. Ofarim and T. Waks, *J. Immunol.* **124**, 775 (1980).
43. N. S. Borges, Y. Kumagai, K. Okumura, N. Hirayama, Z. Ovary and T. Tada, *Immunogenetics* **13**, 499 (1981).
44. M. Utsui, T. Hirano, H. Miyajima, S. Ando, M. Kurimoto, C. Yamaji, T. Matuhashi, Z. Ovary and K. Okumura, *Immunogenetics* **37**, 301 (1993).
45. S. Tonegawa, *Nature* **302**, 575 (1983).
46. A. R. Venkitaraman, G. T. Williams, P. Dariavach and M. S. Neuberger, *Nature* **352**, 777 (1991).
47. T. Honjo, *Ann. Rev. Immunol.* **1**, 499 (1983).
48. E. A. v Berhring and S. Kitasato, *Deutsche Med. Wochenschr.* **16**, 1145 (1890).
49. M. Heidelberger and F. E. Kendall, *J. Exp. Med.* **62**, 697 (1935).
50. At the 5th International Congress of Immunology, Bill Paul, who knew that I was a close friend of Tomio Tada (I showed him the marvels of Italy when we went there in the summer each year for 10 years), asked me to speak with Tomio, the organizer of this Congress. He asked that a work should be accepted for presentation by a young researcher, though it was not submitted in time to the Programme Committee, but that it was so sensational, it was worth making an exception. Tada immediately accepted that Mark Davis should present his work on the cloning of a chain of the murine T cell receptor.
51. S. M. Hedrick, D. I. Cohen, E. A. Nielsen and M. Davis, *Nature* **308**, 149 (1984).
52. Y. Yanagi, Y. Yoshikai, H. Leggett, S. P. Clark, I. Aleksander and T. K. Mak, *Nature* **308**, 148 (1984).
53. M. A. Goldsmith and A. Weiss, *Immunol. Today* **9**, 220 (1988).
54. H. Cantor and E. A. Boyse, *J. Exp. Med.* **141** 1376 (1975).
55. R. R. Mossman and R. I. Coffman, *Ann. Rev. Immunol.* **7**, 145 (1989).
56. F. D. Finkelman, I. M. Katona, J. F. Urban Jr, J. Holmes, J. Ohara, A. S. Yung, J. vG. Sampel and W. E. Paul, *J. Immunol.* **141**, 2335 (1988).
57. J. H. Brown, Y. Jardetzky, M. A. Saper, B. Samraoui, P. J. Bjorkman and D. C. Wiley, *Nature* **332**, 845 (1988).
58. J. H. Brown, M. A. Jardetzky, J. C. Gorga, L. J. Stern, R. G. Urban, J. L. Strominger and D. C. Wiley, *Nature* **364**, 33 (1993).
59. R. Shimonkevitz, J. Kappler, P. Marrack and H. Grey, *J. Exp. Med.* **15**, 303 (1983).
60. R. W. Chesnut and H. M. Grey, *J. Immunol.* **126**, 1075 (1981).
61. C. V. Hardin, F. Leyva-Cobian and E. R. Unanue, *Immunol. Rev.* **106**, 79 (1988).
62. T. Hirano, Y. Kumagai, K. Okumura and Z. Ovary, *Proc. Natl Acad. Sci. USA* **80**, 3435 (1983).
63. L. Vernino, L. M. McAnally, J. Ramberg and P. E. Lipsky, *J. Immunol.* **148**, 404 (1992).
64. K. Rajewsky, H. Gu, P. Vieira and I. Forster, *Cold Spring Harbor Symp. Quant. Biol* **54**, 209 (1989).
65. B. Schittek and K. Rajewsky, *Nature* **346**, 749 (1990).
66. F. G. M. Kroese, A. S. Wubbema, J. G. Seijen and P. Nieuwenhuis, *Eur. J. Immunol.* **17**, 1069 (1987).
67. V. K. Tsiagbe, P.-J. Linton and G. J. Thorbecke, *Immunol. Rev.* **126**, 113 (1991).
68. P. J. Linton, D. J. Decker and N. R. Klinman, *Cell* **59**, 1049 (1989).
69. W. E. Paul and J. Ohara, *Ann. Rev. Immunol.* **5**, 429 (1987).
70. E. S. Vitetta, J. Ohara, C. Myers, J. Layton, P. M. Krammer and W. E. Paul, *J. Exp. Med.* **155**, 1726 (1982).
71. F. D. Finkelman, I. M. Katona, J. F. Urban Jr, C. M. Snapper, J. Ohara and W. E. Paul, *Proc. Natl Acad. Sci. USA* **83**, 9675 (1986).
72. M. Azuma, T. Hirano, H. Miajima, N. Watanabe, H. Yagita, S. Enomoto, S. Furusawa, Z. Ovary, T. Kinashi, T. Honjo and K. Okumura, *J. Immunol.* **139**, 2538 (1987).
73. R. L. Coffman and J. A. Carty, *J. Immunol.* **136**, 949 (1986).
74. H. Miajima, T. Hirano, S. Hirose, H. Karasuyama, K. Okumura and Z. Ovary, *J. Immunol.* **146**, 457 (1991).
75. J. Stavnezer-Nordgren and S. Sirlin, *EMBO J.* **5**, 95 (1986).

76. J. Stavnezer, G. Radcliffe, Y. C. Lin, J. Nietupski, L. Berggren, R. Sitia and E. Severinson, *Proc. Natl Acad. Sci. USA* **85**, 7704 (1988).

77. P. Rothman, Y.-Y. Chen, S. Lutzker, S. C. Li, V. Stewart, R. Coffman and F. W. Alt, *Mol. Cell. Biol.* **10**, 1672 (1990).

78. M. Matsuoka, K. Yoshida, Y. Maeda, S. Usuda and H. Sakano, *Cell* **62**, 135 (1990).

79. T. Iwasato, A. Shimizu, T. Honjo, and H. Yamagishi, *Cell* **62**, 143 (1990).

80. K. Yoshida, M. Matsuoka, S. Usuda, A. Mori, K. Ishizaka and H. Sakano, *Proc. Natl Acad. Sci. USA* **87**, 7829 (1990).

81. A. Shimizu, M. C. Nussenzweig, H. Han, M. Sanchez and T. Honjo, *J. Exp. Med.* **173**, 1385 (1991).

82. T. Tada and K. Okumura, *J. Immunol.* **107**, 1682 (1971).

83. T. Itaya and Z. Ovary, *J. Exp. Med.* **150**, 507 (1979).

84. K. Ishizaka, *Int. Arch. Allergy Appl. Immunol.* **88**, 8 (1989).

85. J. F. Marcelletti and D. H. Katzx, *J. Immunol.* **133**, 2845 (1984).

Tumour Immunology

GEORGE KLEIN
Laboratory of Tumour Biology, Microbiology and Tumour Biology Center, Karolinska Institute, S–171 77 Stockholm, Sweden

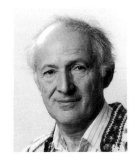

EVA KLEIN
Laboratory of Tumour Biology, Microbiology and Tumour Biology Center, Karolinska Institute, S–171 77 Stockholm, Sweden

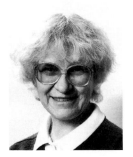

At the International Congress of Immunology in Paris, 1980, one of the editors of this book, Gustav Nossal, circulated a paper entitled 'The case history of Mr T.I: terminal patient or still curable?' (*1*). In his introductory statement, Nossal wrote:

> Mr T.I. is about 25 years old, and at present appears to be in a rather serious state. The chief symptoms are fatigue and confusion, which have followed a period of unusually intense activity. The detailed history reveals that T.I. has never really been free of symptoms, and though his rate of growth was very rapid, especially during his teens, there have been periods of euphoria alternating with depression, and close observers have noted a certain malaise throughout. The laboratory tests have not contributed to the diagnosis, as some appear to suggest robust good health whereas others hint at a terminal state. Mr T.I., whose full name is Tumour Immunology, is thus a diagnostic and prognostic puzzle.

Summarizing the Tumour Immunology section of that same congress, one of us responded to this challenge as follows (*2*):

> In his article, distributed to all Congress participants, Gustav Nossal asks whether Tumour Immunology (Mr TI) is a terminal patient or still curable. Surely, this must

be a case of mistaken identities. TI is not a patient at all. He is still a youngster who had a very complicated childhood. He was born like the hero of Kalevala, the Finnish national epos, the great poet Väinemöinen, after an immensely prolonged pregnancy. Väinemöinen was 600 years old at birth. TI was not that old but, like V, he was regarded old and wise already in the cradle. Expectations were therefore enormous. He was pressured, pushed and pulled in all directions. Oscillations of great praise and even greater blame arrested his development. He became like little Oscar in the Tin Drum of Günther Grass. Sometimes he would scream at the top of his shrill voice so that all windows would break. At other times he would just sit, sullen, sour, and silent. He failed to grow normally.

Actually, Nossal did not end his article on a pessimistic note. He wrote:

> I do not regard Mr TI as a terminal patient. I believe he is curable, but I also think this is an appropriate time to plan his therapy more thoughtfully, more rationally, more conservatively. If this is done, the long-term prognosis is good, and future Grand Rounds should be able to record considerable progress.

In this chapter we will look at some of the early history, prior to the 1980 congress, and note the progress during the ensuing years.

Early History

The question of whether tumour cells are recognized as foreign by the immune system is as old as immunology itself, or at least as old as the distinction between self and non-self. Are tumour cells self or non-self?

Until the late 1950s, this field has been bedevilled by the confusion between tumour and transplantation immunology. It is rarely remembered nowadays that the laws of tissue transplantation were discovered as a by-product of the tumour grafting experiments of the Bar Habor geneticists (3,4). Originally, Little and his colleagues started these experiments in order to study the heredity of cancer susceptibility. It was the lasting contribution of George Snell and Peter Gorer to have ironed out the relationship between genetics and transplantation, graft rejection and tumour acceptance. Peter Gorer pioneered the serology (5,6). Gorer and Snell were a formidable pair of scientists breaking totally new ground, but they were understood and recognized by very few. When I asked George Snell in 1956 how many colleagues understood his work on the H-2 system, he answered that he could easily count them without using all his fingers.

Not that he did very much to become widely understandable. Peter Gorer did even less. Although he was passionately interested in his work, he pretended that he could not care less, as it becomes an English gentleman. At Guy's Hospital where he worked in a small, antiquated laboratory, with the rank of Reader, not Professor, he was known by very few. In his seminars and conference lectures, he did nothing to explain the complicated jargon. We used some of his papers as the acid test to distinguish between truly motivated and less-interested students. Peter was a heavy smoker, as also attested by his tragic early death from lung cancer. Sometimes he lectured with a cigarette in his mouth and occasionally he got a coughing attack just as he was reaching the main point. I do not believe this was affectation – it was more a reflection of scholarly introversion, as far removed from competitive emphasis on success as you can get. He never showed any ambition to enlighten a backward and uncomprehending audience. I watched him chairing the tumour immunology session of the 1958 Cancer Congress in London with much puzzlement. Sitting at the old-fashioned magisterial table in the suffocating heat of a poorly ventilated room in the City Hall of London, with a glass of water and a small heap of headache pills in front of him, Peter called one 10-minute speaker after the other and listened to their misguided claims of having detected specific tumour immunity, not being aware of the fact that they were reporting the violation of major histocompatility barriers by tumour allografts in the first place. Peter never uttered any comment or criticism. He occasionally swallowed a pill and reminded the speakers of their allotted time. After the last talk he exclaimed: 'Open the windows. We need some fresh air.'

How quickly all this has changed! Asking George Snell to approach the King of Sweden to receive his Nobel Prize – which he shared in 1980, when Peter Gorer was no longer alive, with Jean Dausset and Baruj Benacerraf – one of us could say the following (7):

> Your long journey has led you, after many adventures, to . . . the major histocompatibility complex, and through it to this happy event tonight. You have been responsible for turning what at first appeared as an esoteric area of basic research on inbred mice into a major biological system of the greatest significance for the understanding of cell recognition, immune responses and graft rejection. We have the rare esthetic pleasure of seeing a series of fundamental discoveries, coupled with immediate applications in clinical medicine.

Antigenicity of Chemically Induced Tumours

At the time of the London Congress, a change was already in the air among the few *cognoscenti*. It came with the discovery of specific tumour immunity in syngeneic, and even autochthonous, hosts. Foley (8) first found, and Prehn and Main (9) later confirmed, that chemically induced mouse sarcomas, but not spontaneous mammary carcinomas, could elicit a state of immunity in syngeneic mice. The data were persuasive but still not fully convincing. Did chemically induced tumour cells really possess a distinct antigenicity of their own, or did these experiments merely reflect a residual heterozygosis in the inbred strains? It was obvious that the question would be decisively settled if it could be shown that the primary host could be immunized against its own tumour.

Using a combined scheme of tumour induction, operative removal, immunization with irradiated autologous tumour cells, and challenge with graded numbers of viable cells, we could show that methylcholanthrene (MC)-induced sarcoma cells were indeed capable of inducing rejection reactions in the original host (10). Different tumours varied in their immunogenicity over a five log range of cell doses, required to break the state of immunity. Their antigencity was individually distinct, that is, they did not cross-immunize against each other, as also noted by Prehn, Baldwin, and Old (11–13). Immunization of mice with pools of MC-induced sarcomas could not protect them from MC induction of sarcomas, but non-specific immunomodulators had a certain preventive effect, presumably by potentiating the host's own responsiveness (12).

There was a certain connection between the chemical composition of the carcinogen and the immunogenicity of the tumour it induced. MC, benzopyrene and dimethylbenzantracene induced sarcomas with decreasing immunogenicity, in that order. Sarcomas induced by the implantation of cellophane films were hardly immunogenic at all (14). In the rat, Baldwin found that most azo-dye-induced tumours were highly immunogenic, whereas acetylaminofluorene-induced tumours and spontaneous fibrosarcomas were not immunogenic at all (15).

Forty years after their discovery, the biochemistry of the 'tumour specific transplantation antigens' (TSTAs) of the chemically induced tumours is still not understood.

Antigenicity of Virus-Induced Tumours

In 1958, one of us (G.K.) participated in the Canadian Cancer Conference, in Honey Harbor, Ontario. Stewart and Eddy's pioneering work on the polyoma virus was still very new. Most participants were flabbergasted by the number and variety of the tumours that arose after the inoculation of the virus into newborn mice. Burnet was one of them. 'Sir Mac' had recently shifted from virology to immunology. Concurrently, he developed a very negative view on the role of viruses in cancer causation. Basically, he considered all virus-induced tumours as laboratory artefacts. He believed that all viruses were cytopathic, and saw no place for any direct transforming effect. Confronted with the polyoma story for the first time, he formulated immediately a new hypothesis. It was based on the only observation of Stewart and Eddy that turned out to be incorrect. They claimed that polyoma tumours were not transplantable. This was later shown to have been due to the use of heterozygous Swiss mice, as transplant recipients, however. The old 'cardinal sin' was still throwing its shadow over the field.

Burnet, who was not aware of this experimental artefact, suggested that polyoma virus may destroy some unknown, systematic 'growth-controlling centre', a possible 'hypothalamus-like' homeostatic regulator that could influence cell renewal in many different tissues. Destruction of this presumptive regulatory centre would lead to the unbridled growth of cells in many tissues. These tumours would not be transplantable unless the recipient mice would have been similarly conditioned by polyoma virus.

Hans-Olof Sjögren had just started to work with us at this time. Stimulated by Burnet's speculation, I asked him to test the idea by comparing the transplantability of polyoma tumours in unmanipulated and polyoma-infected syngeneic mice. The result was the exact opposite of what was predicted by the hypothesis: the tumours were fully transplantable to untreated mice, while at least the small or moderate-sized inocula that grew in the controls were rejected by virus-inoculated syngeneic mice (16). Graft resistance could be transferred adoptively with lymphocytes but not with serum. Both Karl Habel and our group later showed that antiviral immunity was neither necessary nor sufficient to induce rejection (17,18). Polyoma-induced tumours or transformed cells induced rejection, whether they released virus or not. All polyoma-induced tumours were rejected by the immunized mice, irrespective of tissue origin, but they did not reject tumours induced by other viruses or by chemical agents. We have therefore developed the concept of a polyoma-specific transplantation antigen (TSTA) that was present in all tumours induced by polyoma virus. We and others later found that similar group-specific rejection-inducing antigens were present on other virus-induced tumours (for a review, see Klein (19)). The retrovirus-induced leukaemias permitted the detection of specific serum antibodies, as shown by Old et al. (20), and by our group (19). Moloney-virus-induced lymphomas were particularly useful, since they gave a brilliant membrane fluorescence reaction with the sera of preimmunized, syngeneic animals. Nevertheless, it was not possible to distinguish the rejection-inducing antigen from the proteins associated with virus production. Different Moloney lymphomas induced in the same inbred strain differed in their rejection-inducing potential (21). This study also showed that immunogenicity and immunosensitivity are at least partially independent variables.

For the polyoma tumours, the modern development showed that rejection was directed against MHC class I associated peptides derived from the transformation associated large T and middle T proteins encoded by the virus (22).

Burkitt's Lymphoma

Sometime in the mid-1960s we wanted to use our experience on virus-induced murine lymphomas to examine a human lymphoma with a presumptive viral aetiology. Could we detect group-specific antibodies that would react with the tumour cells? Burkitt's lymphoma was the obvious choice. Its climate-related endemic occurrence in Africa suggested a possible viral aetiology (23,24).

We anticipated similar results as with the retrovirus-induced murine leukaemias, where the diseased animals often lacked antibodies against the virally infected leukaemia cells, in contrast to tumour-free adults exposed to the virus, who had high titres. This hypothesis turned out to be quite wrong, but it was the basis for the sampling of a large number of sera not only from the tumour patients, but also from their tumour-free relatives and neighbours, which turned out to be quite valuable.

We wrote to numerous hospitals in Africa and to international organizations, explaining our project and asking for tumour, blood and serum. We received some polite letters in reply, promises of material, and some lovely stamps which made our son happy. But the material was not forthcoming at all, apart from an occasional shipment that arrived broken or infected. Then I made a mistake. I found the papers of the epidemiologist A. J. Haddow (for a review see Haddow (25)). I thought, wrongly, that the author was my good friend Alexander Haddow, the Director of the Chester Beatty Research Institute in London. I wrote to him, asking for material. He told me about the mistaken identity, but he also advised me to write to Peter Clifford, ENT surgeon at the Kenyatta National Hospital in Nairobi.

We got no letter and no stamps in reply, but the material started coming in a continuous flow. It arrived with unfailing regularity on the single weekly SAS flight from Nairobi, every Tuesday afternoon. Dry-ice boxes carried hundreds of sera, while a wet-ice package contained small bottles with fresh biopsy material in tissue culture medium, accompanied by a long list in Clifford's own handwriting with all the essential patient information and a brief 'good luck' message. Our collaboration started in 1965 and lasted for more than a decade.

Peter Clifford had had a profound interest in Burkitt's lymphoma (BL) ever since he had introduced chemotherapy in the treatment of the disease and became fascinated by the remarkably good regression in the majority of patients (26). The 15–20% 'long-term survivors' turned out to be cured, eventually. Many of them only received incomplete chemotherapy. This was quite different from the effect of chemotherapy on other types of B-cell lymphomas. Clifford was convinced that the immunological response of the patient was decisive for the ultimate outcome of the disease. If there was a strong immune response, even incomplete chemotherapy would induce total and long-lasting remission. Even more effective forms of chemotherapy would ultimately fail if the immune response was inefficient, according to this hypothesis. Peter was pleased that we were looking for antitumour responses in his patients.

We changed our working habits. Every Tuesday night was 'Burkitt night'. It was not difficult to motivate our personnel to work through the night each week. We made living cell suspensions from the fresh tumours, which turned out to be surprisingly easy, we reacted them with the patient's own serum and a panel of other sera, and tried to read the immunofluorescence tests immediately to obtain clues for the continuing work.

Eventually, numerous other laboratories in the USA, England and Japan requested material, and some of them became engaged in collaborative projects.

We could identify a membrane antigen (MA) that was expressed in some Burkitt-lymphoma-derived cultures but not in others (27). When we presented these data at an American Cancer Society conference in Rye, New York, in 1967 (28), Werner Henle gave a talk in the same session. He reported the results of the immunofluorescence test on fixed Burkitt's lymphoma cells that he and Gertrud Henle had just developed, later known as the 'viral capsid antigen' (VCA) test (29). They already knew that the reaction was due to structural antigens of a newly discovered herpesvirus, first seen by Epstein, Barr and Achong under the electron microscope (30) Henle showed that it was antigenically distinct from previously known herpesviruses (31). We decided to call it Epstein–Barr virus (EBV).

The Henles' VCA test and our MA test showed a good concordance. The same lines appeared to react or failed to react in both tests. At the Rye meeting we agreed to collaborate. This initiated a highly productive association that lasted for 20 years, terminated only by Werner Henle's death in 1987.

At the beginning of this work we obtained definite evidence that MA was encoded by EBV (32). It is now known as the major viral envelope glycoprotein. It assembles within the membrane of the virus-producing cells and, after virus release, it can also attach to other cells in the same culture if they carry EBV receptors. With Jondal, Yefenof and Oldstone, we later identified the B-cell-specific C3d (CR2) receptor as the attachment site of the viral glycoprotein (33,34).

By 1970, it was clear that Epstein, the Henles and ourselves had only seen the tip of the iceberg when we looked at viral particles, VCA or MA. They only appeared in virus-producing lines, and only in some of the cells. However, with Harald zur Hausen, in 1970, we found that more than 90% of the African Burkitt's lymphomas (BLs) and all low differentiated or anaplastic nasopharyngeal carcinomas (NPCs) contained multiple EBV genomes per cell, no matter whether they produced virus or not (35). In 1973, together with Beverly Reedman, we found that 100% of the cells in EBV–DNA-positive BL biopsies and cell lines contained EBV-associated and, presumably EBV-encoded, nuclear antigen(s), which we decided to call EBNA (36). Today, we know that EBNA consists of a family of six different proteins (37,38).

Several important discoveries had been made by others in the meanwhile. The Henles, Pope et al. and Nilsson et al. found that EBV could readily immortalize normal B cells in vitro (39–41). Originating with a serendipitous observation of seroconversion in a laboratory assistant in the course of acute infectious mononucleosis, the Henles discovered (42) that EBV is the causative agent of infectious mononucleosis (IM). With Svedmyr, we could readily detect EBNA-positive cells in the peripheral blood of mononucleosis patients (43), and the Henles and George Miller (44) found that the saliva of these patients contained transforming virus. Transformation was thus a natural property of the virus, not a laboratory artefact due to the accidental isolation of a defective strain, as our colleagues in the lytic herpesvirus field initially surmised. Miller and Epstein have also shown that EBV can cause lethal lymphoproliferative disease in immunologically naive marmoset and owl monkeys (45,46).

Mononucleosis appeared as an acute rejection reaction against the virally infected B cells, mounted by the 'immunologically prepared' human host, selectively conditioned by our nearly symbiotic relationship with EBV that must have prevailed over millions of years, as indicated by the existence of close EBV relatives in all Old World (but not New World) primates. Our group has found that the peripheral blood of acute mononucleosis patients contains activated cytotoxic cells that can lyse EBV-carrying and other target cells (47,48). Autologous mixed lymphocyte cultures of EBV-transformed B cells and T cells of EBV seronegative donors generated an equally strong proliferative and cytotoxic response as found in MHC-incompatible allogeneic mixed lymphocyte cultures (MLCs) (49). Later, cell-mediated immunity was analysed in the B-cell immortalization system *in vitro*. When blood lymphocytes of healthy EBV seropositives were explanted in culture, the T cells inhibited the outgrowth of EBV-carrying B-cell lines (50–52). The virus-carrying B cells grew *in vitro* during the first few days, but the proliferation did not continue beyond that. This regression was due to direct cell-mediated cytotoxicity and also to growth-inhibitory lymphokine production and growth inhibition (53). Moss, Rickinson and Pope showed that the autologous mixed cultures generated specific MHC class I-restricted CTLs by repeated stimulation (54). One of us (E.K.) showed, with Sigurbjörg Torsteinsdottir, and Maria Grazia Masucci, that the cytotoxic T lymphocyte (CTL) response was heterogeneous, being directed against different target epitopes (55). This was fully confirmed by the later development, as will be described below.

The hypothesis that T-cell-mediated responses inhibit the proliferation of EBV-carrying B-cells in healthy seropositives and in IM patients *in vivo* was reaffirmed when we found with David Purtilo (56) that most, and perhaps all, lymphoproliferative diseases that appear in congenitally or iatrogenically immunodefective patients, such as children with the X-linked lymphoproliferative syndrome or organ transplant recipients, carry EBV genomes. Hanto, Ho and others later showed that these initially polyclonal immunoblastic proliferations may progress to monoclonal lymphoma (57,58).

While the tumourigenic potential of EBV was clearly established by these and related findings, its lifelong, innocuous latent presence in more than 80% of the people in all human populations has also suggested that disease occurs only as an accident. Even mononucleosis appears as an 'accident' of modern hygienic conditions that have apparently interfered with the normal, disease-free ecology of the virus–host relationship, based on the essentially symptom-free early childhood infection.

For Burkitt's lymphoma, the main accident has been identified as the juxtaposition of the *c*-myc gene to immunoglobulin sequences, as described in the next section. The pathogenesis of nasopharyngeal carcinoma, the most regularly EBV-carrying human tumour, is still not understood.

Oncogene Activation by Chromosomal Translocation

By 1970 it was clear that some important element was missing from the Burkitt's lymphoma scenario. EBV has clearly contributed to the genesis of the high endemic form of the disease, since 97% of the African Burkitt's lymphomas carried the viral genome, whereas non-Burkitt's lymphomas did not (for a review see Klein (59)). Moreover, the prospective study of Geser and de Thé (reviewed by de Thé (60)) showed that children with a high EBV load are at a greater risk to develop Burkitt's lymphoma than their brothers and sisters with a low EBV load, as judged by the anti-viral capsid antigen (VCA) titres.

Since the number of EBV-infected B cells represents only a minor fraction of the total B-cell population even in persons with a high EBV load, the presence of the virus in the majority of the African Burkitt's lymphomas can only be interpreted to mean that an EBV-carrying B cell runs a greater risk of turning into a Burkitt's lymphoma cell under the conditions prevailing in the 'high Burkitt's lymphoma belt' of Africa than does its EBV-negative counterpart. This is to say that EBV contributes to the aetiology of the tumour. But this is still not a satisfactory explanation: some essential element is obviously missing. Burkitt's lymphomas differ from the true EBV-induced proliferations like fatal mononucleosis or the immunoblastomas that occur in organ-transplant recipients, with regard to their phenotype (61). The latter resemble the EBV-transformed B-cell lines of non-neoplastic origin (LCLs). LCLs are permanently growing immunoblasts that express a set of activation markers but not CD10 (CALLA) or CD77 (BLA). Burkitt's lymphoma cells, on the other hand, carry surface antigen and glycoprotein markers that resemble resting B cells, rather than immunoblasts (61,62). They express CALLA and BLA but no activation markers (unless they drift to a more LCL-like phenotype during prolonged cultivation) (63). Gregory et al. have detected normal B cells with a corresponding phenotype in tonsil germinal centres (64).

For the understanding of the pathogenesis Burkitt's lymphoma, it is also important to remember that approximately 3% of the African and 80% of the sporadic Burkitt's lymphomas that occur all over the world are EBV negative. Among the AIDS-associated Burkitt's lymphomas, the incidence of the EBV-carrying form is approximately 40–50%.

The discovery of the 'missing factor' in the 'Burkitt equation' started when Manolov and Manolova reported in 1972 (65) that a 14q+ chromosomal marker was present in about 80% of the tumours. The Manolovs came from Sofia, Bulgaria, to work with us in 1970, at the time when the chromosome-banding technique was discovered by Caspersson and Zech. I suggested that they apply the banding technique to the cytogenetically unexplored Burkitt's lymphoma that kept coming in from Clifford every Tuesday in excellent condition. They agreed rather reluctantly, since they had hoped to learn some immunology. But their cytogenetic work soon picked up momentum, particularly after Albert Levan agreed to guide them. When George Manolov showed me the extra band that he found attached to the distal part of the long arm of one chromosome 14 in a BL biopsy, I first suspected some trivial reason, perhaps a constitutional variation (isochromosome?), and suggested that the Manolovs should take a look at the fibroblasts of the patient. They did and found that the anomaly was totally restricted to the clonal tumour.

After the Manolovs had returned to Bulgaria, we continued the work on the problem with Lore Zech. She soon showed that the 'extra piece' was derived from chromosome 8; the 14q+ marker was thus a product of a reciprocal 8; 14 translocation (66). Several groups found subsequently that approximately 20% of the Burkitt's lymphomas had no 14q+ marker but carried one of two variant translocations instead (for a review see Bernheim *et al.* (67)). Chromosome 8 broke at the same site (8q24) and entered into a reciprocal translocation either with the short arm of chromosome 2 or with chromosome 22. All Burkitt's lymphomas were found to carry one of the three translocations, no matter whether they were high endemic or sporadic, EBV positive or negative. The same translocations were only exceptionally found in non-Burkitt's lymphomas, although 14q+ markers are quite common; they usually arise by reciprocal translocations between chromosome 14 and some other chromosome, with 11 and 18 as the most frequent participants. But Burkitt's-lymphoma-type translocations were also found in B-cell-derived ALL which resembles Burkitt's lymphoma cells phenotypically and is often called 'Burkitt's leukaemia'.

Meanwhile, another, quite independent cytogenetic study, entirely confined to mouse tumour cells, was progressing in our laboratory. It started when the Hungarian–Romanian pathologist Francis Wiener joined our group in 1970. Wiener became interested in the role of chromosome 15 trisomy in mouse T-cell leukaemia. In the late 1970s Wiener also examined a series of pristane-oil-induced mouse plasmacytomas (MPCs), together with a Japanese guest worker, Shinsuke Ohno and in collaboration with Michael Potter's group at the NIH. Our 1979 paper published in *Cell* described the MPC-associated typical (12;15) and variant (6;15) translocations (68).

Mouse plasmacytomas are very different from Burkitt lymphomas. The only common denominator is that both originate from cells of the B-lymphocyte series. We never expected to find anything in common between the two. The fact that two apparently unrelated research projects, carried out by different cytogeneticists, led to the discovery of a common pathogenetic mechanism, based on almost exactly homologous chromosomal translocations, was one of the greatest and most pleasant surprises of our scientific career. It was even more surprising that the highly speculative working hypothesis, formulated to explain the mechanism whereby the translocations contribute to the tumourigenic process, turned out to be essentially correct.

The hypothesis was built on the fact that the recipient murine chromosomes of the dislocated fragment from chromosome 15 were known to carry the IgH (chromosome 12) and the κ (chromosome 6) gene, respectively. Likewise, human chromosome 14 was known to carry the IgH cluster. We have therefore speculated that a proto-oncogene and probably the same proto-oncogene may be localized at the breakpoint of the murine chromosome 15 and the human chromosome 8. Accidental translocation of the putative gene to one of the immunoglobulin loci might have led to its constitutional activation, by analogy to the retroviral activation of the *c*-myc gene by the insertion of an ALV-derived long terminal repeat (LTR) in the chicken bursal lymphoma, as described by Hayward *et al.* (69).

One of us (G.K.) started to expose the hypothesis to the test of peer criticism in 1979. An outstanding molecular biologist who was also a close friend, called it the 'most hair-raising extrapolation from the centimorgans to the kilobases'. It was. Still, the hypothesis was published in *Nature* in 1981 (70), but I was not fully convinced of it myself, until the critical moment during the summer of the same year, when I was waiting for a plane at Washington airport on my way to Tokyo. The waiting hall was full of people, mostly Japanese. There were only two telephones on the inside of the security check. They were busy most of the time. The plane was called up. Finally, one of the telephones was free. I tried to get hold of Philip Leder at the NIH. I wanted to hear whether he knew anything about the chromosomal location of the immunoglobulin light-chain genes in humans. Leder came to the telephone. No, he had not heard anything; it was still unknown. But one of his colleagues had just come back from the Human Chromosome Mapping Meeting in Oslo. If I waited, he would ask if the colleague had heard anything.

'Final call.' The last Japanese walked aboard, and I had to leave. At the moment when I was about to hang up the phone, Leder's voice came back. 'Yes, there were two small reports in Oslo. An English group had found that κ is on chromosome 2. An American group had proved that λ is on chromosome 22.' I ran on board. It was an intoxicating feeling! I knew for certain that the hypothesis was correct.

The molecular confirmation and clarification came in a virtual avalanche during 1982. Taking off from quite different points, Jerry Adams with Susan Cory in Australia and Kenneth Marcu in New York showed for MPC, and Carlo Croce and Phil Leder for Burkitt's lymphoma, that the translocations led to the juxtaposition of donor-chromosome-derived sequences and immunoglobulin gene sequences. Michael Cole's group has identified the transposed gene as *c*-myc (for reviews see Klein (71) and Adams and Cory (72)).

The subsequent development has led to many new insights, but it has also created some puzzles and paradoxes with regard to myc regulation, constitutive activation, and certain details of the timing and regulation of Ig gene rearrangement (for a review see Klein and Klein (73)). With Francis Wiener and Janos Sümegi, we have also found a third Ig/myc translocation carrying tumour (74–76), the spontaneous immunocytoma of the Louvain rat (RIC), developed by Hervé Bazin. A comparison of the translocations in MPC, RIC, and Burkitt's lymphoma at the molecular level revealed more similarities than differences. It would be hard to find a comparable situation in cancer biology where three pathogenetically different tumours that arise from the same cell lineage in three different species show a similarly close pathogenetic mechanism at the molecular level.

The causal, that is rate-limiting, involvement of constitutive myc activation in the genesis of the three tumours was deduced from the regularity of the Ig/myc juxtaposition that extended to cryptic translocations and complex rearrangements, where two or three successive genetic events had occurred (74,77). Further confirmation came from facsimile experiments. Michael Potter and Francis Wiener showed (78) that introduction of an activated myc gene within a retroviral (J3) construct into pristane-oil-treated Balb/c mice induced plasmacytomas that did not carry any translocations, provided they expressed the inserted (v-myc) gene. Adams and Cory's group generated transgenic mice that carried the myc gene coupled to the IgH enhancer (79). The mice developed more than 90% pre-B- or B-cell-derived lymphomas. Using the Australian transgenic mice, we have subsequently found that Abelson virus infection, already known to increase the incidence and shorten the latency period of pristane-oil-induced mouse plasmacytoma, has led to the appearance of plasmacytomas in Eμ-myc transgenic mice (80). The virus has obviated the pristane requirement and lifted the genetic restrictions to MPC susceptibility. These plasmacytomas were also translocation free.

The finding that introduction of an activated myc construct was tumourigenic for B cells and obviated the need for the translocations could only be interpreted to mean that the naturally occurring constitutive activation of myc by the Ig translocations provided an essential, rate-limiting step within the carcinogenic process. But it is not the only step. All tumours were monoclonal, even in the transgenic mice where myc was activated in all B and pre-B cells. Sequential activation of several oncogenes or, alternatively, loss of suppressor genes may provide additional steps. Feedback inhibition by the clone that happens to get the upper hand first would be another alternative.

The Burkitt's lymphoma story has also developed further and has posed some new fascinating questions. We have suggested, for both conceptual and factual reasons, that the Burkitt's lymphoma progenitor is a long-lived B memory cell. In this scenario, antigenically stimulated B-cell clones that have previously expanded as immunoblasts, were in the process of switching their phenotype to CALLA- and BLA-positive, activation-marker-negative memory cells when, upon the waning of the antigenic stimulus, the translocation accident occurred. Due to the linking of myc to a constitutively active Ig locus, the cells were unable to leave the cycling compartment, however.

Phenotype studies have subsequently shown that the translocation carrying 'suspended resting cell' had several additional properties that were potentially competent to facilitate its evasion from immunological control. Certain MHC class I polymorphic specificities were down-regulated in the Burkitt's-lymphoma cells, compared to EBV-transformed B-cell lines of normal origin

(81). Gregory *et al.* showed that the Burkitt's-lymphoma cells also failed to express certain adhesion molecules present on the LCLs or expressed them at a low level (82). Even the EBV-encoded, growth-transformation-associated nuclear and membrane antigens were down-regulated in the Burkitt's-lymphoma cells, with the exception of EBNA-1 (83). This was paralleled by a relative resistance of the Burkitt's-lymphoma cell to CTL-mediated lysis (55).

It thus appears that the myc/Ig translocation promotes the malignant growth of the Burkitt's-lymphoma cell by several mechanisms. This may explain the extraordinary regularity of its presence in all typical Burkitt's lymphomas so far studied.

Immune Surveillance Against DNA Tumour Virus Infected Cells – A Success Story

Polyoma virus in mice, EBV in humans, herpesvirus saimiri and ateles in the squirrel and the spider monkey, respectively, are highly transforming and potentially tumourigenic viruses that do not cause any tumours in their natural host, as a rule, unless the host is immunosuppressed. They can be tumourigenic without immunosuppression in closely related host species that do not carry the same or related viruses. Obviously, the natural host species had been selected for the recognition of transformed tumour precursor cells. The mechanism of this immune surveillance has been analysed most extensively in the EBV system. Eight proteins (EBNA-1 to -6, LMP1 and 2) are expressed in EBV-transformed immunoblasts. Seven of them, all except EBNA-1, generate peptides that can serve as CTL targets, when presented by the appropriate HLA class I molecules. The exceptional status of EBNA-1 may be seen in relation to the key role of this protein in the maintenance of the viral episomes (84) and the associated fact that, in contrast to all other virally encoded, transformation associated EBV proteins, it is regularly expressed in all EBV–DNA-carrying cells (85). For a recent discussion of the cell phenotype dependent differential expression of other EBV proteins and the strategy of the latent virus to escape immune elimination see Klein (86).

Depending on their HLA class I phenotype, healthy EBV-carrying persons tend to generate EBV-specific CTLs upon stimulation with autologous EBV-transformed B cells, characterized by one or a few dominating MHC restrictions. Each restriction reflects the specific association of the 'chosen' MHC with appropriate peptides, derived from one or several of the seven immunogenic growth transformation associated proteins. As shown by the groups of Moss in Australia (87), Rickinson in England (88) and Masucci *et al.* at our laboratory (89), the resulting 'chessboard' of HLA class I specificities and of the seven virally encoded proteins provides our species with a virtually watertight protection against the proliferation of EBV-transformed immunoblasts. The fact that similar protection does not prevail in EBV-susceptible New World primates such as marmosets or owl monkeys that do not harbour EBV-related viruses is consistent with the postulate, already mentioned, that our protective system has been established by selection during our long history of coexistence with what must have been originally a highly pathogenic virus, competent to induce lymphoblastic immunoproliferative disease.

Concomitantly, the virus has evolved a strategy of its own, consisting of an initial, proliferative, and a subsequent, persistently latent, phase. All seven immunogenic proteins are expressed during the temporary proliferation of the virally transformed B blasts during acute mononucleosis. The length of this period, prior to CTL-mediated rejection, is probably critical for viral survival and persistence, as indicated by the finding that immunodominant peptides of EBNA 4 may mutate in key anchorage sites in human populations with a high prevalence of the corresponding HLA class I specificity (90). Such mutations can only provide the virus with a temporary growth advantage, prior to rejection, but that may be all that is needed. Following the rejection of the infected B blasts, the virus persists in the small resting B cells where, as in the Burkitt's lymphoma type I cells, it only expresses the CTL-unrecognized EBNA-1 protein (86).

New Departures From the Impasse

If long-lasting selection is required to establish the potent surveillance systems that prevent the growth of cells transformed by widespread, potentially tumourigenic viruses in their natural hosts, is there no hope for the immune recognition of spontaneously arising, non-viral tumours that evolve by multistep progression? For several decades, it appeared that there was not much hope. More recently, the picture has become brighter again. The non-immunogenicity of tumour cells and the anergy of the host may not be irreversible or unmanipulatable. The development of cellular immunity requires adequate antigen presentation and the proper function of cytokine circuits. In contrast to many cells of the haemopoetic system, such as B cells, macrophages and dendritic cells that are 'professional' antigen presenters, fibroblasts, epithelial cells, and the malignant tumours derived from them are not. Experimental modifications to improve the situation include transfection of tumour cells with genes that enhance the expression of MHC or adhesion molecules, or encode cytokines. Even earlier approaches that have used to induce new antigens by infecting the tumour cells with viruses, by cell hybridization or by mutagenesis may be considered. It has been repeatedly shown that immunization with manipulated cells may prevent or inhibit the growth of both resident and grafted, unmanipulated tumour cells in suitable host–tumour combinations.

The recent developments have been dominated by the important work of Boon et al. (91). They have departed from the observation that non-tumourigenic (tum+) mutants derived from seemingly non-immunogenic tumours of spontaneous origin could immunize against the original tumourigenic (tum+) cell. Subsequently, they have generated tumour-specific CTL clones, directed against the relevant antigenic target. Using these T-cell clones as their reagents, they could eventually isolate the gene encoding the antigen. The same technique was subsequently applied to the detection of human tumour associated antigens and the cloning of their genes. Different categories of antigens were recognized. One type, only identified in experimental (mouse) tumours so far, was the product of a mutated gene (92). Another category, found in human melanoma, was a peptide derived from tyrosinase, a normal-tissue-specific protein (93). A third category includes reactivated embryonic genes that are not expressed in normal adult tissues. The most extensively investigated gene in this category is MAGE-1, expressed on about half of the human melanomas and one-quarter of human breast carcinomas (94). So far, all human melanoma-associated antigens studied belong to the second and third categories, and thus represent improperly activated normal proteins.

Yet another category of tumour rejection antigen, recognized by CTLs on pancreatic and breast tumours, is represented by underglycosylated mucins (95). A repeating motif is recognized by the CTLs in the protein core of the mucin. This reaction shows no MHC restriction, indicating that the reactive cells may have been sensitized to superantigens. The identification of these antigens opens a new phase in specific immunotherapy, as detailed elsewhere (96).

Another biochemically based strategy for identifying tumour antigens recognized by T cells is based on the extraction of peptides from the MHC class I molecules of tumour cells. These are fractionated by high performance liquid chromatography (HPLC), eluted, and tested on a surrogate target cell that expresses the same MHC allele as the tumour, but is not lysed by the tumour-specific CTLs. Analysis of the fractions that confer sensitivity to the killing action of the tumour-specific CTL may identify the antigen (97).

The products of mutated oncogenes or tumour suppressor genes may serve as tumour-specific antigens in some instances. Mutated ras peptides can generate specific CTLs (98–100). Similar findings were made with mutated p53 (101) and the p210 protein product of the bcr/abl fusion gene (102). Heat shock proteins from cancer cells or virus-infected cells may carry bound peptides which can induce T-cell immunity against the specific viral or tumour antigens (103,104).

Taken together, these recent developments indicate that many spontaneous tumours may carry potential CTL targets. Why are they not recognized in the unmanipulated tumour host? Antigen presentation may represent one of the major problems, as already mentioned. Numerous attempts have been reported that may overcome this difficulty. One of them has been to transfect mouse tumour cells with the B7 gene. The B7 protein is normally expressed on antigen presenting cells. CD28, its ligand on T-cells forms a tight complex with B7 (105,106). Another approach that has been successfully used to improve the antigen presentation of otherwise non-immunogenic tumours is based on the introduction of cytokine genes (for a review see Pardoll (107)). A recent, strikingly successful experiment was reported by Dranoff *et al.* (108). They have introduced a whole gamut of cytokine genes into a poorly immunogenic murine melanoma, in order to determine which of the transfectants could generate resistance to the non-transfected tumour. None of the cytokines showed much effect, except GM-CSF. Tumours transfected with the latter were found to induce a virtually complete resistance against their non-transfected parental cell, to which both CD4- and CD8-positive T cells contributed. It was suggested that the effect may be due to mobilization of dendritic and other antigen presenting cells by the, presumably released, GM-CSF.

In view of the fact that cellular antigens are recognized by T cells in the form of MHC class I associated peptides, attempts to increase the expression of MHC and adhesion molecules are also interesting. In one of many experimental tests, the highly metastatic B16-F-10.9 melanoma was treated *in vitro* in γ-interferon (IFN-γ) (109). It induced elevated H-2K^b and H-2D^b expression and rendered the tumour cells immunogenic. They generated CTLs *in vivo* and *in vitro*, and became sensitive to their lytic effect. Pre-exposure of the mice to treated tumours protected them against the growth of grafted tumour cells and prevented the metastatic spread of intravenously injected untreated tumour cells.

We found that *in vitro* treatment with IFN-γ and tumour necrosis factor α (TNF-α) elevated the MHC class I expression of *ex vivo* human carcinomas. Such cells induced a cytotoxic potential in six-day mixed blood lymphocyte–tumour cell cultures. Importantly, the untreated tumour cells were also damaged in a proportion of experiments.

These and similar developments are currently spurring new efforts to develop human cancer vaccines, as summarized by Cohen (110).

Conclusions

In conclusion, tumour immunology is on the ascendance once again. This is the fifth transfiguration of the famous sine curve, first triggered by the false excitement over the strong resistance that could be generated against 'transplantable' tumours, followed by a decline when it was realized that this was merely homograft immunity. A new optimism was generated by the discovery that chemically and virally induced experimental tumours were perceptibly and often fairly strongly immunogenic in syngeneic hosts. This was succeeded by another abrupt fall when spontaneous tumours that have arisen without any experimental interference, failed to provide suitable rejection targets. The most recent developments have led to an increasing understanding of the reasons for this failure. As in many other areas of tumour biology, they directed the searchlight towards the plasticity of tumour-cell populations. The ready appearance of new mutants does not only contribute to tumour progression, that is, escape from homeostatic growth control, but also to escapes from immune surveillance.

Depending on the mechanisms of the latter, the apparent non-immunogencity of tumour cells and/or the anergy of the host may be overcome. Our rapidly increasing understanding of peptide–MHC class I interactions and antigen presentation to T cells that carry the appropriate T-cell receptors, together with the opening of new inroads into the fields of specific and non-specific immune modulators have brought much new encouragement. May new developments, based on the increasing application of genetic engineering to produce more immunogenic cells, lead the way, in spite of all the difficulties (*111*), towards the much coveted clinical applications.

Notes and References

1. G. J. V. Nossal, *Immunol. Today* **1**, 5 (1980).
2. G. Klein, *Prog. Immunol.* **4**, 680 (1980).
3. C. C. Little, *Science* **40**, 904 (1914).
4. G. D. Snell, *J. Genetics* **49**, 87 (1948).
5. P. Gorer, *J. Pathol. Bacteriol.* **44**, 691 (1937).
6. P. A. Gorer and Z. B. Mikulska, *Proc. R. Soc. London, Ser. B.* **151**, 57 (1959).
7. G. Klein, *Les Prix Nobel, 1980*, Nobel Foundation, Stockholm (1981).
8. E. J. Foley, *Cancer Res.* **13**, 835 (1953).
9. R. T. Prehn and J. M. Main, *J. Natl Cancer Inst.* **18**, 769 (1957).
10. G. Klein, H. O. Sjögren, E. Klein and K. E. Hellström, *Cancer Res.* **20**, 1561 (1960).
11. R. W. Baldwin, *Br. J. Cancer* **9**, 652 (1955).
12. L. J. Old, E. A. Boyse, D. A. Clarke and E. A. Carswell, *Ann. NY Acad. Sci.* **101**, 80 (1962).
13. R. T. Prehn, *Ann. NY Acad. Sci.* **101**, 107 (1962).
14. G. Klein, H. O. Sjögren and E. Klein, *Cancer Res.* **23**, 84 (1963).
15. R. W. Baldwin, *Adv. Cancer Res.* **18**, 1 (1973).
16. H. D. Sjögren, I. Hellström and G. Klein, *Cancer Res.* **21**, 329 (1961).
17. K. Habel, *Virology* **18**, 553 (1962).
18. H. O. Sjögren, *J. Natl Cancer Inst.* **32**, 375 (1964).
19. G. Klein, *Ann. Rev. Microbiol.* **20**, 223 (1966).
20. L. J. Old, E. A. Boyse and E. J. Stockert, *J. Natl Cancer Inst.* **31**, 977 (1963).
21. G. Klein, E. Klein and G. Haughton, *J. Natl Cancer Inst.* **36**, 607 (1966).
22. T. Dalianis, *Adv. Cancer Res.* **55**, 57 (1990).
23. D. Burkitt, *Nature* **194**, 232 (1962).
24. D. Burkitt, *J. Natl Cancer Inst.* **42**, 19 (1969).
25. A. J. Haddow, in *Burkitt's Lymphoma* (D. P. Burkitt and D. H. Wright, eds), Livingstone, London (1978), pp. 198–209.
26. P. Clifford, S. Singh, J. Stjernswärd and G. Klein, *Cancer Res.* **27**, 2578 (1967).
27. G. Klein, P. Clifford, E. Klein and J. Stjernswärd, *Proc. Natl Acad. Sci. USA* **55**, 1628 (1966).
28. G. Klein, E. Klein and P. Clifford, *Cancer Res.* **27**, 2510 (1967).
29. G. Henle and W. Henle, *J. Bacteriol.* **91**, 1248 (1966).
30. M. A. Epstein, G. B. Achong and Y. N. Barr, *Lancet* **i**, 702 (1964).
31. G. Henle and W. Henle, *Cancer Res.* **27**, 2442 (1967).
32. G. Klein, G. Pearson, J. S. Nadkarni, J. J. Nadkarni, E. Klein, G. Henle, W. Henle and P. Clifford, *J. Exp. Med.* **128**, 1011 (1968).
33. M. Jondal, G. Klein, M. B. A. Oldstone, V. Bokish and E. Yefenof, *Scand. J. Immunol.* **5**, 401 (1976).
34. E. Yefenof, G. Klein, M. Jondal and M. B. A. Oldstone, *Int. J. Cancer* **17**, 693 (1976).
35. H. zur Hausen, H. Schulte-Holthausen, G. Klein, W. Henle, G. Henle, P. Clifford and L. Santesson, *Nature* **228**, 1056 (1970).

36. B. M. Reedman and G. Klein, *Int. J. Cancer* **11**, 499 (1973).
37. A. Ricksten, B. Kallin, H. Alexander, J. Dillner, R. Fåhraeus, G. Klein, R. Lerner and L. Rymo, *Proc. Natl Acad. Sci. USA* **85**, 995 (1988).
38. J. Dillner and B. Kallin, *Adv. Cancer Res.* **50**, 95 (1988).
39. W. Henle, V. Diehl, G. Kohn, H. zur Hausen and G. Henle, *Science* **157**, 1064 (1967).
40. K. Nilsson, G. Klein, W. Henle and G. Henle, *Int. J. Cancer* **8**, 443 (1971).
41. J. H. Pope, M. K. Horne and W. Scott, *Int. J. Cancer* **3**, 857 (1968).
42. W. Henle and G. Henle, *New Engl. J. Med.* **288**, 263 (1973).
43. G. Klein, E. Svedmyr, M. Jondal and P. O. Persson, *Int. J. Cancer* **17**, 21 (1976).
44. G. Miller, in *Viral Oncology* (G. Klein, ed.), Raven Press, New York (1980), pp. 713–738.
45. M. A. Epstein, R. Hunt and H. Rabin, *Int. J. Cancer* **12**, 309 (1973).
46. T. Shope, D. De Chiaro and G. Miller, *Proc. Natl Acad. Sci. USA* **70**, 2487 (1973).
47. E. Svedmyr and M. Jondal, *Proc. Natl Acad. Sci. USA* **72**, 1622 (1975).
48. E. Klein, I. Ernberg, M. G. Masucci, R. Szigeti, Y. T. Wu, G. Masucci and E. Svedmyr, *Cancer Res.* **41**, 4210 (1981).
49. E. A. Svedmyr, F. Deinhardt and G. Klein, *Int. J. Cancer* **13**, 891 (1974).
50. D. A. Thorley-Lawson, L. Chess and J. L. Strominger, *J. Exp. Med.* **146**, 495 (1977).
51. D. A. Thorley-Lawson, *J. Immunol.* **126**, 829 (1981).
52. D. J. Moss, A. B. Rickinson and J. H. Pope, *Int. J. Cancer* **22**, 662 (1978).
53. M. T. Bejarano, M. G. Masucci, I. Ernberg, G. Klein and E. Klein, *Int J. Cancer* **35**, 327 (1985)
54. D. J. Moss, A. B. Rickinson and J. H. Pope, *Int. J. Cancer* **22**, 662 (1978).
55. S. Torsteinsdottir, M. G. Masucci, B. Ehlin-Henriksson, C. Brautbar, H. Ben-Bassat, G. Klein and E. Klein, *Proc. Natl Acad. Sci. USA* **83**, 5620 (1986).
56. D. T. Purtilo and G. Klein, *Cancer Res.* **41**, 4209 (1981).
57. D. W. Hanto, G. Frizzera, K. J. Gajl-Peczalska, K. Sakamoto, D. T. Purtilo, H. H. Balfour, R. L. Simmons and J. S. Najarian, *N. Engl. J. Med.* **306**, 913 (1982).
58. M. Ho, R. Jaffe, G. Miller, M. K. Breining, J. S. Dummer, L. Makowka, R. W. Atchison, F. Karrer, A. Nalesnik and T. E. Starzl, *Transplantation* **45**, 719 (1988).
59. G. Klein, *Cold Spring Harbor Symp. Quant. Biol.* **39**, 783 (1975).
60. G. de Thé, in *Viral Oncology* (G. Klein, ed.), Raven Press, New York (1980), pp. 769–797.
61. K. Nilsson and G. Klein, *Adv. Cancer Res.* **37**, 319 (1982).
62. B. Ehlin-Henriksson and G. Klein, *Int. J. Cancer* **33**, 459 (1984).
63. M. Rowe, C. M. Rooney, C. F. Edwards, G. M. Lenoir and A. B. Rickinson, *Int. J. Cancer* **37**, 367 (1986).
64. C. D. Gregory, T. Tursz, C. F. Edwards, C. Tetaud, M. Talbot, B. Caillou, A. B. Rickinson and M. Lipinski, *J. Immunol.* **139**, 313 (1987).
65. G. Manolov and Y. Manolova, *Nature* **237**, 33 (1972).
66. H. Zech, U. Haglund, K. Nilsson and G. Klein, *Int. J. Cancer* **17**, 47 (1976).
67. A. Bernheim, R. Berger and G. Lenoir, *Cancer Genet. Cytogenet.* **3**, 307 (1981).
68. S. Ohno, M. Babonits, F. Wiener, J. Spira, G. Klein and M. Potter, *Cell* **18**, 1001 (1979).
69. W. S. Hayward, B. G. Neel and S. M. Astrin, *Nature* **290**, 475 (1981).
70. G. Klein, *Nature* **294**, 313 (1981).
71. G. Klein, *Cell* **32**, 311 (1983).
72. J. M. Adams and S. Cory, *Proc. R. Soc. London, Ser. B* **226**, 59 (1985).
73. G. Klein and E. Klein, *Immunol. Today* **6**, 208 (1985).
74. W. S. Pear, G. Wahlström, S. F. Nelson, H. Axelson, A. Szeles, F. Wiener, H. Bazin, G. Klein and J. Sümegi, *Mol. Cell Biol.* **8**, 441 (1988).
75. J. Sümegi, J. Spira, H. Bazin, J. Szpirer, G. Levan and G. Klein, *Nature* **306**, 497 (1983).
76. F. Wiener, M. Babonits, J. Spira, G. Klein and H. Bazin, *Int. J. Cancer* **29**, 431 (1982).
77. P. D. Fahrlander, J. Sümegi, J. Q. Yang, F. Wiener, K. B. Marcu and G. Klein, *Proc. Natl Acad. Sci. USA* **82**, 3746 (1985).
78. M. Potter, J. F. Mushinski, E. B. Mushinski, S. Brust, J. S. Wax, F. Wiener, M. Babonits, U. R. Rapp and H. C. Morse III, *Science* **235**, 787 (1987).

79. J. M. Adams, A. W. Harris, C. A. Pinkert, L. M. Corcoran, W. S. Alexander, S. Cory, R. D. Palmiter and R. L. Brinster, *Nature* **318**, 533 (1985).
80. H. Sugiyama, S. Silva, Y. Wang, G. Weber, M. Babonits, A. Rosén, F. Wiener and G. Klein, *Int. J. Cancer* **46**, 845 (1990).
81. M. L. Andersson, N. J. Stam, G. Klein, H. L. Ploegh and M. G. Masucci, *Int. J. Cancer* **47**, 544 (1991).
82. C. D. Gregory, C. Edwards and A. B. Rickinson, *J. Exp. Med.* **167**, 1811 (1988).
83. M. Rowe, D. T. Rowe, C. D. Gregory, L. S. Young, P. Farrell, H. Rupani and A. B. Rickinson, *EMBO J.* **6**, 2743 (1987).
84. J. Yates, N. Warren and B. Sugden, *Nature* **313**, 812 (1985).
85. B. A. Contreras-Brodin, M. Anvret, S. Imreh, E. Altiok, G. Klein and M. G. Masucci, *J. Gen. Virol* **72**, 3025 (1991).
86. G. Klein, *Cell* **77**, 791 (1994).
87. R. Khanna, S. Borrows, M. Kurilla, C. Jacob, I. Misko, T. Sculley, E. Kieff and D. Moss, *J. Exp. Med.* **176**, 169 (1992).
88. R. Murray, M. Kurilla, J. Brooks, W. Thomas, M. Rowe, E. Kieff and A. Rickinson, *J. Exp. Med.* **176**, 157 (1992)
89. M. G. Masucci, R. Gavioli, P. O. de Campos-Lima, Q.-J. Zhang, P. Trivedi and R. Dolcetti, *Ann. NY Acad. Sci.* **690**, 86 (1993).
90. P. O. de Campos-Lima, R. Gavioli, Q.-J. Zhang, L. E. Wallace, R. Dolcetti, M. Rowe, A. B. Rickinson and M. G. Masucci, *Science* **260**, 98 (1993).
91. T. Boon, *Adv. Cancer Res.* **58**, 177 (1992).
92. C. Lurguin, A. Van Pel, B. Mariame, E. De Plaen, J. Szikora, P. Janssens, M. Reddehase, J. Lejeune and T. Boon, *Cell* **58**, 293 (1991).
93. V. Brichard, A. Van Pel, T. Wölfel, C. Wölfel, E. De Plaen, B. Lethé, P. Coulie and T. Boon, *J. Exp. Med.* **178**, 489 (1993).
94. P. Van der Bruggen, C. Traversari, P. Chomez, C. Lurquin, E. De Plaen, B. Van den Eynde, A. Knuth and T. Boon, *Science* **254**, 1643 (1991).
95. K. R. Jerome, D. I. Barnd, K. M. Bendt, C. M. Boyer, J. Taylor-Papadimitrou, I. F. C. McKenzie, R. C. Bast Jr and O. J. Finn, *Cancer Res.* **51**, 2908 (1991).
96. G. Klein and T. Boon, *Curr. Opinion Immunol.* **5**, 687 (1993).
97. C. Slingeloff, A. Cox, R. Henderson, D. Hunt and V. Engelhard, *J. Immunol.* **150**, 2955 (1993).
98. D. J. Peace, W. Chen, H. Nelson and M. A. Cheever, *J. Immunol.* **146**, 2059 (1991).
99. J. Skipper and H. J. Strauss, *J. Exp. Med.* **177**, 1493 (1993).
100. T. Gedde-Dahl III, B. Fossum, J. A. Eriksen, E. Thorsby and G. Gaudernack, *Eur. J. Immunol.* **23**, 754 (1993).
101. M. Yanuck, D. R. Carbone, D. C. Pendelton, T. Tsukui, S. F. Winter, J. D. Minna and J. A. Berzofsky, *Cancer Res.* **53**, 3257 (1993).
102. W. Chen, D. J. Peace, D. K. Rovira, S. You and M. A. Cheever, *Proc. Natl Acad. Sci. USA* **89**, 1468 (1992).
103. P. K. Srivastava, *Adv. Cancer Res.* **62**, 154 (1993).
104. Z. Li and P. K. Srivastava, *EMBO J.* **12**, 3143 (1993).
105. L. Chen, S. Ashe, W. A. Brady, I. Hellström, K. E. Hellström, J. A. Ledbetter, P. McGowan and P. S. Linsley, *Cell* **71**, 1093 (1992).
106. S. E. Townsend and J. P Allison, *Science* **259**, 368 (1993).
107. D. M. Pardoll, *Curr. Opinion Immunol.* **5**, 719 (1993).
108. G. Dranoff, E. Jaffe, A. Lazenby, P. Golulmbek, H. Levitsky, K. Brose, V. Jackson, H. Hirofumi, D. Pardoll and R. C. Mulligan, *Proc. Natl Acad. Sci. USA* **90**, 3539 (1993).
109. A. Porgador, B. Brenner, E. Vadal, M. Feldman and L. Eisenbach, *Int. J. Cancer* **6** (Suppl.), 54 (1991).
110. J. Cohen, *Science* **262**, 841 (1993).
111. E. Kedar and E. Klein, *Adv. Cancer Res.* **59**, 245 (1992).

Hepatitis B Virus and Vaccine

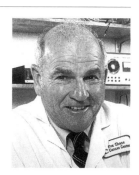

BARUCH S. BLUMBERG
770 Bierholme Avenue, Philadelphia, PA 19111, USA

In this chapter I will describe the studies done by my colleagues and myself at the Fox Chase Cancer Center in Philadelphia, PA, which resulted in the discovery of the hepatitis B virus (HBV) and the invention of the vaccine against it. Immunological techniques and principles were essential to the studies, but few of our group had training in immunology. Only one, Irving Millman, was a microbiologist and the others, W. Thomas London, Alton Sutnick and myself were trained as clinicians and our experience was in clinical research and epidemiology. Our approach was that of amateurs adventuring in a field which we found to be intriguing and mysterious, but not totally familiar. This paper will not, therefore, describe advances in the science of immunology but rather the application of fundamental and long-known principles to discovery and, later, application.

What Was Known About the Subject?

Hepatitis, an inflammation of the liver associated with acute or persistent dysfunction, had been known clinically from the very earliest times, primarily because of the distinctive yellow jaundice which characterizes the illness. Historically, jaundice is associated with poor sanitation and the mass movement of people. It is a common illness of armies and civilians during times of war and much of the early research was by the military. By the mid-1960s it had been shown that many cases of jaundice were infectious and caused by a filterable agent, that is, a virus, and that there were at least two forms of the virus. One was transmitted by the faecal–oral route, that is, contaminated water and food (hepatitis A), and the other in some manner transmitted from the blood of an infected person to that of an uninfected one. Research in the area intensified during World War II and the Korean War, when hepatitis was one of the main causes of morbidity. However, the postulated viruses had not been identified and it was not possible to prevent post-transfusion hepatitis because asymptomatic carriers of the virus could not be identified among blood donors. It was also impossible to protect those at risk by the use of vaccines, and no treatment other than symptomatic treatment was available.

Why Were We Interested in the Problem?

The research which resulted in the discovery of the hepatitis B virus was not, at its start, designed to do so. Rather, it was initiated by a curiosity about inherited differences between people and how these relate to disease susceptibility. My interest in this somewhat esoteric problem began when I was doing field and clinical research in Surinam, South America, in 1949 and 1950 during my last year in medical school. I was based in Moengo an isolated mining town located in the coastal swamps of the northern portion of the country. Living in Moengo were the descendants of several populations (Africans, Indians, Indonesians) who had been brought to or had emigrated to the country to work on the sugar plantations and in other colonial occupations. There were also indigenous native Americans who lived in the nearby jungle. We found a profound difference between several of these populations in their susceptibility to infection with *Wuchereria bancrofti*, the agent of filariasis (elephantiasis). We wanted to study inherited characteristics which might account for the susceptibility differences.

By 1957, when I was completing my doctoral degree in Biochemistry at Oxford University, Oliver Smithies had introduced starch gel electrophoresis. This allowed the detection of serum protein entities which had not previously been separable and some of these constituted inherited polymorphic systems. I use this term in the sense defined by E. B. Ford, the Oxford lepidopterist, that is, the existence in the same region of two or more inherited forms of a trait in such numbers that the form in lowest frequency could not have been maintained by recurrent mutation. This infers that in some of the systems differential selection had been operating. For example, there are several inherited forms of the serum transferrin, an iron transport protein. In some populations several per cent of the less common form may exist in the population. The bearers of the different forms may have no external evidence of their genotype (that is, no disease), although it is likely that subtle survival differences may be associated with the protein heterogeneity. A significant percentage of the human genome is polymorphic and these systems constitute a large portion of the measurable inherited variation in humans and other species. Other examples of polymorphism detectable at the phenotypic level were the red blood cell antigen system, the sickle cell trait, and the HLA or major histocompatibility complex (MHC). Since the development of molecular biology it has been possible to identify polymorphisms at the genic level, by using the restriction fragment length polymorphism (RFLP) and other methods which identify groups of DNA sequences by their comparative length after enzymatic digestion. This has renewed interest in polymorphisms and these approaches are used extensively to locate specific genes associated with diseases.

Results of the Study

During the late 1950s and early 1960s we investigated the distribution of several of the serum protein systems in widely distributed populations and places (Spanish Basques, Nigeria, Marshall Islands, Alaska, etc.) and found interesting patterns of distribution. In the early 1960s, in an effort to identify new polymorphisms, A. C. Allison and I, working at the National Institutes of Health in Bethesda, MD, introduced a method designed to discover immunological inherited (or acquired) variation. We reasoned that if there were serum protein polymorphisms still unknown and that one or more of these were antigenic, then patients who received multiple transfusions would be likely to have been injected with blood containing proteins which they themselves had not acquired or inherited and to develop antibodies against them. We used the microimmunodiffusion technique, in which the serum of a multiply transfused patient was placed in the central well of a pattern cut into agar gel. If a specific antibody were present then it would diffuse into the gel and interact with specific antigen present in sera placed in the peripheral wells. Using this approach we soon discovered an antibody in a much-transfused patient with aplastic anaemia which identified a rich variation of the low-density lipoproteins (the 'Ag' polymorphism). The Ag system, and variants of it have subsequently proven to be of interest in the study of disease related to the mechanism by which the body deals with fats and cholesterol.

Emboldened by this discovery, we continued our search for new antibodies and polymorphic proteins. In 1966 we identified an antigen–antibody system different from Ag. The antiserum was found in the blood of a haemophilia patient from New York and the antigen in an Australian aborigine. Initially, we considered the hypothesis that the 'Australia antigen' system was another serum protein polymorphism, but by 1967 we had evidence that the antigen was on the surface of one of the hypothesized hepatitis viruses and that the antibody had developed in the transfused patient as a consequence of exposure to the virus. It is ironic that the HBV which causes so much human disease was identified using serum from two individuals neither of whom were obviously suffering from hepatitis.

This investigation had started as an esoteric exercise to identify human biochemical variation in relation to susceptibility to disease. The virus was identified because one individual, the haemophilia patient, reacted by developing an antibody, and the second, the Australian aborigine, by becoming a carrier.

There was a polar difference in their immunological responses, and we believed that these differences were, in some complex way, inherited. Later, it was concluded that 'Australia antigen' identified HBV characterized by blood-borne transmission.

The Vaccine

Our decision to go ahead with the development of a vaccine was a consequence, in part, of a directive we had received from the funding agencies of the US Federal government. At the end of the 1960s we were advised that research organizations would be required to find sources of income in addition to the government grants. In particular, patenting and commercialization of the products of their research was recommended.

By coincidence, our discovery of the virus coincided with the arrival of Dr Irving Millman at Fox Chase Cancer Center. Prior to joining us he had worked at Merck, the pharmaceutical company, where he had successfully developed a rubella vaccine. Initially he thought he would be working on inherited serum proteins and their immunological interactions. He was surprised to learn that we believed that Australia antigen was on a virus. His immediate reaction was that the large amounts of viral antigen present in the blood, sufficient to be detected by the insensitive immunodiffusion technique, could not all be whole virus since a load of the magnitude we had found would be deadly. Further, we did not see significant amounts of nucleic acid in the isolated antigen.

An additional finding was epidemiological; in our early studies using immunodiffusion we very rarely detected both Australia antigen and the antibody to it in the same individual. This was consistent with the explanation that the antibody was protective. We then devised a unique method for preparing a vaccine. Based on animal challenge studies, we showed that a highly purified fraction of the blood containing Australia antigen did not transmit hepatitis, but a less purified preparation did. We inferred that in addition to the particles that contained only the Australia antigen there were whole virions containing nucleic acid, which had not yet been detected, and that these could be separated by centrifugation since their densities would be different. Starting with the blood of a carrier, the Australia antigen was separated from other serum proteins and the hypothesized whole virion. In animal experiments we showed that this material was not infectious and that it could induce high titres of antibody. An application for a patent was submitted in 1969 and issued in 1971.

Primary Hepatocellular Carcinoma

Primary hepatocellular carcinoma (PHC) is one of the most common cancers in the world and is a disease of public health importance in parts of Asia,

Oceania, and sub-Saharan Africa. In the 1950s, Payette and others in highly endemic areas had, on pathological grounds, suggested that hepatitis might be the cause of the disease. With the identification of HBV it became possible to show, based on epidemiological, molecular and other studies that HBV is a major cause of PHC. Interest in the application of the vaccine was increased, I believe, because of the great concern engendered by this deadly and difficult to treat cancer.

Publication and Reaction of the Community

By early 1967, we stated that we had identified the hepatitis virus and that we were proceeding to test this hypothesis further. However, we had some difficulty in having our paper accepted. It was submitted to the *Annals of Internal Medicine* and the reviewers initially rejected it, we were told, because there had been many false claims for the discovery of a hepatitis virus, and ours was likely to be another. However, we were successful in publishing the paper by late 1967 and there was a nearly immediate interest in our findings, particularly in the parts of the world where HBV was very common. In order to facilitate confirmation of our discovery, and to advance the research as rapidly as possible, we distributed samples of the antigen and antibody to investigators who requested them. The equipment for doing the studies was very simple and essentially without cost, and it was possible to rapidly reproduce our findings.

Acceptance of the vaccine was slower. Although the patent was issued in 1971, and we informed many of our colleagues, it did not excite very much attention. A vaccine had never been prepared from the blood of a carrier, nor has it been since the hepatitis B vaccine, and it was not surprising that it did not gain acceptance. However, by the mid-1970s several investigators published the results of experimental studies with primates (particularly chimpanzees who were highly susceptible to infection, but who did not show signs of disease) which strongly supported the notion that the vaccine produced from carriers was protective. The Fox Chase Cancer Center licensed the Merck Pharmaceutical Company to develop and produce the vaccine and after a series of successful field trials, particularly those of Wolf Szmuness conducted on male homosexual volunteers from New York, the efficacy (more than 90%) and safety of the vaccine was established. By the early 1980s it was certified for use in the USA and elsewhere. Later, several groups developed a recombinant vaccine, the first (and, so far, the only) such vaccine produced and marketed.

Long-term Impact

Shortly after the discovery, diagnostic techniques for HBV were developed. The detection of occult carriers of the virus among potential blood donors was now possible. Increasingly sensitive methods were introduced; immunodiffusion, electroimmunodiffusion, and radioimmunoassay which had been adapted by Coller, Millman and myself from the established method. Enzyme immuno-assays are currently used. Soon, regulations and legislation were enacted that required the testing of all blood used for transfusion and the manufacture of human blood products. There was a dramatic drop in post-transfusion hepati-tis due to HBV, and in many parts of the world this problem has essentially dis-appeared. This was the first required blood testing for a virus, a practice that has now been extended to several others (HIV, hepatitis C virus, HTLV-1). Since the introduction of screening for hepatitis C there have been even further reduc-tions in post-transfusion hepatitis. There is, however, a residual number of cases due to as yet unidentified blood-borne viruses.

Use of the vaccine began almost immediately after certification, but its spread was delayed by high cost. There were also concerns about the use of a blood-derived vaccine (HIV had recently been discovered), even though it had been shown that the HBV blood-derived vaccine was free of HIV or other known infectious agents. By the early 1980s, a national programme for the vac-cination of the newborn children of carrier mothers was begun in Taiwan and in Japan. This has resulted in dramatic decreases in the frequency of HBV car-riers in the impacted age groups. Soon, other manufacturers began to produce the vaccine – the price dropped, and use increased rapidly.

In 1977, I visited the Peoples' Republic of China at the invitation of the Chinese Medical Association. This was in the period before diplomatic rela-tions between China and the USA had been established and travel was relatively uncommon. However, the Chinese public health officials and physicians were anxious to learn about the vaccine and also the association of HBV and primary hepatocellular carcinoma, one of the most common cancers in China, and the cause of an enormous amount of morbidity and mortality. I spoke to several thousand scientists during a month's travel and described the vaccine, provided them with access to the patent, and put them in contact with the manufactur-ers. At present there are in China factories for the manufacture of the vaccine, originally from carrier blood and more recently by recombinant methods, and the use of the vaccine is widespread.

The World Health Organization (WHO) has included HBV vaccine in the recommended paediatric vaccines and there are national vaccination pro-grammes in more than 40 countries. HBV carriers are much more common in Italy than in most other European countries and universal vaccination pro-grammes have been established in several regions. It was very gratifying to hear from an Italian colleague and friend that prior to the introduction of the vaccine he had to advise carrier mothers to avoid pregnancy. He can now assure them that their newborns can be protected against infection.

It has been predicted that vaccination will considerably decrease cancer of the liver in countries where HBV is the predominant cause, and a long-term sur-veillance project has been established in the Gambia to test this hypothesis. If the vaccine is effective in reducing the incidence of PHC then it would be the first preventive vaccine for cancer and, possibly, a prototype for other viral-caused cancers.

Studies of the molecular biology of HBV in patients with PHC are providing insights into how this virus causes cancer. It may provide a guide to the pathogenesis of this important class of disease and, perhaps, lead to additional treatments and cures for PHC and, by inference, other cancers.

Conclusion

The discovery of the virus was an unexpected consequence of a basic scientific study, and the applications flowed from this. It has resulted in significant improvements in health and the prevention of disease. This is often the case in biological sciences and provides another argument for the support of fundamental scientific inquiry and curiosity-based research.

Studies of Thyroid Autoimmunity: Their Role in Shaping Modern Immunology

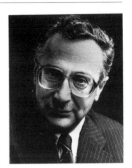

NOEL R. ROSE

Department of Pathology and of Molecular Microbiology and
Immunology, The Johns Hopkins Medical Institutions, 615 North
Wolfe Street, Baltimore, MD 21205, USA

I began my career in immunology in the early 1950s, after completing a Ph.D. in Stuart Mudd's department at the University of Pennsylvania in Philadelphia. I was fortunate to receive an invitation from Ernest Witebsky to join his Department of Bacteriology and Immunology at the University of Buffalo. Witebsky offered me a salaried position as faculty member (permitting me to support my newly acquired wife and soon-to-be-born child), as well as the opportunity to complete my medical studies. He assigned me a small room, which I used as both office and laboratory, and the part-time assistance of a very competent technician, Janet Sciolino. He also suggested a fascinating project for me to work on, namely the organ specificity of thyroglobulin, the major protein constituent of thyroid gland extracts. Organ-specific antigens are not only unique for the particular organ, but frequently cross-react extensively with analogous antigens from many other species, suggesting that these antigens are critical to the specialized function of the organ.

As a young investigator in Heidelberg, Germany, Witebsky had confirmed an earlier report of Hektoen *et al.* (*1*), showing that thyroglobulin is an organ-specific protein (*2*). This finding was quite puzzling to Witebsky who felt that organ-specific antigens were heat-stable, alcohol-soluble 'lipoids' (*3*). The apparent organ specificity of thyroglobulin, Witebsky suggested, was an artefact due to denaturation of the protein in its preparation. Since I had a good background in biochemistry, Witebsky suggested I prepare thyroglobulin carefully and determine its organ specificity.

The experiments that we started in 1952 led directly to the discovery of thyroid autoimmunity in experimental animals and humans in 1956. The results played a significant part in changing the direction of immunological thought and giving rise to contemporary understanding of the laws governing the immune response.

In the early 1950s, two somewhat contradictory dicta were universally accepted by immunologists. The first was related to theories of antibody formation. In his initial proposals, Paul Ehrlich (4) had suggested that antigens bind pre-existing side-chains on cells, causing their extrusion; overproduction of the receptor leads to secretion of circulating antibodies capable of binding the same antigen. Ehrlich's selective side-chain theory seemed to be invalidated by the discoveries, first of Obermaier and Pick (5), and, in much greater depth, by Karl Landsteiner (6), showing that antibodies can be induced by exotic chemical haptens, even some freshly invented by the organic chemist. The only reasonable explanation, it seemed, was that the antigen instructed the cell to produce antibody of a particular specificity. One form of this theory was propounded first by my original mentor, Stuart Mudd (7), who suggested that antigen dictates the sequence of amino acids in the antibody molecule. Similar views were elaborated at the same time by Alexander (8) in Great Britain and Breinl and Haurowitz (9) in Germany. A decade later, the instruction theory was modified by Linus Pauling (10), who suggested that antigen forms a template around which the antibody folds. A direct consequence of instruction or template theories was that antibodies can be produced to any molecule with an established structure. There was no reason why constituents of the host itself would not be antigenic. Autoantibodies were taken up, however, by the corresponding autoantigen, acting as an 'antigen sink', or were overwhelmed by 'immunologic paralysis'.

Paradoxically, the other theory that was generally accepted by immunologists in 1952 was based on Ehrlich's famous dictum of 'horror autotoxicus'. When Ehrlich found that goats would produce antibodies to foreign erythrocytes or even erythrocytes from other goats while failing to produce antibodies to their own erythrocytes, he felt that there must be some basic biological law involved (11). Most later investigators failed to notice that Ehrlich also pointed out that this law of horror autotoxicus might occasionally be violated and account for some human diseases. Ernest Witebsky was a student of Hans Sachs, who, in turn, was one of Ehrlich's two principal protégés. He was, therefore, the inheritor of the Ehrlich mantle and was universally recognized as a vigorous champion of the horror autotoxicus principle.

It was in this setting of instructional theories of antibody production and horror autotoxicus that I began work on the immunological specificity of thyroglobulin. A detailed account of these experiments was recently published (12) and, therefore, will be summarized only briefly here.

My first task was to purify thyroglobulin in the most gentle manner in order to avoid denaturation. I developed a scheme for stepwise addition of ammonium sulphate to thyroid extracts and finally isolated a satisfactory product. It was improved and evaluated by an expert protein chemist in our group, Sidney Shulman, who found that the thyroglobulin seemed to be unaltered in the ultracentrifuge and electrophoresis apparatus. This native protein possessed the same antigenic properties of organ specificity that Hektoen and his colleagues described a quarter of a century previously. Witebsky, however, was still dubious. I, therefore, devised the 'perfect experiment' of preparing thyroglobulin from rabbit thyroids and injecting it into rabbits. The *horror autotoxicus* principle instructed us that undenatured thyroglobulin would fail to elicit a response, whereas the denatured product would. Furthermore, instructional theories of antibody formation stated that antibodies to native rabbit thyroglobulin could be detected by rabbits if their own thyroid glands (the only source of thyroglobulin in the animal) were removed. When we did the requisite experiments, we found that both groups of rabbits, thyroidectomized or non-thyroidectomized, were capable of producing antibodies to rabbit thyroglobulin. After recovering from our astonishment, we had enough sense to examine the thyroids of the immunized, non-thyroidectomized rabbits and found they were markedly inflamed; in fact, they had developed severe thyroiditis. Similar disease, as well as autoantibody production, resulted from immunization of rabbits with their own thyroglobulin (*13,14*). We could only conclude with reluctance that we had induced a true autoimmune disease by experimental immunization, apparently violating the law of *horror autotoxicus*. Our finding that thyroidectomized rabbits produced antibodies as well as non-thyroidectomized rabbits also seemed to contradict the instructional theories of antibody formation. This single series of experiments, therefore, challenged both prevailing dogmas!

Our surgical collaborator, John Paine, remarked one day that the pathological changes seen in the thyroids of immunized rabbits reminded him of human Hashimoto's disease. We therefore set out to collect sera from patients with chronic thyroiditis. Several of the sera contained large amounts of antibodies to human thyroglobulin. Based on the similarity of human thyroiditis and the experimental model, we suggested that chronic thyroiditis is an example of a human autoimmune disease (*15*). The British team of Roitt, Doniach, Campbell and Vaughan Hudson, having seen an abstract of our rabbit studies, carried out parallel investigations in London and came to exactly the same conclusion (*16*). Coincidentally, our first publication on chronic thyroiditis and autoimmunization was awarded the Hektoen Medal by the American Medical Association.

The discovery of thyroid autoimmunity had a profound effect on immunological thought. Soon a large number of human diseases were being attributed to autoimmunity, although often the evidence was quite circumstantial. At the same time, the doctrine of *horror autotoxicus* and tolerance of self-antigens had to be reconfigured. A central tenet of Burnet's clonal selection as a necessary basis for immune tolerance held that in embryonic life the precursors of immunocytes would have a degree of immaturity such that 'contact with any determinant associated with a body component or any foreign determinant artificially introduced results in the elimination of cells carrying such sites, and if all such clones are eliminated full tolerance is established'. Autoimmunity, if this should occur, would depend on 'forbidden clones' that later arose through somatic mutation (17).

In the years since the discovery of thyroid autoimmunity, an entirely new set of premises and concepts has grown up, comprising the modern science of immunology. In the study of self/non-self-discrimination, thyroid autoimmunity has remained a valuable teacher. A number of key discoveries were made using thyroiditis as a model. Thyroiditis can be induced in rabbits, not only by rabbit thyroglobulin, but by thyroglobulins from many foreign species, providing an early example of what is now called 'molecular mimicry' (18,19). Delayed hypersensitivity skin tests are an integral part of the thyroglobulin autoimmune response, and the pathological manifestations of thyroiditis can be transferred adoptively to syngeneic recipients, using T cells (20). The critical role of cell-mediated immunity in many autoimmune diseases is now well accepted.

The association of autoimmune disease with the major histocompatibility complex has had enormous impact on modern research. The first evidence of such an association arose from investigations carried out on experimental thyroiditis. Vladutiu and I examined a large number of inbred mouse strains and found that they differed greatly in their susceptibility to the experimentally induced disease (21). By using congenic strains, we were able to show that the major control resides within the H-2 gene segment. Later investigations revealed that there are two levels of major histocompatibility complex (MHC) regulation of autoimmune thyroiditis in the mouse. The induction of disease depends mainly upon MHC class II genes located at I-A, whereas the severity of lesions is modulated by class I genes at D (22). Additional non-MHC genes also play a role in determining susceptibility to autoimmune thyroiditis (23). In some species, such as the rat, they may actually overshadow the MHC genes (24). The spontaneous development of disease as seen in human patients or in genetically determined thyroiditis in the Obese strain (OS) chicken is due to the influence of a number of MHC and non-MHC genes in the same individual (25,26). The genetic traits conferring susceptibility to autoimmune thyroiditis may act by completely different mechanisms. There are, for example, intrinsic abnormalities in the thyroid gland and in the thymus, in addition to the immune response genes associated with the MHC (27). Autoimmunity occurs spontaneously when a number of these unrelated genetic traits coalesce. Even in animals carrying these predisposing genes, environmental factors are often needed as precipitating agents. For example, methylcholanthrene triggers autoimmune thyroiditis in the genetically predisposed BUF rat (28).

Another important concept based on studies of autoimmune thyroiditis is immunological escalation. It suggests that once an autoimmune process has begun in an organ, other antigens of the same organ are recruited into the autoimmune process. Thus, initial immunization of monkeys with thyroglobulin results eventually in the production of antibodies to a second thyroid antigen, thyroperoxidase (29). Virtually all human autoimmune diseases are characterized by the presence of multiple autoantibodies.

A major challenge of the future is the development of new methods for the treatment or, even better, prevention of autoimmune disease. Two steps are required. The first is to recognize individuals at high risk for developing destructive autoimmunity by means of genetic biomarkers. Although HLA is certainly one such biomarker in the human, many more need to be discovered before we can accurately predict and assess risk. The second step is to silence or extirpate the T cells that are required for initiation of autoimmune responses. In general, this step requires knowing the initiating antigen. In the case of thyroiditis, Silverman and I reported many years ago that thyroiditis can be prevented in the BUF rat if thyroglobulin is injected as a bolus of soluble antigen (without adjuvant) in newborn animals (30). Modern molecular biological methods are bringing us closer to the definition of the actual antigenic determinants involved in the initiation of pathological autoimmune responses (31). We are also learning about the MHC products necessary to present these epitopes as well as the particular T cell receptors required for their recognition. Thus, the tools for specific intervention are coming to hand.

Studies of thyroid autoimmunity have been an important component of the avalanche of research that comprises modern immunology. At their initiation, these studies contributed to the overthrow of two major dogmas of the past, *horror autotoxicus* and instructional theories. They established a paradigm for investigations of human diseases associated with autoimmunity. The studies demonstrated for the first time the important role of major histocompatibility complex genes on autoimmunity. They showed how multiple genes can interact in an additive fashion to build up susceptibility to autoimmune disease and pointed to ways by which this cascade of events might be interrupted. The interaction of environmental agents with intrinsic genetically determined factors has been well illustrated by studies of thyroid autoimmunity.

The most important lesson learned from studies of thyroid autoimmunity has been that the doctrines of the present must constantly be re-evaluated. Immunology has flourished because it is built on the shoulders of giants, including my own esteemed teachers, Stuart Mudd and Ernest Witebsky, but also because it has never accepted their dicta as eternal truths.

Notes and References

1. L. Hektoen, H. Fox and K. Schulhof, *J. Inf. Dis.* **40**, 641 (1927).
2. E. Witebsky, *Naturwissenschaften* **40**, 771 (1927).
3. Even though by this time the protein nature of lens autoantigens was well known.
4. P. Ehrlich, *Proc. R. Soc. London, Ser. B* **66**, 424 (1900).
5. F. Obermayer and E. P. Pick, *Wiener klin Wochenschr.* **19**, 327 (1906).
6. K. Landsteiner, *The Specificity of Serological Reactions*, revised edn, Dover, New York (1962).
7. S. Mudd, *J. Immunol.* **23**, 423 (1932).
8. J. Alexander, *Protoplasma* **14**, 296 (1932).
9. F. Breinl and F. Haurowitz, *Z. Physiol. Chem.* **192**, 45 (1930).

10. L. Pauling, *J. Am. Chem. Soc.* **62**, 2643 (1940).
11. P. Ehrlich and J. Morgenroth, *Berliner klin Wochenschr.* **37**, 453 (1900).
12. N. R. Rose, *Immunol. Today* **12**, 167 (1991).
13. E. Witebsky and N. R. Rose, *J. Immunol.* **76**, 408 (1956).
14. N. R. Rose and E. Witebsky, *J. Immunol.* **76**, 417 (1956).
15. E. Witebsky, N. R. Rose, K. Terplan, J. R. Paine and R. W. Egan, *J. Am. Med. Assoc.* **164**, 1439 (1957).
16. I. M. Roitt, D. Doniach, P. N. Campbell and V. Hudson, *Lancet* **ii**, 820 (1956).
17. F. Burnet, *The Clonal Selection Theory of Antibody Production*, Cambridge University Press, Cambridge (1959), pp. 60–61.
18. E. Witebsky and N. R. Rose, *J. Immunol.* **83**, 41 (1959).
19. K. L. Terplan, E. Witebsky, N. R. Rose, J. R. Paine and R. W. Egan, *Am. J. Pathol.* **36**, 213 (1960).
20. N. R. Rose, J. H. Kite Jr., T. K. Doebbler, R. Spier, F. R. Skelton and E. Witebsky, *Ann. NY Acad. Sci.* **124**, 201 (1965).
21. A. O. Vladutiu and N. R. Rose, *Science* **174**, 1137 (1971).
22. Y. M. Kong, C. S. David, A. A. Giraldo, M. Elrehewy and N. R. Rose, *J. Immunol.* **123**, 15 (1979).
23. K. W. Beisel, Y. M. Kong, K. S. J. Babu, C. S. David and N. R. Rose, *J. Immunogen.* **9**, 257 (1982).
24. N. R. Rose, *Cell Immunol.* **18**, 360 (1975).
25. N. R. Rose, L. D. Bacon, R. S. Sundick, Y. M. Kong, P. Esquivel and P. E. Bigazzi, in *Autoimmunity – Genetic, Immunologic, Virologic, and Clinical Aspects* (N. Talal, ed.), Academic Press, New York (1977), chap. 3.
26. N. R. Rose, L. D. Bacon, R. S. Sundick and W. E. Briles, in *Animal Models of Comparative and Developmental Aspects of Immunity and Disease* (M. E. Gershwin and E. L. Cooper, eds), Pergamon Press, New York (1978), pp. 143–153.
27. N. R. Rose, Y. M. Kong and R. S. Sundick, *Clin. Exp. Immunol.* **39**, 545 (1980).
28. D. A. Silverman and N. R. Rose, *J. Natl Cancer Inst.* **53**, 1721 (1974).
29. J. A. Andrada, N. R. Rose and J. H. Kite Jr, *Clin. Exp. Immunol.* **3**, 133 (1968).
30. D. A. Silverman and N. R. Rose, *Lancet* **i**, 1257 (1974).
31. R. C. Kuppers, H. S. Bresler, C. L. Burek, S. L. Gleason and N. R. Rose, in *Molecular Immunobiology of Self-Reactivity* (C. A. Bona and A. Kaushik, eds), Marcel Dekker, New York (1992), pp. 247–284.

Index

Numbers in *italics* refer to illustrations or tables